Renal Dysfunction in Cardiovascular Pathologies

Adrian Covic • Alexandru Burlacu
Editors

Renal Dysfunction in Cardiovascular Pathologies

Implications for Management

Springer

Editors
Adrian Covic
University of Medicine and Pharmacy
"Grigore T. Popa"
Iasi, Romania

Nephrology Clinic, Dialysis
and Renal Transplant Center – 'C.I. Parhon'
University Hospital
Iasi, Romania

Alexandru Burlacu
Institute of Cardiovascular Diseases
"Prof. Dr. George I.M. Georgescu"
Iasi, Romania

University of Medicine and Pharmacy
"Grigore T. Popa"
Iasi, Romania

ISBN 978-3-032-25433-7 ISBN 978-3-032-25434-4 (eBook)
https://doi.org/10.1007/978-3-032-25434-4

This Springer imprint is published by the registered company Springer Nature Switzerland AG
The registered company address is: Gewerbestrasse 11, 6330 Cham, Switzerland

Scientific progress is built on rigor, but sustained by patience. This work owes its endurance to those whose patience made rigor possible—above all, within the family.

Adrian Covic, Alexandru Burlacu

Contents

Chapter 1
Introduction

Alexandru Burlacu and Adrian Covic

1.1 Why This Book, and Why Now?

The past two decades have witnessed a profound shift in how clinicians and researchers understand the interactions between the heart and the kidneys. No longer viewed as separate entities affected merely by shared risk factors, the cardiovascular and renal systems are now recognised as being tightly interwoven in a bidirectional continuum. Globally, both chronic kidney disease (CKD) and cardiovascular disease (CVD) have reached epidemic proportions, each amplifying the burden of the other and disproportionately affecting ageing populations, individuals with multimorbidity, and socioeconomically vulnerable groups. Cardiovascular mortality remains the leading cause of death among patients with CKD, while even mild renal impairment significantly worsens outcomes across nearly all cardiovascular conditions—from acute coronary syndromes and arrhythmias to heart failure and structural heart disease.

Despite this overwhelming epidemiologic reality, clinical care pathways are still too often siloed. Cardiologists typically focus on haemodynamics, ischaemia, arrhythmias, and ventricular function; nephrologists emphasise electrolyte balance, fluid management, uraemic toxicity, and long-term renal decline. Yet the patient's biology refuses to respect such boundaries. What is urgently needed—and

A. Burlacu (✉)
Institute of Cardiovascular Diseases "Prof. Dr. George I.M. Georgescu", Iasi, Romania

University of Medicine and Pharmacy "Grigore T. Popa", Iasi, Romania
e-mail: alexandru.burlacu@umfiasi.ro

A. Covic
University of Medicine and Pharmacy "Grigore T. Popa", Iasi, Romania

Nephrology Clinic, Dialysis and Renal Transplant Center – 'C.I. Parhon' University Hospital, Iasi, Romania

A. Covic, A. Burlacu (eds.), *Renal Dysfunction in Cardiovascular Pathologies*,
https://doi.org/10.1007/978-3-032-25434-4_1

insufficiently available in the existing literature—is a coordinated, multidisciplinary, and clinically actionable framework that addresses the entire cardio-renal spectrum. This book emerges precisely from this unmet need.

1.2 A Modern Understanding of Cardio–Renal Integration

The conceptual evolution from discrete disorders to an integrated cardio-renal–metabolic continuum is driven by major advances in pathophysiology, imaging, molecular biology, and therapeutics. Inflammation, oxidative stress, endothelial dysfunction, neurohormonal activation (RAAS & SNS), microvascular impairment, and fibrosis operate across organ systems, shaping phenotypes that cannot be adequately explained by organ-specific models. The well-known classification of cardiorenal syndromes remains useful but insufficient to capture the complexity observed in real-world patients. Our understanding has therefore moved towards the concept of renal-cardiac interactions—a bidirectional physiology in which cardiac and renal dysfunction mutually reinforce one another. This book aims to synthesise these mechanisms and translate them into practical frameworks relevant to clinicians across disciplines.

1.3 Persistent Gaps in Diagnosis and Management

Although both cardiology and nephrology benefit from robust, guideline-driven recommendations, important knowledge gaps persist at their intersection. Diagnostic limitations are well-known: serum creatinine lacks sensitivity for early renal impairment; chronic elevations in cardiac biomarkers (particularly troponins) complicate the diagnosis of myocardial infarction in CKD; and current imaging protocols are not always optimised for patients at risk of contrast-related injury. Similarly, the therapeutic landscape presents challenges: drug dosing, the safety of anticoagulation, management of hypertension, and the use of guideline-directed medical therapy for heart failure require nuanced adjustment in renal dysfunction. Even recent breakthroughs—such as the advent of SGLT2 inhibitors or the refinement of non-invasive imaging and interventional strategies—have yet to be fully integrated into cohesive, cross-disciplinary care models. Accordingly, the clinical community continues to seek comprehensive, up-to-date, organ-system–spanning resources such as the present volume.

1.4 A Book Built on Collaboration: Bridging Disciplines for Better Care

If there is one central message underpinning this volume, it is the imperative of collaboration. The management of patients with coexisting cardiovascular and renal dysfunction cannot remain the responsibility of a single speciality. Optimal outcomes require coordination among cardiologists, nephrologists, cardiovascular surgeons, interventionalists, imaging specialists, intensivists, and, often, endocrinologists or geriatricians. Such a 'Heart–Kidney Team' approach mirrors the established Heart Team Paradigm in structural and coronary interventions, demonstrating consistent benefits in complex decision-making. This book is structured deliberately to support collaboration. Its chapters have been authored by experts representing both perspectives and often working at the interface of the two fields. The topics mirror the reality of contemporary clinical practice: episodes of acute cardiorenal deterioration, arrhythmias in CKD, therapeutic anticoagulation in renal dysfunction, challenges of coronary intervention in end-stage kidney disease, cardiac stunning during dialysis, metabolic and haematologic perturbations, vascular calcification, and the surgical management of advanced cardio-renal disease. The volume culminates with discussions on therapeutic adjustments and future directions, reinforcing a unified, forward-looking vision.

1.5 Emerging Paradigms and Future Directions

Rapid scientific progress continues to reshape the cardio-renal landscape. The integration of high-resolution imaging, omics-based profiling, and digital biomarkers holds promise for more precise phenotyping and individualised therapy. Machine learning and artificial intelligence are beginning to influence risk stratification in CKD and CVD, enabling earlier detection of deterioration and better prediction of decompensation events. Interventional cardiology and cardiovascular surgery are evolving to meet the needs of patients with advanced renal impairment, while dialysis technology and peri-dialytic monitoring increasingly recognise the cardiovascular vulnerability inherent in this population. These emerging paradigms suggest that the next decade will bring significant refinement to how we conceptualise and manage the heart–kidney axis. By providing a foundation rooted in current evidence and enriched by multidisciplinary perspectives, this volume seeks not only to synthesise contemporary knowledge but also to facilitate the transition towards the next generation of integrated cardio-renal care.

1.6 Conclusion

This book offers a comprehensive, clinically oriented, and collaboratively authored resource designed to bridge specialties and support practitioners who care for cardio-renal patients—patients whose needs transcend traditional disciplinary boundaries. We hope this work will serve as a valuable reference for clinicians, trainees, and researchers and catalyse further innovation, dialogue, and collaboration within this rapidly evolving field.

Declarations

Competing Interests The author(s) has no competing interests to declare that are relevant to the content of this manuscript.

Ethics Approval The author(s) declares that this manuscript does not include primary research with human participants.

The author(s) declares that this manuscript does not include primary studies involving animals.

Chapter 2
Epidemiology of Cardio-Renal Syndrome

Dimitrios Kirmizis

2.1 Introduction

Cardiorenal syndrome (CRS) refers to a spectrum of clinical disorders in which acute or chronic dysfunction of the heart and kidneys are interdependent, such that injury to one organ precipitates or accelerates injury to the other through complex hemodynamic, neurohormonal, inflammatory, and metabolic pathways [1–4]. Chronic heart failure and chronic kidney disease (CKD) frequently coexist, and large observational cohorts consistently demonstrate that approximately one-third to one-half of patients with heart failure have concomitant CKD, while cardiovascular disease represents the leading cause of death in advanced CKD [5–9]. The bidirectional relationship between the heart and kidneys is mediated by reduced cardiac output, venous congestion, activation of the renin–angiotensin–aldosterone system (RAAS), sympathetic nervous system overactivity, endothelial dysfunction, oxidative stress, and chronic systemic inflammation [1–4, 10]. These maladaptive responses promote progressive myocardial and renal fibrosis, fluid retention, and metabolic derangement, leading to a vicious cycle of organ dysfunction. As a result, CRS should be viewed not as a late complication of isolated organ disease but as a central pathophysiological driver of morbidity, mortality, and healthcare utilization across cardiovascular and renal populations [3, 4, 7].

From a public health perspective, CRS reflects the epidemiological convergence of the most prevalent non-communicable diseases worldwide: cardiovascular disease, CKD, diabetes mellitus, hypertension, obesity, and population ageing [6–9, 11–13]. Heart failure affects more than 64 million individuals globally [11], while CKD affects over 800 million people, accounting for approximately 10% of the global population [6, 7]. Hypertension affects ~1.28 billion adults worldwide [12,

D. Kirmizis (✉)
East Suffolk and North Essex NHS Foundation Trust, Colchester, UK

A. Covic, A. Burlacu (eds.), *Renal Dysfunction in Cardiovascular Pathologies*,
https://doi.org/10.1007/978-3-032-25434-4_2

13], and diabetes mellitus affected ~537 million adults in 2021, with projections indicating further rapid increases [14].

Over the past two decades, epidemiological evidence has firmly established CRS as a population-level phenomenon rather than a niche or tertiary-care condition [3, 4, 6]. Its rising prevalence reflects demographic ageing, improved survival from acute cardiovascular events, expansion of metabolic disease, and broader recognition of renal dysfunction in cardiovascular cohorts [5–9]. Understanding the epidemiology of CRS is therefore essential for clinical decision-making, health-system planning, and public-health policy development [3, 4, 7].

Epidemiologically, CRS remains challenging to quantify precisely. Variable definitions, evolving AKI diagnostic criteria (RIFLE/AKIN to KDIGO), inconsistent heart failure phenotyping (HFrEF, HFmrEF, HFpEF), and heterogeneity in biomarker availability complicate comparisons across studies and regions [15, 16]. Nevertheless, the adoption of standardized definitions—particularly the KDIGO AKI guideline—has improved epidemiological precision and enhanced comparability across cohorts. Importantly, CRS is still rarely coded explicitly in routine datasets; thus, much of the epidemiology is inferred from heart failure, CKD, and AKI registries rather than from CRS-specific registries. The most widely used CRS framework is the five-type classification proposed by Ronco and colleagues [1], which is clinically useful but epidemiologically imperfect because most datasets do not consistently stratify or code by CRS subtype. Heart failure registries preferentially capture types 1 and 2; CKD registries emphasize type 4 outcomes; intensive care datasets often reflect type 5 physiology; and systemic conditions (e.g., sepsis, diabetes) further blur boundaries [1, 4].

2.2 Global Burden of CRS: Scope and Significance

2.2.1 Intersection of Two Global Epidemics: Heart Failure and CKD

The burden of CRS is fundamentally driven by the overlapping epidemics of heart failure and CKD. The global prevalence of heart failure (~64 million) and CKD (>800 million) forms the epidemiological foundation of CRS [6–8]. Given the high rates of co-prevalence, the potential CRS population is enormous. Heart failure prevalence ranges from 1–2% in the general adult population to >10% in individuals older than 70 years, with HFpEF now accounting for nearly half of all heart-failure cases in high-income countries [17–19]. CKD prevalence similarly increases with age, reaching 20–25% in adults older than 65 years, and up to 50% in high-risk populations such as those with diabetes or hypertension [6–9].

CKD is a powerful independent risk factor for cardiovascular disease, heart failure, and sudden cardiac death [7–9]. Conversely, heart failure is a major determinant of CKD progression, particularly in patients with recurrent congestion and repeated hospitalizations. As a consequence, up to 60% of patients with chronic heart failure exhibit some degree of renal dysfunction, and the prevalence of CRS rises in parallel with heart-failure severity [4, 18, 20].

2.2.2 *Indirect Estimation of CRS Burden*

Because CRS is rarely coded explicitly in administrative datasets, its epidemiological burden is commonly inferred through multiple complementary approaches, including:

- Co-prevalence of heart failure and CKD in population-based cohorts and registries [4–9].
- Incidence of AKI or worsening renal function during hospitalizations for acute heart failure [17, 21–23].
- Increased risk of heart-failure hospitalization and cardiovascular mortality following AKI [24–26].
- Cardiovascular mortality rates and structural heart disease prevalence in CKD cohorts [7–9, 27].
- High prevalence of left ventricular hypertrophy and sudden cardiac death in dialysis populations [28–31].

Integration of these data strongly suggests that CRS affects hundreds of millions of individuals worldwide, directly or indirectly, and contributes substantially to global cardiovascular and renal mortality [6–9, 27].

2.3 Prevalence and Incidence Across CRS Types

2.3.1 *CRS Type 1: Acute Cardiorenal Syndrome*

CRS type 1, defined by acute cardiac dysfunction leading to AKI, is among the most clinically relevant and prognostically severe CRS phenotypes. Across major acute-heart-failure registries, 25–40% of patients hospitalized with acute decompensated heart failure develop AKI, with reported rates approaching 50% when sensitive biomarkers or KDIGO criteria are applied [17]. Risk factors include advanced age, pre-existing CKD, hypotension, severe venous congestion, arrhythmias, exposure to nephrotoxic agents, and aggressive diuretic or invasive hemodynamic therapies [21–23]. Importantly, worsening renal function in acute heart failure is associated with three- to eight-fold higher in-hospital mortality, prolonged hospitalization, and a marked increase in 30-day readmission rates, particularly when renal deterioration is accompanied by persistent congestion [17, 22–24].

2.3.2 CRS Type 2: Chronic Cardiorenal Syndrome

CRS type 2 reflects progressive renal dysfunction in the setting of chronic heart failure. CKD is present in 40–55% of patients with chronic heart failure, with prevalence increasing as heart-failure severity worsens [4, 6, 20]. HFpEF patients exhibit slightly higher CKD prevalence than HFrEF patients, consistent with their older age, higher burden of metabolic disease, and greater prevalence of systemic inflammation [17–19]. Longitudinal studies demonstrate an annual incidence of new or progressive CKD of approximately 10–15% among heart-failure patients, particularly among elderly individuals, those with diabetes, and patients with recurrent hospitalizations [4, 20]. Progressive decline in eGFR is one of the strongest predictors of mortality in chronic heart failure, with 5-year mortality exceeding 50% in patients with combined HF and CKD [18, 20].

2.3.3 CRS Type 3: Acute Renocardiac Syndrome

CRS type 3 describes acute cardiac dysfunction following AKI. AKI induces cardiac injury through inflammatory cytokine release, oxidative stress, electrolyte disturbances, volume overload, and uremic toxin accumulation. Among hospitalized patients with AKI, 13–25% develop acute heart failure or major cardiac complications, while 10–15% experience clinically significant arrhythmias [24–26]. Survivors of AKI have a two- to five-fold increased risk of subsequent heart-failure hospitalization and cardiovascular mortality, even after apparent renal recovery [26, 32]. Imaging studies suggest persistent subclinical myocardial fibrosis following AKI, underscoring the long-term cardiovascular consequences of acute renal injury [25, 32].

2.3.4 CRS Type 4: Chronic Renocardiac Syndrome

CRS type 4 is the most prevalent CRS phenotype globally. CKD promotes cardiac injury via hypertension, anaemia, uremic toxins, arterial stiffness, mineral-bone disorder, and chronic inflammation [7–9, 27]. Between 25% and 50% of patients with CKD stages 3–5 have clinical heart failure, and left ventricular hypertrophy is present in more than 75% of dialysis patients [28–31]. Heart-failure risk increases progressively as eGFR declines, rising approximately two-fold in CKD stage 3 and five- to ten-fold in stages 4–5 [7–9]. Cardiovascular disease accounts for >50% of deaths in advanced CKD and dialysis populations, with sudden cardiac death representing a major cause of mortality [29–31].

2.3.5 CRS Type 5: Secondary Systemic CRS

CRS type 5 arises from systemic disorders such as sepsis, diabetes mellitus, autoimmune disease, amyloidosis, cirrhosis, and critical illness [3, 4]. In sepsis, AKI develops in approximately 50% of patients, and concurrent cardiac dysfunction occurs in 20–30% [33–35]. Diabetes mellitus alone accounts for 40–50% of global CKD cases and confers a two- to three-fold increased risk of heart failure, making it a dominant upstream driver of CRS worldwide [14, 36].

2.3.6 CRS in Dialysis Populations

Dialysis patients represent the most severe expression of type 4 CRS. Structural cardiac disease is highly prevalent—LV hypertrophy affecting ~75% of incident dialysis patients—and arrhythmic risk is high [19–21]. Sudden cardiac death is a leading cause of death in haemodialysis, frequently accounting for ~25% of overall mortality in many series [20–23]. These epidemiological realities drive the need for integrated cardio-renal strategies in dialysis pathways.

2.4 Risk Factors and Demographic Variations

CRS risk is strongly age-dependent. Ageing reduces renal reserve, increases vascular stiffness, and amplifies multimorbidity; heart failure prevalence rises steeply with age, and CKD prevalence similarly increases, creating the substrate for CRS expansion. CRS prevalence doubles approximately every decade after the age of 50. Individuals aged ≥70 years have a two- to three-fold higher CRS risk and exhibit slower renal recovery after CRS events [6–9]. The shift toward HFpEF in ageing and metabolic populations further intensifies CRS burden [14].

Sex differences are evident: men more frequently develop ischemic heart disease–driven CRS and experience faster CKD progression, whereas women are overrepresented in HFpEF and may be underdiagnosed or undertreated, particularly in older age groups [17–19]. Racial and ethnic disparities are also pronounced, with individuals of African ancestry exhibiting higher CKD progression risk—partly related to APOL1 variants—while South Asian populations experience rapidly rising diabetes-driven CRS at younger ages. Lower socioeconomic status is consistently associated with delayed diagnosis, higher hospitalization rates, faster CKD progression, and reduced access to disease-modifying therapies such as SGLT2 inhibitors and ARNIs [6, 9, 36]. Hypertension and diabetes prevalence and control vary widely across regions and socioeconomic strata, and structural barriers limit access to early diagnosis and disease-modifying therapy in underserved populations [9–11]. These inequalities are central to CRS's public health impact.

Significant geographical variations are also observed globally. In high-income countries, higher recorded CRS prevalence may reflect better detection (laboratory access, imaging, biomarkers), older population structure, and improved survival from cardiovascular events, which increases the pool living with chronic HF and CKD [8, 14, 24]. In low- and middle-income countries, rapid growth of diabetes and hypertension—often coupled with delayed diagnosis, limited access to specialists, and constrained kidney replacement therapy—yields a high CRS burden with earlier onset and higher mortality [9–11, 24]. This disparity highlights CRS as both a clinical and equity challenge.

Beyond traditional risk factors (hypertension, diabetes, dyslipidaemia, smoking, obesity), emerging contributors include chronic inflammation, mineral metabolism abnormalities (e.g., FGF-23 pathway disturbances), gut microbiome dysbiosis, environmental exposures, and repeated nephrotoxic insults [4–7]. While these are harder to quantify at the population level, they may explain regional variability and residual risk.

2.5 Mortality, Morbidity, and Healthcare Utilization

Across all CRS subtypes, mortality is markedly elevated compared with isolated heart or kidney disease. CRS type 1 confers three- to eight-fold higher in-hospital mortality, while CRS type 4 accounts for the majority of cardiovascular deaths in CKD and dialysis populations [7–9, 18, 29]. CRS patients experience high healthcare utilization, including prolonged hospital stays, frequent readmissions, increased ICU use, and healthcare costs two- to four-fold higher than heart failure alone [23, 37]. Dialysis and advanced heart-failure therapies contribute disproportionately to health-system expenditure [37].

2.6 Public Health Implications and Trends

CRS is a major and growing public health challenge whose impact extends beyond individual outcomes to health systems, economic sustainability, workforce productivity, and health equity. It sits at the intersection of global disease burdens: cardiovascular disease, CKD, diabetes, and hypertension [5–11]. This convergence has produced:

- An increasing CRS prevalence, particularly chronic phenotypes (types 2 and 4).
- Earlier onset in low- and middle-income settings.
- Prolonged survival with chronic, resource-intensive disease states.

CRS populations exhibit high hospital use: longer stays, higher ICU admissions, and frequent readmissions, especially in acute heart failure settings complicated by renal deterioration [7, 17, 18].

2.6.1 *Shifting Trends*

Three broad forces are likely to drive CRS epidemiology over the next two decades:

1. *Ageing and multimorbidity expansion*, increasing co-prevalence of HF and CKD [5–8, 14].
2. *HFpEF growth*, tightly linked to obesity, diabetes, and CKD [14].
3. *Therapeutic advances* that improve survival (thereby increasing prevalence of chronic CRS while potentially slowing progression and reducing events) [3, 4].

These trends collectively predict substantial growth in CRS prevalence and healthcare system demand unless prevention and integrated care pathways scale effectively. Without coordinated prevention, early detection, and integrated cardio-renal care pathways, CRS prevalence is projected to increase by 30–50% over the next two decades, with widening global inequities [6–9, 36, 37].

2.7 Conclusions

CRS is an expanding global epidemiological challenge driven by ageing populations, the rising burden of metabolic disease, and complex bidirectional interactions between cardiac and renal dysfunction. Although precise quantification remains difficult due to heterogeneity in definitions and coding, convergent evidence from heart failure, CKD, AKI, and dialysis cohorts shows that CRS is common, prognostically severe, and resource-intensive. Standardized surveillance, harmonized definitions, prevention strategies, and integrated cardio-renal models of care are essential to mitigate its future burden.

Declarations

Competing Interests The author(s) has no competing interests to declare that are relevant to the content of this manuscript.

Ethics Approval The author(s) declares that this manuscript does not include primary research with human participants.

The author(s) declares that this manuscript does not include primary studies involving animals.

References

1. Ronco C, Di Lullo L. Cardiorenal syndrome. Heart Fail Clin. 2014;10(2):251–80.
2. Ronco C, McCullough P, Anker SD, et al. Cardio-renal syndromes: report from the consensus conference of the Acute Dialysis Quality Initiative. Eur Heart J. 2010;31(6):703–11.
3. Rangaswami J, Bhalla V, Blair JEA, et al. Cardiorenal syndrome: classification, pathophysiology, diagnosis, and treatment strategies. Circulation. 2019;139(16):e840–78.

4. Bikbov B, Purcell CA, Levey AS, et al.; GBD Chronic Kidney Disease Collaboration. Global, regional, and national burden of chronic kidney disease, 1990–2017: a systematic analysis for the Global Burden of Disease Study. Lancet. 2020; 395(10225):709–733.
5. Matsushita K, van der Velde M, Astor BC, et al, CKD Prognosis Consortium. Association of estimated glomerular filtration rate and albuminuria with all-cause and cardiovascular mortality. Lancet. 2015;386(10003):1248–1260.
6. Kovesdy CP. Epidemiology of chronic kidney disease: an update 2022. Kidney Int Suppl. 2022;12(1):7–11.
7. Herrington WG, Smith M, Bankhead C, et al. Epidemiology of chronic kidney disease: a global perspective. Lancet. 2023;402(10399):786–802.
8. Savarese G, Lund LH. Global public health burden of heart failure. Cardiovasc Res. 2017;113(1):7–11.
9. Roth GA, Mensah GA, Johnson CO, et al. Global burden of cardiovascular diseases and risk factors, 1990–2019. J Am Coll Cardiol. 2020;76(25):2982–3021.
10. Heidenreich PA, Albert NM, Allen LA, et al. Forecasting the impact of heart failure in the United States. Circ Heart Fail. 2013;6(3):606–19.
11. Borlaug BA. Evaluation and management of heart failure with preserved ejection fraction. New Engl J Med. 2020;382(17):1609–20.
12. Shah SJ, Katz DH, Selvaraj S, et al. Phenomapping for novel classification of heart failure with preserved ejection fraction. Circulation. 2015;131(3):269–79.
13. ADHERE Scientific Advisory Committee. Relationship between renal dysfunction and outcomes in hospitalized patients with heart failure. J Am Coll Cardiol. 2005;45(4):631–7.
14. Metra M, Cotter G, Davison BA, et al. Worsening renal function in patients hospitalized for acute heart failure. Eur J Heart Fail. 2012;14(1):68–75.
15. KDIGO. Clinical practice guideline for acute kidney injury. Kidney Int Suppl. 2012. Available at: https://kdigo.org/wp-content/uploads/2016/10/KDIGO-2012-AKI-Guideline-English.pdf?utm_source=chatgpt.com. Accessed 10/08/2025.
16. Khwaja A. KDIGO clinical practice guidelines for AKI. Nephron Clin Pract. 2012;120(4):c179–84.
17. Testani JM, Chen J, McCauley BD, Kimmel SE, Shannon RP. Potential effects of aggressive decongestion during the treatment of decompensated heart failure on renal function. Circulation. 2010;122(3):265–72.
18. Coca SG, Singanamala S, Parikh CR. Chronic kidney disease after acute kidney injury: a systematic review and meta-analysis. Kidney Int. 2012;81(5):442–8.
19. Chawla LS, Eggers PW, Star RA, Kimmel PL. Acute kidney injury and chronic kidney disease as interconnected syndromes. N Engl J Med. 2014;371(1):58–66.
20. Go AS, Chertow GM, Fan D, McCulloch CE, Hsu CY. Chronic kidney disease and the risks of death, cardiovascular events, and hospitalization. N Engl J Med. 2004;351(13):1296–305.
21. McCullough PA, Chan CT, Weinhandl ED, Burkart JM, Bakris GL. Intensive hemodialysis, left ventricular hypertrophy, and cardiovascular disease. Am J Kid Dis. 2016;68(5 Suppl 1):S5–S14.
22. Green D, Roberts PR, New DI, Kalra PA. Sudden cardiac death in hemodialysis patients. Am J Kid Dis. 2011;58(6):921–9.
23. de Bie MK, van Dam B, Gaasbeek A, et al. The current status of sudden cardiac death in dialysis patients. Eur Heart J. 2012;33(22):2744–52.
24. Poston JT, Koyner JL. Sepsis associated acute kidney injury. Clin Chest Med. 2019;40(4):675–84.
25. Kellum JA, Lameire N, KDIGO AKI Guideline Work Group. Diagnosis, evaluation, and management of acute kidney injury. Kidney Int Suppl. 2012;2(1):1–138.
26. NCD Risk Factor Collaboration (NCD-RisC). Worldwide trends in hypertension prevalence, awareness, treatment, and control, 1990–2019. Lancet. 2021;398(10304):957–80.
27. World Health Organization. Hypertension. Fact sheet. Geneva: WHO; 2021.
28. International Diabetes Federation. IDF diabetes atlas. 10th ed. Brussels: IDF; 2021.

29. Stanifer JW, Muiru A, Jafar TH, Patel UD. Chronic kidney disease in low- and middle-income countries. Lancet. 2016;387(10015):123–36.
30. Himmelfarb J, Ikizler TA. Hemodialysis. N Engl J Med. 2010;363(19):1833–45.
31. Himmelfarb J, Vanholder R, Mehrotra R, et al. The current and future landscape of dialysis. Nat Rev Nephrol. 2020;16(10):573–85.
32. Smith GL, Lichtman JH, Bracken MB, et al. Renal impairment and outcomes in heart failure. J Am Coll Cardiol. 2006;47(10):1987–96.
33. Herzog CA, Asinger RW, Berger AK, et al. Cardiovascular disease in chronic kidney disease. Circulation. 2011;123(12):e267–72.
34. Makar MS, Pun PH. Sudden cardiac death among hemodialysis patients. Kidney Int. 2017;91(5):1139–53.
35. Charytan DM, Foley R, McCullough PA, et al. Arrhythmia and sudden death in hemodialysis patients: protocol and baseline characteristics of the monitoring in dialysis study. Clin J Am Soc Nephrol. 2016;11(4):721–34.
36. Peerapornratana S, Manrique-Caballero CL, Gómez H, Kellum JA. Acute kidney injury from sepsis: current concepts. Nat Rev Nephrol. 2019;15(9):528–42.
37. Himmelfarb J, Ikizler TA. Chronic kidney disease, dialysis, and transplantation: a global public health challenge. Lancet. 2020;395(10225):709–33.

Chapter 3
The Pathophysiology of Cardio-Renal Interactions

Sidar Copur and Mehmet Kanbay

3.1 Introduction

The cardiovascular-kidney-metabolic (CKM) syndrome, an extension of what was formerly known as cardio-renal syndrome (CRS), is a novel concept highlighting the importance and fundamental role of metabolic risk factors including peripheral insulin resistance, hypertension, oxidative stress, and dyslipidemia in the pathophysiology and progression of cardio-renal syndrome [1]. Congestive heart failure (CHF) affects more than 60 million people globally, with even higher rates of chronic kidney disease (CKD) in the CHF population reaching up to 50% [2]. A large-scale meta-analysis study conducted by Damman and colleagues in 2014 involving a total of 85 studies with more than 1.1 million patients has revealed that 32% of CHF patients suffer from CKD while 23% suffered from worsening renal function during the follow-up period. Moreover, both moderate and severe renal impairment are shown to be independent predictors of mortality ($p < 0.001$), emphasizing not only the high prevalence of kidney disease in the CHD population but also its prognostic significance [2]. Even a slight decline in renal function in such a vulnerable population may translate into higher morbidity and mortality rates with a definitive need for acute and chronic management strategies. However, the diagnosis, classification and underlying pathophysiological mechanisms of CKM syndrome are not that straightforward and require careful consideration. Even though serum creatinine and N-terminal pro B-type natriuretic peptide (NT-proBNP) are the two most employed biomarkers in the diagnosis and follow-up of patients

S. Copur (✉)
Department of Internal Medicine, Koc University School of Medicine, Istanbul, Turkey
e-mail: scopur14@ku.edu.tr

M. Kanbay
Department of Internal Medicine and Nephrology, Koc University, School of Medicine, Istanbul, Türkiye

A. Covic, A. Burlacu (eds.), *Renal Dysfunction in Cardiovascular Pathologies*,
https://doi.org/10.1007/978-3-032-25434-4_3

Table 3.1 The currently accepted model for classification of cardio-renal syndrome

Types of CRS	Features
Type I	Acute heart failure leading to acute kidney injury
Type II	Chronic heart failure and/or cardiac dysfunction leading to chronic kidney disease
Type III	Acute kidney injury leading to acute cardiac dysfunction
Type IV	Chronic kidney disease leading to chronic cardiac dysfunction
Type V	Acute or chronic systemic disorders leading to concomitant kidney and cardiac dysfunction

Abbreviations: *CRS* cardiorenal syndrome

Table 3.2 The currently accepted model for the classification of cardiovascular-kidney-metabolic syndrome by the American Heart Association (37807924)

Stages	Features
Stage 0	Absence of CKM risk factors
Stage 1	Excess and/or dysfunctional adiposity
Stage 2	Presence of metabolic risk factors and/or moderate-to-high risk CKD
Stage 3	Subclinical cardiovascular disease in patients with either excess or dysfunctional adiposity, metabolic risk factors, or CKD
Stage 4	Clinical cardiovascular disease in patients with either excess or dysfunctional adiposity, metabolic risk factors, or CKD

Abbreviations: *CKM* cardiovascular-kidney-metabolic, *CKD* chronic kidney disease

suffering from CHF and CKM syndrome, there is a strong need for novel biomarkers with better predictive and prognostic power. Novel kidney injury biomarkers including interleukin-18, N-acetyl-β-D-glycosaminidase, kidney injury molecule-1, neutrophil gelatinase-associated lipocalin and cardiac biomarkers including troponin T, myeloperoxidase and mid-regional proadrenomedullin and galectin-3 have been proposed as potential biomarkers for CKD syndrome [3]. Cardiorenal syndrome was classified into five subtypes based upon the severity, acuity and direction of renal and cardiovascular system involvement (Table 3.1) while CKM syndrome has been categorized at five stages (Table 3.2) [1].

3.2 Pathophysiological Link

The underlying pathophysiological events linking the cardiovascular system and kidneys are not a simple bi-directional relationship but rather a complex interplay between various neurohormonal and signaling pathways.

3.2.1 Congestion

Acute decompensated heart failure and/or CHF has been associated with a hypervolemic state and an increase in central venous pressure (CVP) mediated through multiple mechanisms including salt and water retention via the renin-angiotensin-aldosterone system (RAAS) and anti-diuretic hormone upregulation, and activation of the sympathetic nervous system. Such venous congestion and hypervolemic state may impair kidney function through: (a) reduction of effective kidney perfusion as venous hypertension translates into reduction of arterio-venous pressure gradient; (b) intrarenal congestion translating into elevated interstitial pressure leading to reduction of glomerular filtration rate; (c) upregulation of tubuloglomerular feedback mechanisms in response to lower sodium reaching to macula densa that causes afferent arteriolar vasoconstriction [4]. A large-scale meta-analysis study has demonstrated the statistically significant association between elevated CVP and higher risk for acute kidney injury (AKI), with a 1 mm Hg increase in CVP leading to 6% increase in AKI incidence, and all-cause mortality among critically ill patients [5]. Even though such meta-analysis study is not specific for decompensated heart failure cases, a similar pattern may also appear in those cases, as well, since sepsis and critically ill state are also associated with a hyperdynamic state of heart failure.

Another crucial concept in such hypervolemic state with elevated CVP is the intra-abdominal hypertension, referring to intra-abdominal pressure at or over 12 mm Hg, and abdominal compartment syndrome, referring to intra-abdominal pressure at or over 20 mm Hg accompanied by organ dysfunction [6]. Abdominal compartment syndrome has not only led to compression of renal vasculature and parenchyma but also impaired cardiac output and index in response to elevated afterload [7]. A prospective observational study from a specialized heart failure intensive care unit involving 40 consecutive patients admitted with acute decompensated heart failure has demonstrated that 60% of patients suffered from elevated intra-abdominal pressure, which was associated with poor renal function ($p = 0.009$), along with improvements in hemodynamic parameters following intensive medical therapy. However, inclusion of patients with admission left ventricular ejection fraction ≤30% rather than traditional cut-off of 40% for heart failure with reduced ejection fraction or exclusion of patients with heart failure with either preserved ejection fraction or mildly reduced ejection fraction disabled the generalizability of results. Transvesical method was utilized for intra-abdominal pressure measurement while a cutoff value of 8 mm Hg to identify patients with intra-abdominal hypertension was utilized, potentially overestimating the true incidence as the currently accepted cut-off value is 12 mm Hg [8]. However, similarly high rates were reported in other observational studies as well [9, 10]. Another crucial aspect of such issue is the strong association between intra-abdominal hypertension and poorer diuretic response, as evident from a prospective cohort study involving 30 patients hospitalized for acute decompensated heart failure, demonstrating poorer diuretic response among patients with intra-abdominal hypertension despite receiving similar doses of loop diuretic therapy [9]. Such association is confirmed in another clinical study along with the illustration of longer hospital stay and 1-year all-cause mortality rates if elevated intra-abdominal pressure persisted over 72 h [10]. Additional cardiovascular implications of abdominal compartment syndrome on the cardiovascular system include reduction of preload due to vena cava inferior compression, elevation of afterload due to vasoconstriction in response to reduced cardiac output, elevated intrathoracic pressure due to upward displacement of diaphragm and atelectasis, the elevation of pulmonary artery pressure due to upregulated pulmonary vascular resistance [11]. Therefore, congestion in cardiorenal syndrome appears to be a central core of underlying pathology along with potential prognostic significance.

The therapeutic approaches targeting congestion in cardiorenal syndrome are highly heterogeneous, with diuretic therapy, mostly loop and thiazide-class diuretics, and ultrafiltration modalities being the most employed methodologies.

Sodium-Glucose Cotransporter-2 Inhibitors The cardiorenal beneficial effects of SGLT-2 inhibitor therapy are well-established in major clinical trials with substantial place in both the American Heart Association/American College of Cardiology, the European Society of Cardiology and the KDIGO guidelines. Such beneficiary effects of SGLT-2 inhibitor therapy include but not limited to: (a) osmotic diuresis and natriuresis mediated reduction of congestive load; (b) reduction of both systolic and diastolic blood pressure without endangering intravascular fluid volume; (c) weight loss and improved glycemic control correcting a major risk factor for both cardiac and renal diseases independently; (d) reduction of albuminuria and kidney fibrosis by decline in intraglomerular filtration pressure and hyperfiltration state; (e) uricosuria leading to correction of another major cardiorenal risk factor; (f) restoration of erythropoietin release from kidney and improvement of hematocrit levels and therefore oxygen supply; (g) production of ketone bodies leading to alteration of cardiac energy metabolism; (h) anti-inflammatory, anti-fibrotic and anti-oxidant effects through various signaling pathways; (i) inhibition of NHE1 channels leading to improved calcium homeostasis in cardiomyocytes [12–14]. Even though no pre-specified large-scale clinical trial has evaluated the effects of SGLT-2 inhibitor therapy in cardiorenal syndrome, indirect evidence emerges from published data from two major studies, the DAPA-HF and EMPEROR-Reduced trials. A pre-specified meta-analysis of those two studies has revealed that SGLT-2 inhibitor therapy leads to a significant decline in both cardiac and renal outcomes among patients with baseline heart failure and chronic kidney disease [15]. Moreover, a recent meta-analysis study encompassing four randomized clinical trials with a total of 32,471 patients has illustrated that SGLT-2 inhibitor therapy is associated with a reduction of all-cause mortality ($p = 0.008$) and lower rates of major adverse cardiovascular events ($p = 0.0015$) compared to placebo, along with a decline in reduced hospitalizations for heart failure episodes and cardiovascular mortality [16]. However, the need for dedicated clinical trials specifically on patients with cardiorenal syndrome is clear for the establishment of strong evidence for routine clinical utilization.

Tolvaptan As approximately one third of heart failure patients are classified as diuretic resistant, defined as inadequate urine output despite receiving standard dose diuretic therapy [17], there is a strong need for therapeutic alternatives relieving such congestive state without upregulating potentially detrimental compensatory mechanisms, including the sympathetic system and RAAS. Tolvaptan is a selective antagonist for V2 type receptors of vasopressin, leading to inducing enuresis without affecting the reabsorption of sodium or other electrolytes [18]. A prospective observational cohort study including 174 patients with acute decompensated heart failure has investigated the efficacy and safety of tolvaptan therapy as an add-on to conventional diuretic therapy ($n = 44$). Patients receiving tolvaptan as an add-on therapy demonstrated higher urine output at first 24 ($p = 0.001$) and 48-h period ($p < 0.001$), along with the reduction of worsening renal function incidence (22.7% vs. 41.4%, $p = 0.04$) and persistence of such an outcome after logistic regression analysis for potential confounding factors [19]. Similarly, another prospective cohort study involving 50 consecutive hospitalized patients with acute decompensated heart failure with baseline EF of at least 45% had illustrated that tolvaptan as an add-on therapy to conventional diuretic therapy was linked to decline in worsening kidney function incidence (12% vs. 42%, $p = 0.02$) compared to conventional diuretic therapy with no significant difference in urine output in first 24- or 48-h period [20]. A 2020 meta-analysis study over 5,577 patients hospitalized for acute decompensated heart failure over twelve randomized controlled trials has identified statistically significant improvement in urine output, serum sodium concentration, relief of dyspnea and peripheral edema with add-on tolvaptan therapy, along with significantly lower rates of AKI [21]. However, no beneficial effects on re-hospitalization or mortality rates have been reported in another large-scale meta-analysis study with 5,945 patients from 14 clinical studies [22]. Therefore, tolvaptan therapy at low doses (15–75 mg/day) appears to be a valid add-on therapeutic option for patients with heart failure patients leading to significant improvement in short-term clinical outcomes. However, there is a lack of data on the long-term use of tolvaptan therapy, as an add-on or alternative to conventional diuretic therapy, among CHF patients.

Another significant aspect to be considered in the utilization of tolvaptan therapy on acute decompensated heart failure patients is the potential role of such therapeutic alternative in case of baseline CKD status, a frequent clinical scenario in CHF patients. An open-label parallel-group study has evaluated the effectiveness of such an approach over 33 stage 3–5 CKD patients presenting with fluid retention under 20–100 mg/day furosemide therapy. Patients were divided into two groups with receipt of 15 mg/day tolvaptan therapy or additional 100 mg/day furosemide over seven-day period. Add-on tolvaptan therapy has led to higher increase in urine volume (637 ml vs. 119 ml, $p < 0.05$) and lower incidence of worsening kidney function (18.8% vs. 58.8%, $p < 0.05$) compared to higher dose loop diuretic therapy [23]. Similar pattern of improvements in urine output and kidney outcomes was also reported in a meta-analysis study over seven clinical studies evaluating tolvaptan therapy among patients with CKD and heart failure [24]. Thus, addition of tolvaptan therapy instead of dose up-titration for diuretic therapy appears to be effective and safe for patients with heart failure irrespective of their baseline kidney functional status.

3.2.2 Pump Failure

Two crucial components of hemodynamic assessment in patients with heart failure include cardiac output, referring to the volume of blood pumped by heart within a minute, and cardiac index, referring to cardiac output in relation to body surface area. CRS may impair cardiac index and output through various mechanisms: (a) congestive state leading to higher afterload may impair stroke volume; (b) reduction of cardiac output may upregulate renin-angiotensin-aldosterone system through activation of the juxtaglomerular apparatus and release of renin; (c) cardiac output reduction may introduce a state of pre-renal AKI [25]. The association of low cardiac output on AKI risk was established in a prospective observational cohort study involving 145 patients hospitalized for decompensated heart failure, illustrating a significant correlation between baseline cardiac index and kidney function [26]. Similar patterns were also reported even among patients presenting with cardiogenic shock [27].

However, cases of CHF are not exclusively at a low cardiac output state, with a considerable proportion of patients presenting at a high cardiac output state, including sepsis or patients with heart failure with preserved ejection fraction. Moreover, kidneys exhibit strong adaptive ability to maintain glomerular filtration rate constantly despite a considerable decline in renal plasma flow through vasoconstriction of efferent arterioles via renin release to upregulate filtration fraction [28]. A large-scale cohort study involving more than 100,000 patients from the Acute Decompensated Heart Failure National Registry has illustrated similar rates of AKI among patients with either preserved or reduced ejection fraction [29], highlighting the complex interplay of cardiorenal syndrome. Therefore, the low cardiac output state and associated pre-renal AKI state are not the sole predictors of kidney injury in CRS.

3.2.3 Pro-inflammatory Status

Pro-inflammatory status and imbalance between pro- and anti-inflammatory mechanisms are leading mechanisms underlying the pathophysiology of almost all major comorbidities while CKM syndrome is not an exception. Inflammation has been indicated as a non-traditional risk factor for major adverse cardiovascular events, as evident from a statistically significant association with high C-reactive protein levels [30]. Clinical studies have illustrated approximately five times higher serum levels of certain pro-inflammatory cytokines, including interleukin-6, among patients with type I CRS compared to isolated heart failure patients while such upregulation has also been linked to poor clinical outcomes, including kidney failure and all-cause mortality [31, 32]. However, the exact role of inflammation in the pathogenesis of cardiorenal syndrome is yet to be discovered. The central role of disrupted monocyte and macrophage function in CKD was well-established with upregulated production of pro-inflammatory cytokines and signs of oxidative stress [33]. Reactive oxygen species-induced NF-κB pathway and the NLRP2 inflammasome are the predominant regulators of pro-inflammatory status [34].

Cellular membranes of myocardium are enriched with arachidonic acid, which are hydrolyzed by phospholipase A2. The metabolism of eicosanoids is mediated via three major enzyme groups, including cyclooxygenases (COX), lipoxygenases (LOX) and cytochrome p450 enzyme system [35]. COX-1 and COX-2 mediated release of prostaglandins mediate pro and anti-inflammatory pathways, though both are involved in cardiac homeostasis involved in cardiac protection whereas disruption induced by ischemia-reperfusion injury leads to imbalances [36]. On the other hand, LOX-mediated release of hydroxyeicosatrienoic derivatives is involved in cardiac fibrosis and hypertrophy, myocyte apoptosis [37]. The downregulation of cytochrome p450-mediated epoxyeicosatrienoic acids, a vasodilatory and anti-inflammatory metabolite, release and upregulation of 20-hydroxyeicosatetraenoic acid, a vasoconstrictive and pro-inflammatory metabolite, production has involved in the pathogenesis of cardiotoxicity, renal injury and hypertension [38].

Inflammation in the pathogenesis of CKD, CHF and cardiorenal syndrome has raised the potential role of anti-inflammatory therapies in the management. Sodium-glucose cotransporter-2 inhibitors, mineralocorticoid receptor antagonists such as finerenone and colchicine have all illustrated anti-inflammatory benefits in CKD and congestive heart failure patients [39, 40].

Ziltivekimab Ziltivekimab, a novel, humanized IgG1 targeting anti-interleukin-6, has gained interest in the management of CKD-associated anemia and patients with high atherosclerotic risk factors. A phase I/II multicenter double-blind placebo-controlled RCT has evaluated the efficacy of such an option among hemodialysis patients with the baseline hemoglobin level of 8.5–11 g/dl, ferritin over 300 ng/ml and transferrin saturation of 15–30% with erythropoietin stimulating agent resistance. All participants have high serum levels of IL-6 indicating pro-inflammatory status and potential underlying cause of anemia as systemic inflammation. Ziltivekimab therapy has been shown to lead improvements in anemia parameters including hemoglobin, transferrin saturation and serum iron, reduction of ESA requirements accompanied by the downregulation of pro-inflammatory status as evident from decline in hsCRP, serum amyloid A and fibrinogen levels [41]. Similar beneficiary effects of ziltivekimab on anemia of chronic illness among CKD patients with baseline eGFR of 10–60 ml/min/1.73 m^2 have been illustrated in another phase II RCT [42]. Such improvements in iron parameters and chronic inflammation-associated anemia status with ziltivekimab therapy has raised whether such beneficiary effects may reflect cardiovascular benefits. A large-scale phase II placebo-controlled double-blind clinical trial over 264 CKD patients with high baseline hsCRP level and eGFR of 10–60 ml/min/1.73 m^2 has illustrated significant dose-dependent decline in lipoprotein a levels along with suppression of inflammatory biomarkers [43]. Even though the highly atherogenic role of lipoprotein (a) in atherosclerotic cardiovascular diseases is a well-established phenomenon, the reduction in lipoprotein (a) level with ziltivekimab therapy over a short period of time is not simply an indicator of decline in major adverse cardiovascular events, requiring future clinical trials with longer follow-up periods. Similarly, reduction of N-terminal pro-brain natriuretic peptide levels with ziltivekimab therapy was demonstrated in another clinical trial [44]. N-terminal pro-brain natriuretic peptide is a highly sensitive and specific indicator of congestive heart failure with crucial prognostic value during follow-up period, though it is unclear whether such a decline over short period of follow-up may translate into clear clinical benefits. There are multiple ongoing clinical trials investigating the efficacy and safety of such anti-IL6 based therapeutic option for atherosclerosis (NCT06118281, NCT07276282, NCT07301034) and congestive heart failure (NCT06200207).

Canakinumab Canakinumab is a fully humanized monoclonal antibody targeting interleukin-1β that is utilized in the treatment of various auto-inflammatory conditions with promising anti-inflammatory effects [45]. Recent studies have investigated whether such intriguing anti-inflammatory benefits translate into clinical outcomes including cardiovascular disorders. A large-scale randomized clinical trial involving a total of 10,061 patients with previous myocardial infarction and high baseline hsCRP has illustrated that 150 mg canakinumab therapy every 3 months is associated with lower rates of recurrent cardiovascular events without any improvement in lipid profile [46]. However, such improvements are not without major consequences, including higher rates for fatal infectious disorders. A subgroup analysis of that trial involving a total of 1,875 patients with baseline eGFR below 60 ml/min/1.73 m^2 has revealed that such cardiovascular benefits persist in CKD patients, a subgroup with high cardiovascular disease risk, with the largest benefits achieved in patients achieving hsCRP levels below 2 mg/l. On the other hand, no benefits or harms were observed in terms of eGFR or albuminuria during a median follow-up period of 3.7 years [47]. Similarly, canakinumab therapy has illustrated potentially beneficial effects on peripheral artery disease as well [48].

3.2.4 Mitochondrial Dysfunction

Both kidneys and cardiac muscle tissue are characterized by an abundance of mitochondria in accordance with their high metabolic demands involved in tubular reabsorption and secretion in kidney tissue and maintenance of cardiac contraction in the heart [49]. Disruption of mitochondrial oxidative phosphorylation, the primary method for ATP production, has potentially detrimental effects on cardiorenal function and may promote cardiorenal syndrome progression. CKD has been associated with significant disruption of mitochondrial function including: (a) disruption of oxidative phosphorylation and ATP production via defects at either respiratory chain molecules of components of tricarboxylic acid cycle [50]; (b) decline in the generation of new mitochondria and impaired removal [51]; (c) formation of reactive oxygen species without proper anti-oxidant response leads to damage towards mitochondrial proteins including enzymes and DNA [52]. Similar pathways are also involved in mitochondrial dysfunction observed in congestive heart failure and cardiorenal syndrome, along with an additional role of lipotoxicity induced by the accumulation of toxic lipids that induce progressive mitochondrial damage, inflammation and oxidative stress [53]. Impaired energy metabolism and mitochondrial dysfunction in both systems are not independent mechanisms but are co-dependent pathways induced by similar pathophysiological processes. Furthermore, such pathways are also involved in the regulation of pro-inflammatory pathways, oxidative stress, peripheral insulin resistance, various signaling pathways, and other pathophysiological mechanisms underlying cardiorenal syndrome [54].

As mitochondrial dysfunction is the central event linking cardiac and renal dysfunction, proper targeting of such defect is a promising therapeutic alternative. Szeto Schiller-31, mitochondria-targeting anti-oxidants, binds to cardiolipin at the inner mitochondrial membrane and prevents structural damage and oxidative stress [55]. Administration of SS-31 has offered promising beneficial effects in mice models of sepsis-induced AKI [56] and rat models of unilateral urinary tract obstruction [57]. The beneficiary effects include balancing anti-oxidant mechanisms, prevention of cellular apoptosis and tubulointerstitial injury and improvement of renal hemodynamics in diabetic or renovascular disease models [49]. However, currently no clinical data is yet available for the effects of SS-31 treatment in human models with a limited number of ongoing clinical trials (NCT01755858, NCT02436447). Moreover, multiple other pharmacotherapeutic options, including mitochondrial fission inhibitors, biogenesis activators, resveratrol, anti-oxidants, and coenzyme Q10, have been proposed to target kidney injury in pre-clinical models, though none has come close to clinical application so far.

Recent studies have also indicated potential mitochondrial protective effects of certain anti-diabetic medications, including sodium-glucose cotransporter (SGLT)-2 inhibitors and glucagon-like peptide (GLP)-1 receptor agonists. Pre-clinical models have indicated that GLP-1 receptor agonist therapy leads to: (a) upregulation of SIRT-1, an anti-fibrotic, anti-inflammatory, and anti-apoptotic peptide, expression [58]; (b) reduction of oxidative stress and autophagy mediated via AMPK-mTOR signaling pathway [59]. On the other hand, potential beneficiary effects of SGLT-2 inhibitor therapy on mitochondrial function include, but are not limited to, (a) promotion of mitochondrial fission and fusion (33677060); decline in reactive oxygen species production [60]; downregulation of BCL-2 mediated apoptotic pathways [61]. However, despite the widespread utilization of those anti-diabetic medications, their effects on mitochondrial dysfunction have been poorly described.

3.2.5 Signaling Pathways

As discussed previously, chronic pro-inflammatory and pro-fibrotic status and oxidative stress are essential components of the CKM syndrome. Certain signaling pathways underlie those processes, creating a vicious cycle.

NF-κB Pathway Chronic inflammatory state and peripheral insulin resistance are two well-established mechanisms underlying the CKM syndrome. Hyperinsulinemia and recruitment of macrophages to the pancreatic tissue to clear dysfunctional and apoptotic pancreatic beta-cells are physiological responses to metabolic stress while macrophage-derived release of tumor necrosis factor-alpha is involved in the disruption of peripheral insulin sensitivity [62]. The analysis of publicly available human RNA-sequencing datasets has illustrated upregulation of the NF-κB pathway along with higher levels of mitochondrial reactive oxygen species, while oxidative stress towards mitochondria, leading to NF-κB pathway activation, is involved in the polyubiquitination and clearance of damaged mitochondria, fundamentally a beneficial evolutionary process [63]. Furthermore, pharmacological inhibition of the NF-κB pathway has been shown to attenuate peripheral insulin resistance and therefore slow the progression of type II diabetes mellitus in vivo and pre-clinical models [64, 65]. Additionally, the activation of both canonical and non-canonical NF-κB pathways has been linked to the promotion of kidney inflammation and fibrosis, two critical components in both AKI and CKD progression (28604386). Similarly, upregulation of the NF-κB pathway is involved in endothelial dysfunction and induced by the atherosclerotic state, resulting in the release of pro-inflammatory cytokines such as IL-6 and tumor necrosis factor-alpha and adhesion molecules such as E-cadherin [66]. Such pre-clinical data is further supported by NF-κB essential modulator-deficient, a key regulatory factor involved in the upregulated expression of NF-κB, mice models in which mice models were resistant towards the infiltration of atherosclerotic plaques by macrophages and T-lymphocytes [67]. To conclude, the NF-κB signaling pathway is involved in the initiation and progression of both kidney and cardiovascular diseases through the induction of inflammation and fibrosis and therefore provides a potential target for future therapeutic clinical trials.

PI3K-AKT Pathway The PI3K-AKT signaling pathway is involved in the regulation of cellular proliferation, differentiation, migration and metabolism, with a significant role in the limitation of inflammatory responses to provide a limiting state for uncontrolled inflammation [68]. Visceral adipose tissue is involved in the secretion of various pro-inflammatory cytokines including IL-1, IL-6 and tumor necrosis factor-alpha, which further upregulate other kinases including MAPK and mTOR in which the downregulation of PI3K-AKT pathways plays a considerable role [69]. Additionally, the PI3K-AKT signaling pathway is involved in the peripheral effects of insulin including: (a) facilitating both glucose uptake and glycogenogenesis in skeletal muscle in response to insulin [70]; upregulation of peripheral insulin resistance mediated via Surt1 [71]; induction of inflammation and fibrosis at kidney tissue mediated via upregulated NF-κB pathway [72]; protective effects towards mitochondrial reactive oxygen species formation and oxidative stress [73]. Moreover, the inhibition of the PI3K-AKT pathway via lupeol may have protective effects towards cardiovascular and kidney diseases, while such an effect is attenuated when co-administered with PI3K-AKT agonist 740Y-P on rat models [74]. However, there is a clear need for future large-scale clinical trials targeting the PI3K-AKT signaling pathway in the prevention and treatment of CKM syndrome following the promising outcomes demonstrated in pre-clinical studies.

Wnt/β-Catenin Pathway The Wnt signaling pathway is crucial in the regulation of cellular proliferation, differentiation, and migration. Animal models have illustrated the role of Wnt pathways in the differentiation and development of adipocytes and fibroblasts, two fundamental cells involved in visceral adiposity and tissue fibrosis [75]. Similarly, mutations at genes regulating the activity of the Wnt/β-catenin pathway, such as leucine-rich repeat-containing G protein-coupled receptor 4 (LGR4), have been linked to obesity and metabolic syndrome in humans [76, 77]. Moreover, the role of the Wnt signaling pathway in atherosclerosis is evident from studies indicating upregulated expression of Wnt in atherosclerosis that leads to the release of pro-inflammatory cytokines [78, 79]. Nonetheless, further pre-clinical and clinical trials are needed for a better understanding of the role of the Wnt signaling pathway in CKM syndrome.

Additionally, there are multiple pre-clinical studies regarding the role of various other signaling pathways, namely JAK-STAT and PPARs, on the pathophysiology of CKM syndrome. However, there is scarce data on such a topic.

3.2.6 Multi-Omics Perspective

The utilization of pre-clinical models adjusted to mimic all types of cardiorenal syndrome is of utmost importance in the understanding of the underlying pathophysiology. A mouse model for type I cardiorenal syndrome in which acute cardiac decompensation results in acute kidney injury has been investigated to examine the alterations in gene expression patterns following a sudden cardiac arrest and successful resuscitation. Their models illustrated the intrinsic cellular reprogramming in kidney tissue following an acute cardiac failure, most notably at proximal tubules and distal convoluted tubules, and emphasized the significant differences between type I cardiorenal syndrome and purely renal injuries in terms of gene expression patterns involving immune and inflammatory pathways [80]. Similarly, another study in which rat models with chronic heart failure due to a hypervolemic state induced by the generation of aorto-caval fistula has illustrated a decline in renal perfusion accompanied by modest albuminuria after 21 weeks. Proteomics analysis had revealed altered expression of 67 genes, most of which were involved in either the renin-angiotensin-aldosterone system or fibrosis such as >20-fold elevation in angiotensin-converting enzyme, seven-fold elevation in periostin, and 14-fold elevation in receptor for advanced glycation end-products expression [81]. Such pre-clinical model is significant by enabling the identification of altered gene expression patterns in type II cardiorenal syndrome even without the disease state with worsened glomerular filtration rate.

Pre-clinical models for type III and IV cardiorenal syndrome have also been developed to evaluate the effects of acute or chronic kidney failure on gene expression patterns in cardiac tissue. A pre-clinical model for type IV cardiorenal syndrome has revealed altered expression of 76 genes in the cardiac tissue of a mouse model of chronic kidney injury induced by unilateral ureteral obstruction. Most such genes are involved in the pathways regulating inflammation and fibrosis, cell cycle and proliferation [82]. Specifically, the upregulation of vimentin expression, a mesenchymal cell biomarker, may indicate the proliferation of fibroblasts and cardiac fibrosis, whereas downregulation of genes involved in mitochondrial oxidative phosphorylation and fatty acid metabolism may indicate the altered cellular metabolism at cardiac tissue following a renal insult [82]. Furthermore, such altered gene expression patterns have been illustrated at the microRNA level, as well, by Chade and colleagues in which pig models of chronic kidney disease leading to left ventricular dysfunction [83]. To conclude, pre-clinical models for all cardiorenal syndrome subtypes indicated similar patterns of altered gene expression, including a shift toward a pro-fibrotic state and regulated energy metabolism irrespective of the injury direction. Even though such models are fundamental to comprehending the underlying pathophysiology and histopathological alterations, there is a clear need for human trials to confirm. However, such studies on human subjects are highly limited due to unavailability of biopsy specimens in most cases of cardiorenal syndrome, the presence of multiple confounding factors and heterogeneity between subjects.

Petra and colleagues have evaluated the urinary peptidome of cardiorenal syndrome ($n = 353$) in comparison to age and gender-matched controls ($n = 356$) and identified differential excretion of 559 peptides, 193 peptides specifically found, in urine among cardiorenal syndrome patients. Most of those peptides were products of protein cleavage of extracellular matrix proteins while cleavages were mostly mediated via matrix metalloproteases-2/9/13 [84], highlighting the significance of extracellular matrix regulation in cardiorenal syndrome pathology. Moreover, such a study is clinically crucial for identifying unique peptides for cardiorenal syndrome compared to either isolated heart or kidney failure cases. Moreover, pro-inflammatory state associated with cardiorenal syndrome was established in another observational cohort study, revealing higher levels of IL-6, IL-18, lipopolysaccharides, a marker of gut-derived endotoxins, compared to isolated heart failure cases [85].

Despite confirming the multi-omics studies on animal models for cardiorenal syndrome regarding the altered gene expression patterns involving genes on cell cycle, inflammation, and fibrosis and cellular energy metabolism, human multi-omics or proteomics studies are considerably premature and limited to reaching a definitive conclusion. There is a clear need for future large-scale clinical data on such issues for a better understanding, as cardiorenal syndrome is not a single entity, but rather a heterogeneous phenomenon.

3.3 Conclusion

The interaction and underlying pathophysiology in between cardiovascular system and kidneys are highly complex and require careful consideration from various perspectives, though, proper understanding and addressing of such complex interactions may enable the development of various therapeutic alternatives and may result in superior clinical outcomes for patients with heart failure and/or kidney dysfunction (Fig. 3.1). Even though major progress has been made in the field of cardiorenal medicine, there is still a large-scale unmet need necessitating future pre-clinical and clinical studies to improve diagnostics and therapeutics.

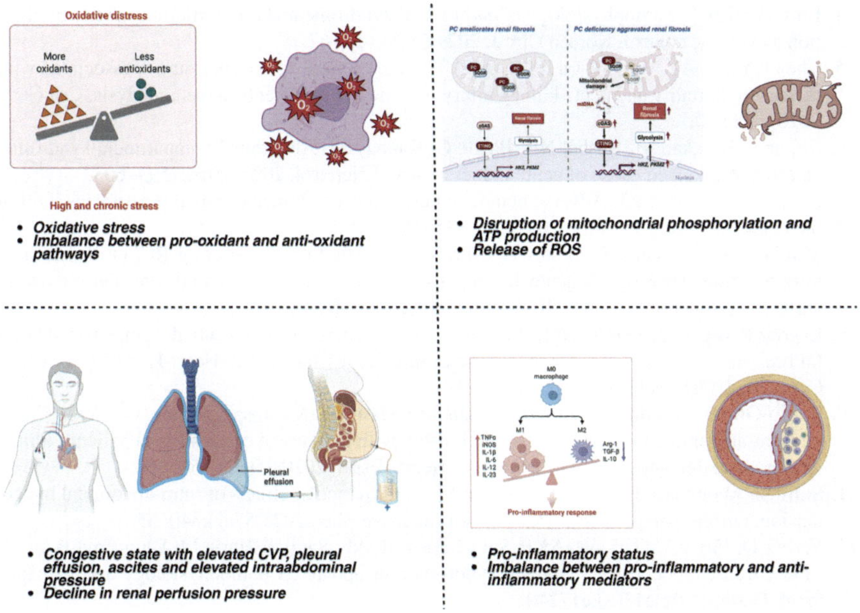

Fig. 3.1 The pathophysiological mechanisms of cardiorenal syndrome including pro-inflammatory and pro-oxidant status, congestive and hypervolemic state and mitochondrial dysfunction. (Abbreviations: CVP central venous pressure, ROS reactive oxygen species)

Declarations

Competing Interests The author(s) has no competing interests to declare that are relevant to the content of this manuscript.

Ethics Approval The author(s) declares that this manuscript does not include primary research with human participants.

The author(s) declares that this manuscript does not include primary studies involving animals.

References

1. Ndumele CE, Neeland IJ, Tuttle KR, Chow SL, Mathew RO, Khan SS, et al. A synopsis of the evidence for the science and clinical Management of Cardiovascular-Kidney-Metabolic (CKM) syndrome: a scientific statement from the American Heart Association. Circulation. 2023;148(20):1636–64.
2. Damman K, Valente MA, Voors AA, O'Connor CM, van Veldhuisen DJ, Hillege HL. Renal impairment, worsening renal function, and outcome in patients with heart failure: an updated meta-analysis. Eur Heart J. 2014;35(7):455–69.
3. Zhao BR, Hu XR, Wang WD, Zhou Y. Cardiorenal syndrome: clinical diagnosis, molecular mechanisms and therapeutic strategies. Acta Pharmacol Sin. 2025;46(6):1539–55.
4. Lim SY, Kim S. Pathophysiology of cardiorenal syndrome and use of diuretics and ultrafiltration as volume control. Korean Circ J. 2021;51(8):656–67.
5. Chen CY, Zhou Y, Wang P, Qi EY, Gu WJ. Elevated central venous pressure is associated with increased mortality and acute kidney injury in critically ill patients: a meta-analysis. Crit Care. 2020;24(1):80.
6. Copur S, Berkkan M, Hasbal NB, Basile C, Kanbay M. Abdominal compartment syndrome: an often overlooked cause of acute kidney injury. J Nephrol. 2022;35(6):1595–603.
7. Rosin D, Rosenthal RJ. Adverse hemodynamic effects of intraabdominal pressure- is it all in the head? Int J Surg Investig. 2001;2(5):335–45.
8. Mullens W, Abrahams Z, Skouri HN, Francis GS, Taylor DO, Starling RC, et al. Elevated intra-abdominal pressure in acute decompensated heart failure: a potential contributor to worsening renal function? J Am Coll Cardiol. 2008;51(3):300–6.
9. Lagosz P, Biegus J, Zymlinski R. Intra-abdominal hypertension in acute decompensated heart failure - an overlooked piece in the puzzle of diuretic resistance. Eur Heart J Acute Cardiovasc Care. 2024;13(Supplement_1):zuae036-073.
10. Rubio-Gracia J, Giménez-López I, Sánchez-Marteles M, Josa-Laorden C, Pérez-Calvo JI. Intra-abdominal pressure and its relationship with markers of congestion in patients admitted for acute decompensated heart failure. Heart Vessel. 2020;35(11):1545–56.
11. Soliman Aboumarie H, Nasa P, Malbrain M. Cardiovascular effects of intra-abdominal hypertension: current perspectives. Anaesthesiol Intensive Ther. 2025;57(1):340–55.
12. Verma D, Firoz A, Garlapati SKP, Sai Charaan Reddy Sathi T, Haris M, Dhungana B, et al. Emerging treatments of cardiorenal syndrome: an update on pathophysiology and management. Cureus. 2021;13(8):e17240.
13. Gajjar A, Raju AK, Gajjar A, Menon M, Shah SAY, Dani S, et al. SGLT2 inhibitors and GLP-1 receptor agonists in cardiovascular-kidney-metabolic syndrome. Biomedicine. 2025;13(8):1924.
14. Hou YC, Zheng CM, Yen TH, Lu KC. Molecular mechanisms of SGLT2 inhibitor on cardiorenal protection. Int J Mol Sci. 2020;21(21):7833.

15. Zannad F, Ferreira JP, Pocock SJ, Anker SD, Butler J, Filippatos G, et al. SGLT2 inhibitors in patients with heart failure with reduced ejection fraction: a meta-analysis of the EMPEROR-reduced and DAPA-HF trials. Lancet. 2020;396(10254):819–29.
16. Paolillo S, Marzano F, Bruzzese D, Di Santo M, Nardi E, Asile G, et al. Effects of dapagliflozin on mortality across the spectrum of cardiovascular-kidney-metabolic syndrome: a meta-analysis. Nutr Metab Cardiovasc Dis. 2026;36(2):104366.
17. Ravnan SL, Ravnan MC, Deedwania PC. Pharmacotherapy in congestive heart failure: diuretic resistance and strategies to overcome resistance in patients with congestive heart failure. Congest Heart Fail. 2002;8(2):80–5.
18. Hirano T, Yamamura Y, Nakamura S, Onogawa T, Mori T. Effects of the V(2)-receptor antagonist OPC-41061 and the loop diuretic furosemide alone and in combination in rats. J Pharmacol Exp Ther. 2000;292(1):288–94.
19. Matsue Y, Suzuki M, Seya M, Iwatsuka R, Mizukami A, Nagahori W, et al. Tolvaptan reduces the risk of worsening renal function in patients with acute decompensated heart failure in high-risk population. J Cardiol. 2013;61(2):169–74.
20. Tamaki S, Sato Y, Yamada T, Morita T, Furukawa Y, Iwasaki Y, et al. Tolvaptan reduces the risk of worsening renal function in patients with acute decompensated heart failure and preserved left ventricular ejection fraction—prospective randomized controlled study. Circ J. 2017;81(5):740–7.
21. Luo X, Jin Q, Wu Y. Tolvaptan add-on therapy in patients with acute heart failure: a systematic review and meta-analysis. Pharmacol Res Perspect. 2020;8(3):e00614.
22. Kansara T, Gandhi H, Majmundar M, Kumar A, Patel JA, Kokkirala A, et al. Tolvaptan add-on therapy and its effects on efficacy parameters and outcomes in patients hospitalized with heart failure. Indian Heart J. 2022;74(1):40–4.
23. Komiya S, Katsumata M, Ozawa M, Haze T, Kawano R, Ohki Y, et al. Efficacy of tolvaptan on advanced chronic kidney disease with heart failure: a randomized controlled trial. Clin Exp Nephrol. 2022;26(9):851–8.
24. Kumar A, Iqbal U, Amin SB, Arsal SA, Ali SMS, Shafique MA, et al. Evaluating the safety and effectiveness of tolvaptan in patients with heart failure and renal impairment: a systematic review and meta-analysis. Eur J Clin Pharmacol. 2025;81(2):203–16.
25. Lo KB, Rangaswami J. Mechanistic insights in cardiorenal syndrome. NEJM evidence. 2022;1(9):EVIDra2200053.
26. Mullens W, Abrahams Z, Francis GS, Sokos G, Taylor DO, Starling RC, et al. Importance of venous congestion for worsening of renal function in advanced decompensated heart failure. J Am Coll Cardiol. 2009;53(7):589–96.
27. Tarvasmäki T, Haapio M, Mebazaa A, Sionis A, Silva-Cardoso J, Tolppanen H, et al. Acute kidney injury in cardiogenic shock: definitions, incidence, haemodynamic alterations, and mortality. Eur J Heart Fail. 2018;20(3):572–81.
28. Merrill AJ. Edema and decreased renal blood flow in patients with chronic congestive heart failure: evidence of "forward failure" as the primary cause of edema. J Clin Invest. 1946;25(3):389–400.
29. Adams KF Jr, Fonarow GC, Emerman CL, LeJemtel TH, Costanzo MR, Abraham WT, et al. Characteristics and outcomes of patients hospitalized for heart failure in the United States: rationale, design, and preliminary observations from the first 100,000 cases in the Acute Decompensated Heart Failure National Registry (ADHERE). Am Heart J. 2005;149(2):209–16.
30. Ridker PM, Stampfer MJ, Rifai N. Novel risk factors for systemic atherosclerosis: a comparison of C-reactive protein, fibrinogen, homocysteine, lipoprotein(a), and standard cholesterol screening as predictors of peripheral arterial disease. JAMA. 2001;285(19):2481–5.
31. Virzì GM, Breglia A, Brocca A, de Cal M, Bolin C, Vescovo G, et al. Levels of proinflammatory cytokines, oxidative stress, and tissue damage markers in patients with acute heart failure with and without cardiorenal syndrome type 1. Cardiorenal Med. 2018;8(4):321–31.
32. Linhart C, Ulrich C, Greinert D, Dambeck S, Wienke A, Girndt M, et al. Systemic inflammation in acute cardiorenal syndrome: an observational pilot study. ESC Heart Fail. 2018;5(5):920–30.

33. Watral J, Formanowicz D, Perek B, Kostka-Jeziorny K, Podkowińska A, Tykarski A, et al. Comprehensive proteomics of monocytes indicates oxidative imbalance functionally related to inflammatory response in chronic kidney disease-related atherosclerosis. Front Mol Biosci. 2024;11:1229648.
34. Sun Y, Sun H, Zhang Z, Tan F, Qu Y, Lei X, et al. New insight into oxidative stress and inflammatory responses to kidney stones: potential therapeutic strategies with natural active ingredients. Biomed Pharmacother. 2024;179:117333.
35. Jenkins CM, Cedars A, Gross RW. Eicosanoid signalling pathways in the heart. Cardiovasc Res. 2009;82(2):240–9.
36. Shinmura K, Tang XL, Wang Y, Xuan YT, Liu SQ, Takano H, et al. Cyclooxygenase-2 mediates the cardioprotective effects of the late phase of ischemic preconditioning in conscious rabbits. Proc Natl Acad Sci USA. 2000;97(18):10197–202.
37. Wen Y, Gu J, Peng X, Zhang G, Nadler J. Overexpression of 12-lipoxygenase and cardiac fibroblast hypertrophy. Trends Cardiovasc Med. 2003;13(4):129–36.
38. Kingma JG, Simard D, Rouleau JR, Drolet B, Simard C. The physiopathology of cardiorenal syndrome: a review of the potential contributions of inflammation. J Cardiovasc Dev Dis. 2017;4(4):21.
39. Koshino A, Neuen BL, Jongs N, Pollock C, Greasley PJ, Andersson EM, et al. Effects of dapagliflozin and dapagliflozin-saxagliptin on erythropoiesis, iron and inflammation markers in patients with type 2 diabetes and chronic kidney disease: data from the DELIGHT trial. Cardiovasc Diabetol. 2023;22(1):330.
40. Tanaka A, Vaduganathan M, Imai T, Okada Y, Sonoda S, Torimoto K, et al. Effects of finerenone on arterial stiffness and cardiorenal biomarkers in patients with type 2 diabetes and chronic kidney disease: a randomised placebo-controlled mechanistic trial (FIVE-STAR). Cardiovasc Diabetol. 2025;24(1):454.
41. Pergola PE, Devalaraja M, Fishbane S, Chonchol M, Mathur VS, Smith MT, et al. Ziltivekimab for treatment of anemia of inflammation in patients on hemodialysis: results from a phase 1/2 multicenter, randomized, double-blind, placebo-controlled trial. J Am Soc Nephrol. 2021;32(1):211–22.
42. Pergola PE, Davidson M, Jensen C, Mohseni Zonoozi AA, Raj DS, Andreas Schytz P, et al. Effect of ziltivekimab on determinants of hemoglobin in patients with CKD stage 3-5: an analysis of a randomized trial (RESCUE). J Am Soc Nephrol. 2024;35(1):74–84.
43. Müller N, Schulte DM, Türk K, Freitag-Wolf S, Hampe J, Zeuner R, et al. IL-6 blockade by monoclonal antibodies inhibits apolipoprotein (a) expression and lipoprotein (a) synthesis in humans. J Lipid Res. 2015;56(5):1034–42.
44. Wada Y, Jensen C, Meyer ASP, Zonoozi AAM, Honda H. Efficacy and safety of interleukin-6 inhibition with ziltivekimab in patients at high risk of atherosclerotic events in Japan (RESCUE-2): a randomized, double-blind, placebo-controlled, phase 2 trial. J Cardiol. 2023;82(4):279–85.
45. Canakinumab. Drugs and lactation database (LactMed®). Bethesda (MD): National Institute of Child Health and Human Development; 2006.
46. Ridker PM, Everett BM, Thuren T, MacFadyen JG, Chang WH, Ballantyne C, et al. Antiinflammatory therapy with canakinumab for atherosclerotic disease. N Engl J Med. 2017;377(12):1119–31.
47. Ridker PM, MacFadyen JG, Glynn RJ, Koenig W, Libby P, Everett BM, et al. Inhibition of interleukin-1β by canakinumab and cardiovascular outcomes in patients with chronic kidney disease. J Am Coll Cardiol. 2018;71(21):2405–14.
48. Russell KS, Yates DP, Kramer CM, Feller A, Mahling P, Colin L, et al. A randomized, placebo-controlled trial of canakinumab in patients with peripheral artery disease. Vasc Med. 2019;24(5):414–21.
49. Tanriover C, Copur S, Ucku D, Cakir AB, Hasbal NB, Soler MJ, et al. The mitochondrion: a promising target for kidney disease. Pharmaceutics. 2023;15(2):570.

50. Zhang L, Miao M, Xu X, Bai M, Wu M, Zhang A. From physiology to pathology: the role of mitochondria in acute kidney injuries and chronic kidney diseases. Kidney Dis (Basel). 2023;9(5):342–57.
51. Jia X, Zhu L, Zhu Q, Zhang J. The role of mitochondrial dysfunction in kidney injury and disease. Autoimmun Rev. 2024;23(6):103576.
52. Ho HJ, Shirakawa H. Oxidative stress and mitochondrial dysfunction in chronic kidney disease. Cells. 2022;12(1):88.
53. Cojocaru K-A, Luchian I, Goriuc A, Antoci L-M, Ciobanu C-G, Popescu R, et al. Mitochondrial dysfunction, oxidative stress, and therapeutic strategies in diabetes, obesity, and cardiovascular disease. Antioxidants. 2023;12(3):658.
54. Vasquez F, Tiscornia C, Lorca-Ponce E, Aicardi V, Vasquez S. Cardiorenal syndrome: molecular pathways linking cardiovascular dysfunction and chronic kidney disease progression. Int J Mol Sci. 2025;26(15):7440.
55. Zhu Y, Luo M, Bai X, Li J, Nie P, Li B, et al. SS-31, a mitochondria-targeting peptide, ameliorates kidney disease. Oxidative Med Cell Longev. 2022;2022:1295509.
56. Sun M, Ma J, Ye J, Fan H, Le J, Zhu J. Protective effect of mitochondria-targeted antioxidant peptide SS-31 in sepsis-induced acute kidney injury. Zhonghua Wei Zhong Bing Ji Jiu Yi Xue. 2021;33(12):1418–22.
57. Liu ZR, Chen SQ, Zou YW, Wu XY, Li HY, Wang XQ, et al. Hypochlorite modified albumins promote cell death in the tubule interstitium in rats via mitochondrial damage in obstructive nephropathy and the protective effects of antioxidant peptides. Free Radic Res. 2018;52(5):616–28.
58. Kume S, Kitada M, Kanasaki K, Maegawa H, Koya D. Anti-aging molecule, Sirt1: a novel therapeutic target for diabetic nephropathy. Arch Pharm Res. 2013;36(2):230–6.
59. Yang S, Lin C, Zhuo X, Wang J, Rao S, Xu W, et al. Glucagon-like peptide-1 alleviates diabetic kidney disease through activation of autophagy by regulating AMP-activated protein kinase-mammalian target of rapamycin pathway. Am J Physiol Endocrinol Metab. 2020;319(6):E1019–e30.
60. Hatanaka T, Ogawa D, Tachibana H, Eguchi J, Inoue T, Yamada H, et al. Inhibition of SGLT2 alleviates diabetic nephropathy by suppressing high glucose-induced oxidative stress in type 1 diabetic mice. Pharmacol Res Perspect. 2016;4(4):e00239.
61. Nilsson LM, Zhang L, Bondar A, Svensson D, Wernerson A, Brismar H, et al. Prompt apoptotic response to high glucose in SGLT-expressing renal cells. Am J Physiol Renal Physiol. 2019;316(5):F1078–f89.
62. Baker RG, Hayden MS, Ghosh S. NF-κB, inflammation, and metabolic disease. Cell Metab. 2011;13(1):11–22.
63. He F, Huang Y, Song Z, Zhou HJ, Zhang H, Perry RJ, et al. Correction: Mitophagy-mediated adipose inflammation contributes to type 2 diabetes with hepatic insulin resistance. J Exp Med. 2025;222(7):e2020141606022025c.
64. Xie F, Zhu J, Hou B, Wang Y, Meng F, Ren Z, et al. Inhibition of NF-κB activation improves insulin resistance of L6 cells. Endocr J. 2017;64(7):685–93.
65. Cyphert TJ, Morris RT, House LM, Barnes TM, Otero YF, Barham WJ, et al. NF-κB-dependent airway inflammation triggers systemic insulin resistance. Am J Physiol Regul Integr Comp Physiol. 2015;309(9):R1144–52.
66. Yan B, Yu X, Cai X, Huang X, Xie B, Lian D, et al. A review: the significance of toll-like receptors 2 and 4, and NF-κB signaling in endothelial cells during atherosclerosis. Front Biosci (Landmark Ed). 2024;29(4):161.
67. Gareus R, Kotsaki E, Xanthoulea S, van der Made I, Gijbels MJ, Kardakaris R, et al. Endothelial cell-specific NF-kappaB inhibition protects mice from atherosclerosis. Cell Metab. 2008;8(5):372–83.
68. Acosta-Martinez M, Cabail MZ. The PI3K/Akt pathway in meta-inflammation. Int J Mol Sci. 2022;23(23):15330.

69. Tanti JF, Ceppo F, Jager J, Berthou F. Implication of inflammatory signaling pathways in obesity-induced insulin resistance. Front Endocrinol (Lausanne). 2012;3:181.
70. DeFronzo RA, Tripathy D. Skeletal muscle insulin resistance is the primary defect in type 2 diabetes. Diabetes Care. 2009;32(Suppl 2):S157–63.
71. Nelson VL, Jiang YP, Dickman KG, Ballou LM, Lin RZ. Adipose tissue insulin resistance due to loss of PI3K p110α leads to decreased energy expenditure and obesity. Am J Physiol Endocrinol Metab. 2014;306(10):E1205–16.
72. Lei L, Zhao J, Liu XQ, Chen J, Qi XM, Xia LL, et al. Wogonin alleviates kidney tubular epithelial injury in diabetic nephropathy by inhibiting PI3K/Akt/NF-κB signaling pathways. Drug Des Devel Ther. 2021;15:3131–50.
73. Wang M, Hu R, Wang Y, Liu L, You H, Zhang J, et al. Atractylenolide III attenuates muscle wasting in chronic kidney disease via the oxidative stress-mediated PI3K/AKT/mTOR pathway. Oxid Med Cell Longev. 2019;2019:1875471.
74. Li D, Guo YY, Cen XF, Qiu HL, Chen S, Zeng XF, et al. Lupeol protects against cardiac hypertrophy via TLR4-PI3K-Akt-NF-κB pathways. Acta Pharmacol Sin. 2022;43(8):1989–2002.
75. Zeve D, Seo J, Suh JM, Stenesen D, Tang W, Berglund ED, et al. Wnt signaling activation in adipose progenitors promotes insulin-independent muscle glucose uptake. Cell Metab. 2012;15(4):492–504.
76. Wang J, Liu R, Wang F, Hong J, Li X, Chen M, et al. Ablation of LGR4 promotes energy expenditure by driving white-to-brown fat switch. Nat Cell Biol. 2013;15(12):1455–63.
77. Styrkarsdottir U, Thorleifsson G, Sulem P, Gudbjartsson DF, Sigurdsson A, Jonasdottir A, et al. Nonsense mutation in the LGR4 gene is associated with several human diseases and other traits. Nature. 2013;497(7450):517–20.
78. Al-Aly Z. Arterial calcification: a tumor necrosis factor-alpha mediated vascular Wnt-opathy. Transl Res. 2008;151(5):233–9.
79. Kim J, Kim J, Kim DW, Ha Y, Ihm MH, Kim H, et al. Wnt5a induces endothelial inflammation via beta-catenin-independent signaling. J Immunol. 2010;185(2):1274–82.
80. Burfeind KG, Funahashi Y, Su XT, Lackey AE, Hagen MW, Blanche S, et al. Kidney cell response to acute cardiorenal and isolated kidney ischemia-reperfusion injury. Physiol Genomics. 2025;57(4):266–78.
81. Melenovsky V, Cervenka L, Viklicky O, Franekova J, Havlenova T, Behounek M, et al. Kidney response to heart failure: proteomic analysis of cardiorenal syndrome. Kidney Blood Press Res. 2018;43(5):1437–50.
82. Munguia-Galaviz FJ, Gutierrez-Mercado YK, Miranda-Diaz AG, Portilla de Buen E, Flores-Soto ME, Echavarria R. Cardiac transcriptomic changes induced by early CKD in mice reveal novel pathways involved in the pathogenesis of cardiorenal syndrome type 4. Heliyon. 2024;10(6):e27468.
83. Chade AR, Eirin A. Cardiac micro-RNA and transcriptomic profile of a novel swine model of chronic kidney disease and left ventricular diastolic dysfunction. Am J Physiol Heart Circ Physiol. 2022;323(4):H659–69.
84. Petra E, He T, Lygirou V, Latosinska A, Mischak H, Vlahou A, et al. Urine peptidome analysis in cardiorenal syndrome reflects molecular processes. Sci Rep. 2021;11(1):16219.
85. Virzì GM, Breglia A, Ankawi G, Bolin C, de Cal M, Cianci V, et al. Plasma lipopolysaccharide concentrations in cardiorenal syndrome type 1. Cardiorenal Med. 2019;9(5):308–15.

Chapter 4
Chronic Kidney Disease in Cardiovascular Pathologies

Bogdan Obrişcă and Gener Ismail

4.1 Kidney Dysfunction in Heart Failure (Cardiorenal Syndrome)

4.1.1 Definition, Classification and Epidemiology of Cardiorenal Syndrome

The *cardiorenal syndrome* (CRS) incorporates a spectrum of different disorders related to the heart and kidney in which an acute or chronic dysfunction in one organ induces an acute or chronic dysfunction in the other organ [1]. The current phenotypical classification of CRS is overly simplified from a clinical and pathophysiological perspective as we must recognize the difficulty in establishing the primary process, the possibility of significant overlapping between different CRS subtypes and the transition of one CRS subtype to another (Table 4.1) [1].

In the Swedish Heart Failure Registry, among 40,230 patients with heart failure (HF) enrolled between 2000 and 2013, 8875 (22%) were classified as HF with preserved EF (HFpEF), 8374 (21%) with HF with mid-range EF (HFmrEF), and 22,981 (57%) with HF with reduced EF (HFrEF) [2]. The prevalence of chronic kidney disease (CKD) was higher in patients with HFpEF than in those with HFmrEF and HRrEF (56% vs. 48% vs. 45%, $p < 0.001$) [2]. Nonetheless, irrespective of the HF phenotype, the mortality rate was increased in those with CKD by comparison to

B. Obrişcă (✉)
Department of Nephrology, "Carol Davila" University of Medicine and Pharmacy, Bucharest, Romania
e-mail: bogdan.obrisca@umfcd.ro

G. Ismail (✉)
Department of Nephrology, Fundeni Clinical Institute, Bucharest, Romania
e-mail: gener.ismail@umfcd.ro

A. Covic, A. Burlacu (eds.), *Renal Dysfunction in Cardiovascular Pathologies*,
https://doi.org/10.1007/978-3-032-25434-4_4

Table 4.1 Current phenotype-based classification of CRS [1]

Phenotype	Denomination	Description	Clinical scenarios
Type 1 CRS	Acute cardiorenal syndrome	Acute worsening of cardiac function leading to acute kidney injury	Cardiogenic shock, acute decompensated heart failure
Type 2 CRS	Chronic cardiorenal syndrome	Chronic abnormalities in cardiac function leading to chronic kidney disease	Chronic congestive heart failure
Type 3 CRS	Acute renocardiac syndrome	Acute worsening of renal function leading to acute heart failure	Hypervolemia, electrolyte abnormalities in AKI that can result in acute heart failure
Type 4 CRS	Chronic renocardiac syndrome	Chronic kidney disease leading to chronic heart failure	Left ventricular hypertrophy associated with hypertension, CKD-associated cardiomyopathy
Type 5 CRS	Secondary cardiorenal syndrome	Systemic disorders leading to both cardiac and renal injury	Amyloidosis

Abbreviations: *CKD* chronic kidney disease, *AKI* acute kidney injury, *CRS* cardiorenal syndrome

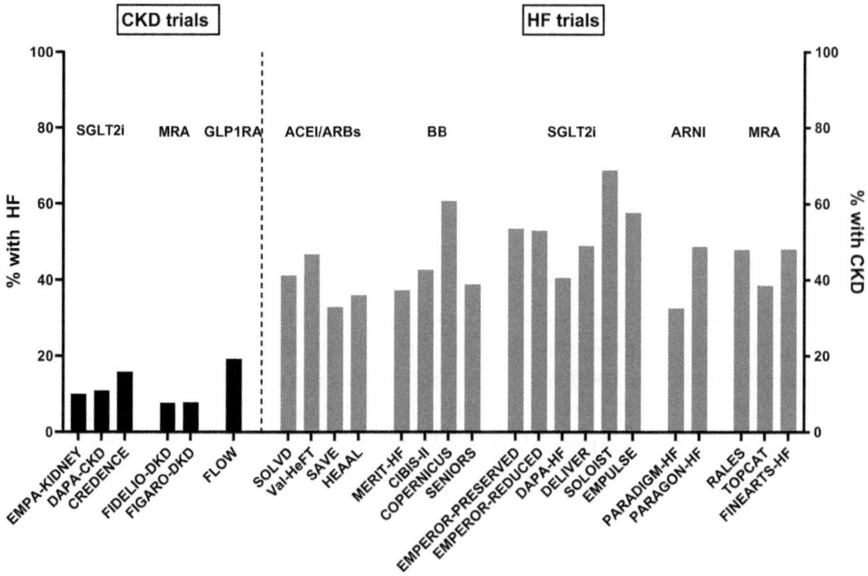

Fig. 4.1 Prevalence of HF in CKD-RCTs and of CKD in HF-RCTs

those without CKD [1-year mortality: 22.6% vs. 13.4% in HFpEF patients, 22.4% vs. 7.8% in HFmrEF, 23% vs. 8% in HFrEF] [2]. In a different setting, among the 105,388 patients hospitalized with acute decompensated heart failure (ADHF) that were enrolled in the ADHERE Registry, 30% had a history of CKD, with 21% and 9% having a serum creatinine over 2 mg/dL and 3 mg/dL, respectively, while 5% were on dialysis [3]. On the contrary, in randomized controlled trials (RCTs) of patients with CKD the prevalence of patients with HF ranged from 7.7% to 19.2% (Table 4.3, Fig. 4.1), while in RCTs of patients with HF the prevalence of patients with CKD ranged from 32.6% to 68.9% (Table 4.4, Fig. 4.1).

Thus, the current classification of CRS possesses challenges in estimating the true prevalence of kidney dysfunction in heart failure, as one patient may transit between different CRS phenotypes (e.g., a patient with a true type 2 CRS may transit to a type 1 CRS in the setting of an acute decompensated heart failure episode or to a type 3 CRS in the setting of a nephrotoxic acute kidney injury, while, over time, type 2 CRS and type 4 CRS may intersect in the same patient).

Accordingly, a recent classification proposes a stepwise approach to cardiovascular-kidney-metabolic (CKM) syndrome, taking into account the progressive pathophysiology. This approach allows us to better integrate a stepwise therapeutic algorithm from addressing metabolic, cardiovascular and chronic kidney disease risk factors towards full implementation of guideline-directed medical therapy. Thus, the CKM syndrome evolves over 5 stages [4]:

- Stage 0—no CKM risk factors.
- Stage 1—excess or dysfunctional adiposity.
- Stage 2—metabolic risk factors and CKD.
- Stage 3—subclinical cardiovascular disease in CKM.
- Stage 4—clinical cardiovascular disease in CKM.

Nonetheless, this classification is more cardio-centric and applicable to patients with metabolic syndrome and disregards other patient subtypes (e.g., those with systemic disorders involving both heart and kidney—amyloidosis or Fabry disease, previously defined as type 5 CRS).

4.1.2 The Interplay Between Cardiorenal Syndromes and the Transition from Successful Achievement of Decongestion to the Optimization of Guideline-Directed Medical Therapy

4.1.2.1 Decongestive Strategies—The Concept of Sequential Nephron Blockade

Patients with CKD and HF are at increased risk of rehospitalization and mortality due to high risk of congestion and suboptimal decongestion rates at discharge, significant diuretic resistance and inadequate implementation of guideline-directed medical therapy (GDMT) [5]. The risk of congestion significantly increases with progressive renal function decline, due to perturbances in salt and water handling associated with nephron loss [5–7]. Accordingly, the percentage of patients with acute decompensated heart failure free from clinical congestion at discharge with the use of loop diuretic monotherapy does not exceed 30% [8]. In the Diuretic Optimization Strategies Evaluation (DOSE) trial, only 18% of patients achieved decongestion at 72 h in the high-dose loop diuretics arm [9]. In addition, the trial excluded patients with a serum creatinine over 3 mg/dL, while the mean serum creatinine in the study groups was 1.5 ± 0.5 mg/dL, thus outlining that this trial did not enroll patients with the most advanced CKD with the highest risk of diuretic resistance from a renal standpoint [9]. Although there may be pharmacological differences between different types of loop diuretics, with some favoring torsemide over furosemide in the management of patients with HF, the TRANSFORM-HF trial failed to show a benefit with respect to mortality in patients randomized to torsemide by comparison to furosemide, with approximately 35% of patients having an underlying CKD [10].

The occurrence of diuretic resistance in these patients can be attributed to multiple mechanisms (neurohumoral activation, intravascular fluid depletion and slow plasma refilling rate) [8]. Apart from these, the adaptation to diuretic therapy is mainly mediated through the diuretic-braking phenomenon associated with nephron remodeling [8]. This concept has reignited the interest in overcoming diuretic resistance through sequential nephron blockade in recent years (Table 4.2) [8].

Table 4.2 Sequential nephron blockade in acute decompensated heart failure

Nephron site	Trial	Background diuretics	Additional comparator agent versus placebo	Events assessed	Results
Proximal nephron blockade	EMPA-RESPONSE-AHF [14]	Loop diuretics	Empagliflozin (10 mg)	Change in dyspnea and NT-proBNP, diuretic response, length of stay	Positive impact on urinary output, rehospitalization rates and mortality
	EMPAG-HF [15]	Loop diuretics	Empagliflozin (25 mg)	Urinary output	Positive impact on urinary output, diuretic efficiency and NT-proBNP change
	EMPULSE [16, 17]	Loop diuretics	Empagliflozin (10 mg)	Weight loss, change in NT-proBNP, clinical congestion score	Positive impact on weight loss and decongestion markers
	DIURESIS-CHF [18]	Loop diuretics	Acetazolamide	Natriuresis	Positive impact on loop diuretic efficiency
	ADVOR [19]	Loop diuretics	Acetazolamide	Successful decongestion	Positive impact on successful decongestion, urinary output and natriuresis No impact on mortality and rehospitalization

(continued)

Table 4.2 (continued)

Nephron site	Trial	Background diuretics	Additional comparator agent versus placebo	Events assessed	Results
Distal nephron blockade	CLOROTIC [20]	Loop diuretics	Hydrochlorothiazide	Change in dyspnea and body weight	Positive impact on diuresis and weight loss No impact on dyspnea, mortality or rehospitalization
	ATHENA-HF [21]	Standard therapy	Spironolactone (100 mg)	Change in NT-proBNP	No impact on NT-proBNP, clinical congestion score, dyspnea, urinary output, weight loss, mortality or rehospitalization
	EVEREST [22]	Standard therapy	Tolvaptan	Mortality (all cause and CV) or hospitalization for HF	Positive impact on dyspnea, weight loss and edema No impact on morbidity or mortality
	TACTICS-HF [23]	Loop diuretics	Tolvaptan	Dyspnea improvement	Positive impact on weight loss No impact on dyspnea
	SECRET of CHF [24]	Loop diuretics	Tolvaptan	Change in dyspnea	Positive impact on weight loss and dyspnea at day 3 (but not day 1)

Reviewed by the authors in [8]
Abbreviations: *CV* cardiovascular, *HF* heart failure

Nonetheless, the current clinical guidelines maintain a low level of evidence for the recommendation of adding a second diuretic agent and only after increasing the loop diuretic doses [11–13]. Thus, these challenges arise from the significant heterogeneity across RCTs in terms of the diuretic regimens and the different definitions of decongestion employed [8]. Accordingly, in clinical practice, the approach to sequential nephron blockade should take into account the patient's phenotype, the nephron segment that is suspected to be the main driver of diuretic resistance (proximal versus distal nephron blockade) and the coexisting or anticipated electrolyte and acid-base disturbances associated with diuretic use [8].

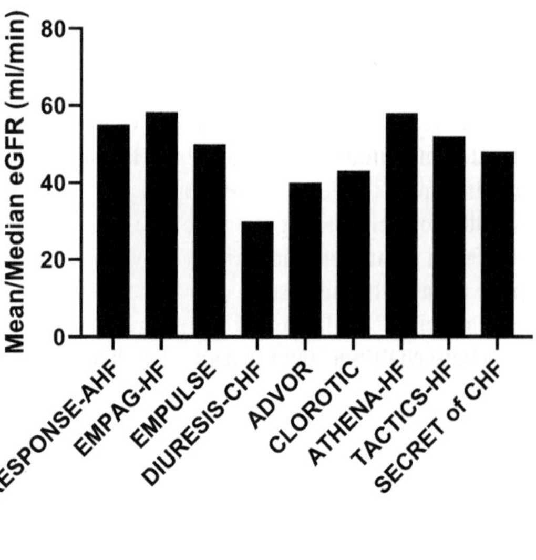

Fig. 4.2 Renal function in the additional diuretic group of the acute decompensated heart failure RCTs [14–21, 23, 24]

A major barrier to adequate implementation of sequential nephron blockade in the cardiorenal patient population remains the representativeness of patients with CKD in the acute decompensated heart failure trials (Fig. 4.2). While few RCTs actually reported the prevalence of CKD, the mean/median estimated glomerular filtration rate (eGFR) ranged from 30 to 58 mL/min/1.73 m^2 in the active arm of the trial (combination of loop diuretics and an additional diuretic agent) (Fig. 4.2). Nonetheless, the prevalence of patients with either defined CKD or an eGFR below 60 mL/min/1.73 m^2 was 20.2%, 80.7% and 85% in the EVEREST, ADVOR and SECRET of CHF trials [19, 22, 24]. In addition, while many trials have excluded patients with more advanced CKD, the EMPULSE and CLOROTIC trials have enrolled 10.2% and 20.2%, respectively, of patients with an eGFR of less than 30 mL/min [16, 17, 20].

The only cardiorenal syndrome dedicated trial (CARRESS-HF trial) randomized patients with acute decompensated heart failure and worsening renal function (increased serum creatinine by at least 0.3 mg/dL within 12 weeks before and up until 10 days after the index admission for heart failure) to ultrafiltration or a diuretic-based stepped pharmacologic therapy [25]. Although the trial excluded patients with a serum creatinine over 3.5 mg/dL, the patient population showed a worse renal function (median serum creatinine ranging from 1.9 to 2.09 mg/dL) by comparison to other diuretic trials [25]. The CARRESS-HF trial showed no difference between a stepped approach to diuretic therapy and ultrafiltration with respect to the primary endpoint that included weight loss at 96 h after randomization [25].

Nonetheless, the assessment of weight change and urinary output (as employed by many trials to up-titrate diuretic doses) has been criticized as being unreliable measures of diuretic efficacy, being influenced by many patient-related and unrelated factors [5]. Accordingly, measuring the urine sodium concentration in a spot urine sample 2 h after the first diuretic doses has been proposed as a more reliable measure of the subsequent natriuretic response [5]. The ENACT-HF was a multicenter, open-label, phase 2 trial that compared the routine standard of care with a standardized natriuresis-guided diuretic protocol in patients with acute heart failure [26]. Briefly, the up-titration of diuretic doses (or adding a thiazide diuretic) was employed if the 2-h urinary sodium concentration was less than 50 mmol/L or the urinary output was less than 100 mL/h. The standardized-guided diuretic approach led to a higher natriuretic response, higher diuresis and shorter length of hospitalization [26]. Similarly, in the PUSH-AHF trial, up-titration of diuretic doses (or adding a second diuretic) was employed if the 2-h urinary sodium concentration was less than 70 mmol/L or the urinary output was less than 150 mL/h [27]. Although the trial did not show an improvement in mortality or rehospitalization for HF, the natriuresis was improved by the natriuretic-guided approach [28]. In addition, 58% of the study cohort had a baseline eGFR below 60 mL/min, with the benefit of the natriuretic-guided approach being identified irrespective of baseline eGFR [29].

4.1.2.2 Guideline-Directed Medical Therapy—Treatment Strategies in Cardiorenal Syndromes

Significant progress has been made during the past decades in improving cardiovascular outcomes in patients with HF and renal outcomes in patients with CKD. Thus, the guideline-directed medical therapy (GDMT) in patients with HFrEF includes the following classes of medication: sodium-glucose cotransporter 2 inhibitors (SGLT2i), angiotensin receptor blockers/neprilysin inhibitor (ARNI), mineralocorticoid receptor antagonists (MRAs) and β-adrenergic receptor blockers (BB) (Fig. 4.3) [11]. Similarly, patients with CKD and diabetes mellitus rely on four treatment pillars: SGLT2i, nonsteroidal MRAs (nsMRAs), angiotensin-converting enzyme inhibitors (ACEi) or angiotensin-receptor blockers (ARBs) and glucagon-like peptide-1 receptor agonist (GLP1RA) (Fig. 4.3) [30]. Nonetheless, dedicated RCTs in patients with cardiorenal syndromes are lacking and data regarding the efficacy of therapies in patients with both comorbidities must be extracted from the HF population enrolled in CKD trials or from CKD population enrolled in HF trials, where available (Figs. 4.4 and 4.5, Tables 4.3 and 4.4). However, these data must be interpreted in the context of differences in the composite cardiovascular or renal outcomes across studies, lack of statistical power in post-hoc analyses restricted to patients with both CKD and HF and in the view that the phenotype of CRS cannot be defined in these patients.

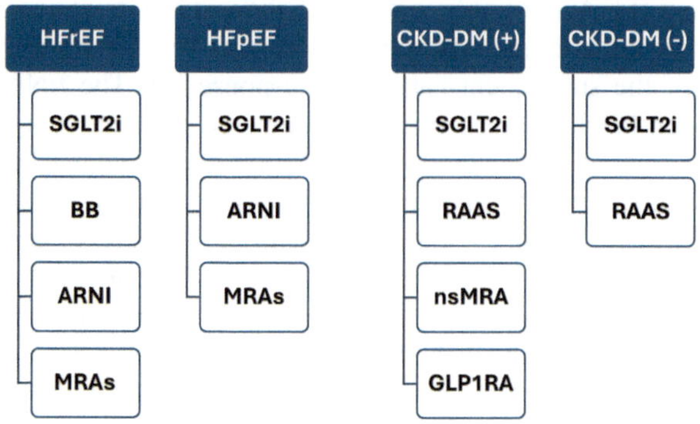

Fig. 4.3 Guideline-directed medical therapies in heart failure and chronic kidney disease [11, 30]

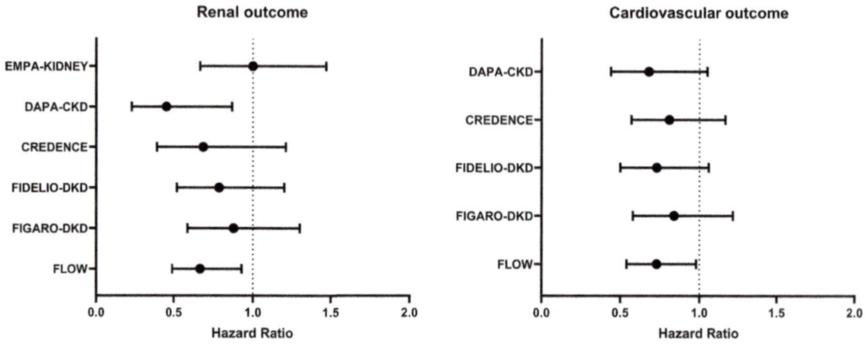

Fig. 4.4 Guideline-directed medical therapies in patients with chronic kidney disease and heart failure—renal and cardiovascular outcomes from CKD randomized controlled trials

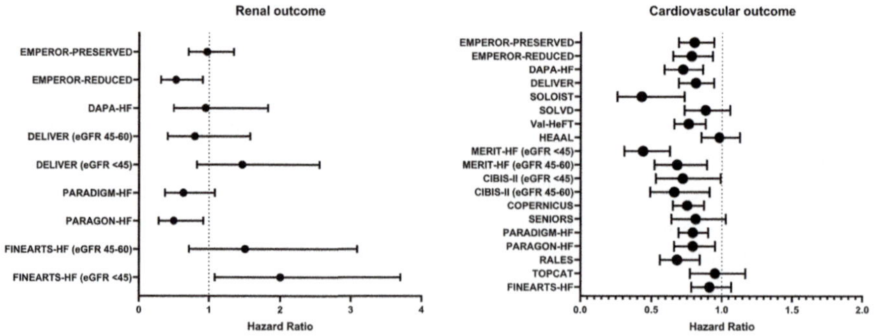

Fig. 4.5 Guideline-directed medical therapies in patients with heart failure and chronic kidney disease—renal and cardiovascular outcomes from HF randomized controlled trials

Table 4.3 Post-hoc analysis of HF population in CKD trials

Class	Trial	Medication	% HF	Renal outcome	Cardiovascular outcome	Ref.
SGLT2i	EMPA-KIDNEY	Empagliflozin vs. Placebo	9.95%	Progression of kidney disease (defined as ESKD, a sustained decrease in eGFR to <10 ml/min/1.73 m^2, a sustained decrease in eGFR of ≥40% from baseline, or death from renal causes) or death from CV causes: HR, 1.00 (95%CI, 0.67–1.47)	N/A	[52]
	DAPA-CKD	Dapagliflozin vs. Placebo	10.9%	More than 50% decline in estimated glomerular filtration rate, end-stage kidney disease, or death from renal causes: HR, 0.45 (95%CI, 0.23–0.87)	CV death or HF hospitalization: HR, 0.68 (95% CI, 0.44–1.05)	[53]
	CREDENCE	Canagliflozin vs. Placebo	15.8%	ESKD, doubling of serum creatinine or death from renal causes: HR, 0.69 (95%CI, 0.39–1.21)	CV death or HF hospitalization: HR, 0.81 (95%CI, 0.57–1.17)	[54]
MRAs	FIDELIO-DKD	Finerenone vs. Placebo	7.7%	Kidney failure, a sustained decrease of at least 40% in the eGFR, death from renal causes: HR, 0.79 (95%CI, 0.52–1.20)	CV death, nonfatal myocardial infarction, nonfatal stroke, or hospitalization for HF: HR, 0.73 (95%CI, 0.5–1.06)	[55]

(continued)

Table 4.3 (continued)

Class	Trial	Medication	% HF	Renal outcome	Cardiovascular outcome	Ref.
	FIGARO-DKD	Finerenone vs. Placebo	7.8%	Kidney failure (ESKD or an eGFR <15 mL/min/1.73 m^2 sustained for ≥4 weeks), a sustained ≥57% decrease in eGFR from baseline for ≥4 weeks, or renal death: HR, 0.88 (95%CI, 0.59–1.3)[a]	CV death or first hospitalization for HF: HR, 0.84 (95%CI, 0.58–1.22)	[56, 57]
	FINE-HEART pooled analysis (FIGARO-DKD, FIDELIO-DKD, FINEARTS-HF)	Finerenone vs. Placebo	36.9%	N/A	CV death: HR, 0.92 (95%CI, 0.78–1.08)	[58]
GLP1RA	FLOW	Semaglutide vs. Placebo	19.2%	Kidney failure (dialysis, transplantation, or an eGFR of <15 mL per minute per 1.73 m^2), at least a 50% reduction in the eGFR from baseline, or death from kidney-related or cardiovascular causes: HR, 0.67 (95%CI, 0.49–0.93)	Time to first new onset or worsening of HF or CV death: HR, 0.73 (95%CI, 0.54–0.98)	[33, 59]

Abbreviations: *CV* cardiovascular, *HF* heart failure, *ESKD* end-stage kidney disease, *eGFR* estimated glomerular filtration rate, *HR* hazard ratio, *SGLT2i* sodium-glucose co-transporter 2 inhibitors, *MRAs* mineralocorticoid receptor antagonists, *GLP1RA* glucagon-like peptide-1 receptor agonist

[a]Analysis included all patients with a history of cardiovascular disease (not restricted to patients with a history of heart failure)

Table 4.4 Post-hoc analysis CKD population in HF trials

Class	Trial	Medication	Renal function exclusion	% CKD	CV endpoint	Renal endpoint	Ref.
ACEI/ ARBs	SOLVD	Enalapril vs. Placebo	SCr > 2.5	41.2%	All-cause mortality: HR, 0.88 (95%CI, 0.73–1.06) Death from CV causes: HR, 0.84 (95%CI, 0.69–1.02) Hospitalization for HF: 0.96 (95%CI, 0.7–1.31)	Long-term eGFR slope: −0.84 ml/min/y (−1.24 to −0.43) for enalapril vs. −1.36 ml/min/y (−1.77 to −0.94) for placebo. Enalapril to Placebo difference: 0.52 (−0.06 to 1.09), $p = 0.08$[a]	[60, 61]
	Val-HeFT	Valsartan vs. Placebo	SCr > 3.4	46.8%	Death from CV causes or hospitalization for HF: HR, 0.76 (95%, 0.66–0.88)	N/A	[62]
	SAVE	Captopril vs. Placebo	SCr > 2.5	32.9%	All-cause mortality: RR, 28% (6–45) Death from CV causes: RR, 31% (14–45)	N/A	[63]
	HEAAL	High-dose losartan vs. Low-dose losartan	SCr > 2.5	36%	Death or hospitalization from HF: HR, 0.98 (0.85–1.13)	N/A	[64, 65]
BB	MERIT-HF	Metoprolol vs. Placebo	None	37.3%	All-cause mortality or hospitalization for HF: eGFR <45 ml/min: HR, 0.44 (95%CI, 0.31–0.63) eGFR 45–60 ml/min: HR, 0.68 (95%CI, 0.52–0.89)	N/A	[66]

(continued)

Table 4.4 (continued)

Class	Trial	Medication	Renal function exclusion	% CKD	CV endpoint	Renal endpoint	Ref.
	CIBIS-II	Bisoprolol vs. Placebo	SCr > 3.4	42.7%	All-cause mortality or hospitalization for HF: eGFR <45 ml/min: HR, 0.72 (95%CI, 0.53–0.99) eGFR 45–60 ml/min: HR, 0.66 (95%CI, 0.49–0.91)	N/A	[67]
	COPERNICUS CAPRICORN	Carvedilol vs. Placebo	None	60.8%	Death from CV causes or hospitalization for HF: HR, 0.75 (95%CI, 0.65–0.87)	N/A	[68]
	SENIORS	Nebivolol vs. Placebo	eGFR < 30	38.9%	All-cause mortality or CV hospitalization: HR, 0.81 (95%CI, 0.64–1.03)	N/A	[69]
SGLT2i	EMPEROR-PRESERVED	Empagliflozin vs. Placebo	eGFR < 20	53.5%	Death from CV causes or hospitalization for HF: HR, 0.80 (95% CI, 0.69–0.94)	Dialysis, kidney transplant, sustained reduction of ≥40% eGFR or sustained eGFR <15 ml/min/1.73 m^2: HR, 0.97 (95% CI, 0.71–1.34).	[70, 71]
	EMPEROR-REDUCED	Empagliflozin vs. Placebo	eGFR < 20	53%	Death from CV causes or hospitalization for HF: HR, 0.78 (95% CI 0.65–0.93)	Dialysis, kidney transplant, sustained reduction of ≥40% eGFR or sustained eGFR <15 ml/min/1.73 m^2: HR, 0.53 (95%CI, 0.31–0.91)	[72, 73]
	DAPA-HF	Dapagliflozin vs. Placebo	eGFR < 30	40.6%	Worsening heart failure or death from CV causes: HR, 0.72 (95%CI, 0.59–0.86)	A sustained decline in the eGFR of 50% or greater, ESKD, or renal death: HR, 0.95 (0.5–1.82)	[74, 75]

	DELIVER	Dapagliflozin vs. Placebo	eGFR < 25	49%	Worsening heart failure or death from CV causes: HR, 0.81 (0.69–0.94)	A sustained decline in the eGFR of 50% or greater, ESKD, or renal death: HR, 0.80 (95% CI, 0.41–1.57) for eGFR 45 to <60 mL/min/1.73m^2; HR, 1.46 (95% CI, 0.83–2.56) for eGFR <45 mL/min/1.73 m^2	[76, 77]
	SOLOIST	Sotagliflozin vs. Placebo	eGFR < 30	68.9%	CV death and hospitalizations and urgent visits for HF (first and subsequent events): HR: 0.43 (95%CI, 0.26–0.73)	N/A	[78]
	EMPULSE	Empagliflozin vs. Placebo	N/A	57.7%	The primary outcome of the trial was clinical benefit, defined as a hierarchical composite of death from any cause, number of HF events and time to first HF event, or a 5-point or greater difference in change from baseline in the KCCQ-TSS at 90 days: HR, 1.38 (95%CI, 1.04–1.83)	N/A	[16]
ARNI	PARADIGM-HF	Sacubitril/ Valsartan vs. Enalapril	eGFR < 30	32.6%	Death from CV causes or hospitalization for HF: HR, 0.79 (95%CI, 0.69–0.9)	A 50% decline in the eGFR, a 30% decline in eGFR to less than 60 ml/ min or ESKD: HR, 0.64 (95%CI, 0.37–1.08)	[79, 80]

(continued)

Table 4.4 (continued)

Class	Trial	Medication	Renal function exclusion	% CKD	CV endpoint	Renal endpoint	Ref.
	PARAGON-HF	Sacubitril/ Valsartan vs. Valsartan	eGFR < 30	48.8%	Death from CV causes or hospitalization for HF: HR, 0.79 (95%CI, 0.66–0.95)	A 50% decline in the eGFR, ESKD or death from renal causes: HR, 0.5 (95%CI, 0.28–0.92)	[81, 82]
MRAs	RALES	Spironolactone vs. Placebo	SCr > 2.5	48%	All-cause mortality: HR, 0.68 (95%CI, 0.56–0.84)	N/A	[83]
	TOPCAT	Spironolactone vs. Placebo	eGFR < 30	38.6%	Death from CV causes, aborted cardiac arrest, or hospitalization for the management of HF: HR, 0.95 (95%CI, 0.77–1.17)	N/A	[84]
	FINEARTS-HF	Finerenone vs. Placebo	eGFR < 25	48.1%	Total worsening HF events and death from CV causes: HR, 0.91 (95%CI, 0.78–1.07)	Sustained decrease in the eGFR of 50% or greater, a sustained decline in the eGFR to less than 15 ml/min, or ESRD: HR, 1.50 (95% CI, 0.72–3.09) for eGFR 45 to <60 mL/min/1.73m^2; HR, 2.00 (95% CI, 1.08–3.70) for eGFR <45 mL/min/1.73 m^2	[85, 86]

Abbreviations: *CV* cardiovascular, *HF* heart failure, *ESKD* end-stage kidney disease, *eGFR* estimated glomerular filtration rate, *HR* hazard ratio, *SGLT2i* sodium-glucose co-transporter 2 inhibitors, *MRAs* mineralocorticoid receptor antagonists, *GLP1RA* glucagon-like peptide-1 receptor agonist, *ARNI* angiotensin receptor blockers/neprilysin inhibitor, *ACEI* angiotensin-converting enzyme inhibitors, *ARBs* angiotensin-receptor blockers

[a]Analysis included all patients (not restricted to the CKD population)

In RCTs of the CKD population, treatment with SGLT2i, nonsteroidal MRAs or GLP1RA consistently improved both renal and cardiovascular outcomes in the subgroup of patients with CKD and HF (Fig. 4.4, Table 4.3). Although, the initial trials with ACEI/ARBs either did not specifically enroll patients with HF (e.g., RENAAL trial) or did not report findings in this population subgroup, they remain the backbone of therapy in both CKD and HF patients as all future RCTs required patients to be treated with a maximum tolerated dose of ACEI/ARBs for several weeks prior to study enrollment [31–33]. The implementation of a quadruple GDMT has not been evaluated yet in patients with CKD and type 2 diabetes, while the use of GLP1RA is currently under evaluation in nondiabetic CKD patients in the FIND-CKD trial [34]. Nonetheless, in the FIDELITY pooled analysis, 6.7% of patients were treated with an SGLT2i at baseline (887 out of 13,026 patients) [35]. The use of both finerenone and SGLT2i was associated with 33% (HR, 0.67; 95%CI, 0.42–1.07) and 58% (HR, 0.42; 95%CI, 0.16–1.08) reduction in the risk of the cardiovascular composite and renal composite endpoint, respectively, by comparison to a reduction of 13% (HR, 0.87; 95%CI, 0.79–0.96) and 20% (HR, 0.80; 95%CI, 0.69–0.92) in those with finerenone without SGLT2i [35]. Similarly, the annualized eGFR change was improved with the combination of finerenone and SGLT2i (−1.92 ml/min/year vs. −2.54 ml/min/year) [36]. These initial observations were further formally tested in the CONFIDENCE trial, in which, the combination of finerenone and empagliflozin led to a 29% and 32% greater reduction in urinary albumin-to-creatinine ratio by comparison to finerenone alone and to empagliflozin alone, respectively [37].

In RCTs of the HF population, the prevalence of CKD (as defined by an eGFR below 60 mL/min) ranged from 32.6% to 68.9%, while most studies excluded patients with either an eGFR below 30 mL/min or a serum creatinine over 2.5 mg/dL (Table 4.4). While the cardiovascular outcomes were consistently improved in the population of patients with HF and CKD across different classes of medication, the renal outcomes were mainly improved in the EMPEROR-REDUCED, PARADIGM-HF and PARAGON-HF trials (Fig. 4.5 and Table 4.4). Accordingly, the risk of the composite renal endpoint was reduced by 47% with empagliflozin in the EMPEROR-REDUCED trial, while the use of ARNI reduced the risk of the composite renal endpoint by 36–50% in the PARADIGM-HF and PARAGON-HF trials (Table 4.4).

Nonetheless, while the renal outcome of this patient subgroup is not consistently reported and the definition of these endpoints may vary across different RCTs, there is a rationale that patients with both comorbidities (HF and CKD) will likely benefit from the uptitration of GDMT. The STRONG-HF trial (Safety, tolerability, and efficacy of up-titration of guideline-directed medical therapies for acute heart failure) evaluated the impact of a rapid up-titration of GDMT to 100% of recommended doses within 2 weeks of discharge by comparison to usual local practice. The risk of heart failure readmission or all-cause mortality by 180 days was significantly reduced (by 34%) among patients receiving rapid up-titration of GDMT [38]. In addition, STRONG-HF trial may truly outline the situation where the disease continuum between the initial achievement of decongestion in acute decompensated heart failure allows the transition to adequate implementation of GDMT in order to significantly impact the mortality of these patients.

However, in real-world clinical practice, the uptitration and adequate implementation of GDMT in patients with HF and CKD remains suboptimal, mainly due to concerns of hyperkalemia and/or worsening of renal function. In a population-based time-series analysis, the rates of spironolactone prescription in patients hospitalized for heart failure increased from 34 per 1000 patients in the period preceding the RALES trial to 149 per 1000 patients after the publication of the RALES trial [39]. In line with these findings, the rates of hospitalization due to hyperkalemia rose from 2.4 to 11 per 1000 patients and the associated mortality rose from 0.3 to 2 per 1000 patients [39]. Thus, the initial 30% reduction in mortality with spironolactone seen in the RALES trial was subsequently offset in real-world clinical practice by the associated hyperkalemia risk [39, 40]. In another population-based analysis that comprised 205,108 patients with different comorbidities (CKD, HF, diabetes mellitus), less than 30% (ranging 19–26%) of individuals received maximum doses of RAAS inhibitors, while the majority (58–65%) received submaximum doses [41]. In addition, even in the case of a mild hyperkalemia event (potassium from 5.1 to 5.4 mEq/L), only 52% of patients on previously maximum RAAS inhibitor dose maintained the same dose, while 16% and 22% of patients either down-titrated to a submaximum dose or completely discontinued the RAAS inhibitor [41]. Furthermore, use of suboptimal RAAS inhibition (submaximal doses or discontinuation) translated into a 2–three fold higher risk of mortality in different patient subgroups [41]. The risk of adverse events was higher in the STRONG-HF trial in the high-intensity group, with hyperkalemia and renal impairment occurring in 18 (3%) and 14 (3%) of patients, respectively, by comparison to none of the patients experiencing hyperkalemia and 1 patient with renal impairment in the usual care group [38]. Nonetheless, even in the setting of an RCT, only 55% of patients from the high-intensity group had been up-titrated to full doses of RAAS inhibitors, 49% to full doses of BBs and 84% to full doses of MRAs [38].

The risk of hyperkalemia in this patient subpopulation may be successfully mitigated following the introduction of SGLT2 inhibitors in the GDMT. While at the start of the STRONG-HF trial, SGLT2 inhibitors were not widely approved and, consequently, not included as part of GDMT, subsequent post-hoc analyses of major RCTs of SGLT2 inhibitors outlined the significant reduction in the risk of hyperkalemia associated with their use. Thus, in a recent meta-analysis conducted on patients with type 2 diabetes at high cardiovascular risk or with CKD that were enrolled in the major RCTs with SGLT2i, the risk of serious hyperkalemia (serum potassium $\geq$6 mmol/L) decreased by 16% with SGLT2i treatment [HR, 0.84 (95%CI, 0.76–0.93) [42]. Accordingly, the ability to better control the hyperkalemia risk may successfully allow the optimal implementation of angiotensin-receptor blockers or angiotensin-converting enzyme inhibitors and even MRAs. Thus, in a pooled survival analysis of two SGLT2i trials (CANVAS and CREDENCE), two nonsteroidal MRAs trials (FIDELIO-DKD and FIGARO-DKD) and eight GLP-1 receptor agonists trials, SGLT2i treatment determined a 37% reduction in the risk of CKD progression (HR, 0.63; 95%CI, 0.53–0.77) and 15% reduction in all cause-mortality (HR, 0.85; 95%CI, 0.75–0.96), while nonsteroidal MRAs were associated with a 23% reduction in the risk of CKD progression (HR, 0.77; 95%CI, 0.67–0.88) and 11% reduction in all cause-mortality (HR, 0.89; 95%CI, 0.79–1.00) [43]. By comparison, the combination of SGLT2i and nonsteroidal MRAs further improved the cardiorenal outcomes, with a 51% reduction in the risk of CKD progression (HR, 0.49; 95%CI, 0.38–0.61) and 24% reduction in all-cause-mortality (HR, 0.76; 95%CI, 0.64–0.90) [43].

Furthermore, if the implementation of GDMT in nondialysis CKD population remains suboptimal due to concerns regarding hyperkalemia and increasing serum creatinine risk, the use of these therapeutic classes in patients undergoing dialysis is even more limited by the lack of data from RCTs and the requirement for adequate pharmacokinetic profiles that evaluate either accumulation or excessive removal of drugs [44]. In a post hoc analysis from the DAPA-CKD trial, those patients that initiated dialysis and continued dapagliflozin had a lower all-cause mortality (8.6 events per 100 patient-years) by comparison to placebo-treated patients (13.4 events per 100 patient-years) [45]. Although this is mainly hypothesis-generating, several studies evaluating the SGLT2i in the dialysis population are awaited [44]. For the β-blockers, the HDPAL study showed that treatment with atenolol in hemodialysis patients with left ventricular hypertrophy and hypertension reduced the cardiovascular morbidity (myocardial infarction, stroke, heart failure) and all-cause hospitalization rates by comparison to lisinopril [46]. Nonetheless, β-blockers dialyzability varies significantly across different agents, ranging from high hemodialysis clearance (atenolol and metoprolol) to negligible dialyzability (carvedilol) [47]. For MRAs, the initial experience suggested a benefit from spironolactone in terms of reducing cardiovascular morbidity and mortality among hemodialysis patients, but recent, more extensive RCTs have failed to confirm the cardiovascular benefit of spironolactone in these patients [48–51].

4.2 Kidney Dysfunction in Ischemic Heart Disease

Similar to heart failure, the relation between chronic kidney disease and ischemic heart disease (IHD) is bidirectional, with CKD being a well-known risk factor for IHD, while patients with IHD have a high prevalence of CKD. In a population-based study that included 13,826 individuals from two longitudinally monitored datasets, the Atherosclerosis Risk in Communities (ARIC) Study and the Cardiovascular Health Study (CHS), the prevalence of cardiovascular disease (CVD) was 12.9% (defined as stroke, angina, claudication, transient ischemic attack, coronary angioplasty or bypass, and recognized or silent myocardial infarction) [87]. Among these patients, the risk of future kidney function decline was 70% higher compared to patients without CVD (prevalence, 7.2% versus. 3.3%) [87]. On the contrary, there is an increasing acknowledgment that CKD must be considered a coronary heart disease equivalent. In an analysis the Kaiser Permanente Renal Registry from Northern California (n = 1,120,295 adults), the risk of hospitalization, cardiovascular events or death increasingly steeply with worsening renal function [88]. Thus, by comparison to patients with an eGFR of at least 60 ml/min, the risk of cardiovascular events was 1.4-fold, two-fold, 2.8-fold and 3.4-fold higher in those with an eGFR of 45–59 ml/min, 30–44 ml/min, 15–29 ml/min and <15 ml/min, respectively [88]. Similarly, the mortality risk increased by 1.2-fold, 1.8-fold, 3.2-fold and 5.9-fold in patients with an eGFR of 45–59 ml/min, 30–44 ml/min, 15–29 ml/min and <15 ml/min, respectively, as compared to those with an eGFR over 60 ml/min [88]. Moreover, other reports have outlined that the risk of mortality after myocardial infarction is higher in those with CKD and diabetes as compared to patients with a previous myocardial infarction, further highlighting the risk of future coronary artery events in patients with CKD [89]. Furthermore, in a recent analysis from the UK Biobank, the risk of sudden cardiac death increased by 1.77-fold in CKD stage 1–3 patients, by 7.46-fold in CKD stage 4 and by 6.15-fold in CKD stage 5 compared to non-CKD individuals [90]. The real-world clinical data is paralleled by observations from RCTs. The VALIANT (Valsartan in Acute Myocardial Infarction Trial) trial randomized patients to receive valsartan, captopril or both after myocardial infarction [91]. Of the 14,527 patients with available serum creatinine assessments, 38.3% had an eGFR of at least 75 ml/min, 28.3% an eGFR of 60–74.9 ml/min, 22.2% an eGFR of 45–59.9 ml/min and 11.3% an eGFR below 45 ml/min [91]. The study assessed mortality as the primary event and a composite endpoint consisting of death from cardiovascular causes, reinfarction, congestive heart failure, resuscitation after cardiac arrest and stroke. Thus, the percentage of patients that died or reached one of the events of the composite endpoint increased progressively from 14.1% and 26.5%, respectively, in the subgroup of patients with an eGFR of at least 75 ml/min towards to 45.5% and 59.9%, respectively, in the subgroup of patients with an eGFR below 45 ml/min [91].

When addressing therapeutic needs of patients with CKD and CVD, one must acknowledge the complex kidney-heart crosstalk that incorporates CKD-specific factors (inflammation, oxidative stress, fluid overload, anemia, mineral and bone disorders, uremic toxins with significant cardiac and vascular toxicity, vascular smooth muscle cell phenotype change toward osteoblast and promotion of vascular calcification) along traditional cardiovascular risk factors (hypertension, diabetes, dyslipidemia) [92]. Accordingly, the effectiveness of primary and secondary prevention strategies varies significantly across the eGFR spectrum, especially regarding antiplatelet and statin therapy in CVD.

Thus, given that the majority of RCTs have excluded patients with moderate or advanced CKD, there is an ongoing debate regarding the benefit versus hemorrhagic risk for antiplatelet therapy for primary prevention of ischemic vascular events. The KDIGO 2024 Clinical Practice Guideline for the Evaluation and Management of Chronic Kidney Disease recommends low-dose aspirin for secondary prevention in patients with CKD and established ischemic cardiovascular disease [30].

In a recent Cochrane Database meta-analysis, 90 studies (40,597 CKD participants) compared an antiplatelet agent with placebo or no treatment, and 29 studies (11,805 CKD participants) directly compared one antiplatelet agent with another [93]. As compared to placebo or no treatment, antiplatelet therapy reduced the overall risk for fatal or nonfatal myocardial infarction (RR, 0.88; 95%CI, 0.79–0.99), the effect being observed only in nondialysis CKD population (RR, 0.85; 0.74–0.99) and not in patients on hemodialysis (RR, 0.83; RR, 0.49–1.41). Nonetheless, antiplatelet therapy did not reduce the risk of fatal or nonfatal stroke (RR, 1.01; 0.64–1.59) or all-cause mortality (RR, 0.94; 95%CI, 0.84–1.06), as compared to placebo or no treatment [93]. In terms of hemorrhagic risk, antiplatelet therapy increased the risk for major bleeding events (RR, 1.35; 95%CI, 1.1–1.65) and minor bleeding events (RR, 1.55; 1.27–1.9), with a potential to increase the risk for fatal bleeding (RR, 1.39; 0.1–19.48) or hemorrhagic stroke (RR, 1.22; 0.69–2.17) [93]. The HOT (Hypertension Optimal Treatment) trial was one of the largest primary prevention trials, randomizing 18,790 patients with diastolic hypertension to two distinct interventions in a multifactorial design: aspirin 75 mg daily or a matching placebo, and to 1 of 3 diastolic pressure targets (≤90, ≤85, or ≤80 mm Hg) [94]. The trial had no exclusion criteria regarding the renal function, and included 16.6% ($n = 3083$) and 2.9% ($n = 536$) patients with an eGFR of 45–59 mL/min and <45 mL/min, respectively. Patients in the lowest eGFR category (<45 ml/min) showed the greatest benefit with a risk reduction of 66% for major cardiovascular disease (HR, 0.34; 95%CI, 0.17–0.67), 69% for myocardial infarction (HR, 0.31; 95%CI, 0.11–0.85), 79% for stroke (HR, 0.21; 95%CI, 0.06–0.75) and 64% for cardiovascular mortality (HR, 0.36; 95%CI, 0.14–0.9), by comparison to a lower impact on cardiovascular events with higher eGFR categories [94]. In parallel, the risk of any bleeding was greater with an eGFR <45 mL/min (HR, 2.76; 95%CI, 1.08–7.05) [94].

In terms of statin therapy, there is a consensus recommendation (1A) for treatment initiation in patients over 50 years with an eGFR below 60 mL/min, but not undergoing dialysis [30]. The SHARP (Study of Heart and Renal Protection) trial randomized 9270 patients with CKD (3023 on dialysis and 6247 not), without a history of myocardial infarction or coronary revascularization, to a combination of simvastatin 20 mg/ezetimibe 10 mg or matching placebo [95]. There was a significant 25% (RR, 0.75; 95%CI, 0.6–0.94) and 21% (RR, 0.79; 95%CI, 0.68–0.93) reduction in the risk of nonhemorrhagic stroke and revascularization procedures, respectively, but only a nonsignificant trend towards a reduction by 8% (RR, 0.92; 95%CI, 0.76–1.11) in the risk for fatal or nonfatal coronary events [95]. Furthermore, the effect on major atherosclerotic events was retained in nondialysis CKD patients (RR, 0.78; 95%CI, 0.67–0.91), but not in those undergoing dialysis (RR, 0.9; 95%CI, 0.75–1.08) [95]. Similarly, in another trial of 1255 patients with type 2 diabetes mellitus, treatment with 20 mg of atorvastatin did not reduce the risk of a primary composite endpoint (cardiovascular death, nonfatal myocardial infarction and stroke) or its individual components, further highlighting that the pathogenesis of atherosclerosis in patients with advanced CKD (including those on dialysis) implies the coexistence of additional, nontraditional, risk factors that are not substantially influenced by the classical statin therapy [96]. Regarding the benefits of revascularization, many trials have excluded patients with advanced CKD, mainly due to the perceived risk of contrast-related nephrotoxicity. The ISCHEMIA-CKD trial included 777 patients with advanced CKD (eGFR less than 30 mL/min) and moderate to severe ischemia on stress test [97]. Patients were randomized to undergo either an initial invasive strategy (consisting of coronary angiography and revascularization in addition to medical therapy) or an initial conservative approach (medical therapy with angiography being reserved in cases of medical therapy failure) [97]. The median eGFR was 23 mL/min in those not receiving dialysis, while 53.4% of the study cohort was undergoing dialysis at the time of randomization [97]. The risk of the primary outcome, death or nonfatal myocardial infarction, was not reduced by an initial invasive approach, nor was the angina-related health status [97, 98].

Declarations

Competing Interests The author(s) has no competing interests to declare that are relevant to the content of this manuscript.

Ethics Approval The author(s) declares that this manuscript does not include primary research with human participants.

The author(s) declares that this manuscript does not include primary studies involving animals.

References

1. Rangaswami J, Bhalla V, Blair JEA, Chang TI, Costa S, Lentine KL, Lerma EV, Mezue K, Molitch M, Mullens W, Ronco C, Tang WHW, McCullough PA, American Heart Association Council on the Kidney in Cardiovascular Disease and Council on Clinical Cardiology. Cardiorenal syndrome: classification, pathophysiology, diagnosis, and treatment strategies: a scientific statement from the American Heart Association. Circulation. 2019;139(16):e840–78.
2. Löfman I, Szummer K, Dahlström U, Jernberg T, Lund LH. Associations with and prognostic impact of chronic kidney disease in heart failure with preserved, mid-range, and reduced ejection fraction. Eur J Heart Fail. 2017;19(12):1606–14.
3. Adams KF, Fonarow GC, Emerman CL, LeJemtel TH, Costanzo MR, Abraham WT, et al. Characteristics and outcomes of patients hospitalized for heart failure in the United States: rationale, design, and preliminary observations from the first 100,000 cases in the Acute Decompensated Heart Failure National Registry (ADHERE). Am Heart J. 2005;149(2):209–16.
4. Ndumele CE, Rangaswami J, Chow SL, Neeland IJ, Tuttle KR, Khan SS, Coresh J, Mathew RO, Baker-Smith CM, Carnethon MR, Despres JP, Ho JE, Joseph JJ, Kernan WN, Khera A, Kosiborod MN, Lekavich CL, Lewis EF, Lo KB, Ozkan B, Palaniappan LP, Patel SS, Pencina MJ, Powell-Wiley TM, Sperling LS, Virani SS, Wright JT, Rajgopal Singh R, Elkind MSV, American Heart Association. Cardiovascular-kidney-metabolic health: a presidential advisory from the American Heart Association. Circulation. 2023;148(20):1606–35.
5. Lo KB, Janakiraman A, Rangaswami J. Kidney dysfunction in heart failure: core curriculum 2025. Am J Kidney Dis. 2025;86(1):109–24.
6. Zoccali C, Levin A, Mallamaci F, Giugliano R, De Caterina R. Decongestion in patients with advanced chronic kidney disease coexisting with heart failure. Clin Kidney J. 2025;18(7):sfaf185.
7. Méndez AB, Azancot MA, Olivella A, Soler MJ. New aspects in cardiorenal syndrome and HFpEF. Clin Kidney J. 2022;15(10):1807–15.
8. Frățilă GV, Obrişcă B, Ismail G. A practical approach to sequential nephron blockade in acute decompensated heart failure. Rom J Cardiol. 2023;33:83–92.

9. Felker GM, Lee KL, Bull DA, Redfield MM, Stevenson LW, Goldsmith SR, et al. Diuretic strategies in patients with acute decompensated heart failure. N Engl J Med. 2011;364(9):797–805.
10. Mentz RJ, Anstrom KJ, Eisenstein EL, Sapp S, Greene SJ, Morgan S, Testani JM, Harrington AH, Sachdev V, Ketema F, Kim DY, Desvigne-Nickens P, Pitt B, Velazquez EJ, TRANSFORM-HF Investigators. Effect of torsemide vs furosemide after discharge on all-cause mortality in patients hospitalized with heart failure: the TRANSFORM-HF randomized clinical trial. JAMA. 2023;329(3):214–23.
11. Heidenreich PA, Bozkurt B, Aguilar D, Allen LA, Byun JJ, Colvin MM, Deswal A, Drazner MH, Dunlay SM, Evers LR, Fang JC, Fedson SE, Fonarow GC, Hayek SS, Hernandez AF, Khazanie P, Kittleson MM, Lee CS, Link MS, Milano CA, Nnacheta LC, Sandhu AT, Stevenson LW, Vardeny O, Vest AR, Yancy CW, ACC/AHA Joint Committee Members. 2022 AHA/ACC/HFSA Guideline for the Management of Heart Failure: a report of the American College of Cardiology/American Heart Association Joint Committee on Clinical Practice Guidelines. Circulation. 2022;145(18):e895–e1032.
12. McDonagh TA, Metra M, Adamo M, Baumbach A, Böhm M, Burri H, et al. 2021 ESC Guidelines for the diagnosis and treatment of acute and chronic heart failure. Eur Heart J. 2021;42(36):3599–726.
13. Ezekowitz JA, O'Meara E, McDonald MA, Abrams H, Chan M, Ducharme A, et al. 2017 comprehensive update of the Canadian Cardiovascular Society Guidelines for the Management of Heart Failure. Can J Cardiol. 2017;33(11):1342–433.
14. Damman K, Beusekamp JC, Boorsma EM, Swart HP, Smilde TDJ, Elvan A, et al. Randomized, double-blind, placebo-controlled, multicentre pilot study on the effects of empagliflozin on clinical outcomes in patients with acute decompensated heart failure (EMPA-RESPONSE-AHF). Eur J Heart Fail. 2020;22(4):713–22.
15. Schulze PC, Bogoviku J, Westphal J, Aftanski P, Haertel F, Grund S, et al. Effects of early empagliflozin initiation on diuresis and kidney function in patients with acute decompensated heart failure (EMPAG-HF). Circulation. 2022;146(4):289–98.
16. Voors AA, Angermann CE, Teerlink JR, Collins SP, Kosiborod M, Biegus J, et al. The SGLT2 inhibitor empagliflozin in patients hospitalized for acute heart failure: a multinational randomized trial. Nat Med. 2022;28(3):568–74.
17. Biegus J, Voors AA, Collins SP, Kosiborod MN, Teerlink JR, Angermann CE, et al. Impact of empagliflozin on decongestion in acute heart failure: the EMPULSE trial. Eur Heart J. 2023;44(1):41–50.
18. Verbrugge FH, Martens P, Ameloot K, Haemels V, Penders J, Dupont M, et al. Acetazolamide to increase natriuresis in congestive heart failure at high risk for diuretic resistance. Eur J Heart Fail. 2019;21(11):1415–22.
19. Mullens W, Dauw J, Martens P, Verbrugge FH, Nijst P, Meekers E, et al. Acetazolamide in acute decompensated heart failure with volume overload. N Engl J Med. 2022;387(13):1185–95.
20. Trullàs JC, Morales-Rull JL, Casado J, Carrera-Izquierdo M, Sánchez-Marteles M, Conde-Martel A, et al. Combining loop with thiazide diuretics for decompensated heart failure: the CLOROTIC trial. Eur Heart J. 2023;44(5):411–21.
21. Butler J, Anstrom KJ, Felker GM, Givertz MM, Kalogeropoulos AP, Konstam MA, et al. Efficacy and safety of spironolactone in acute heart failure: the ATHENA-HF randomized clinical trial. JAMA Cardiol. 2017;2(9):950–8.
22. Konstam MA, Gheorghiade M, Burnett JC Jr, Grinfeld L, Maggioni AP, Swedberg K, Udelson JE, Zannad F, Cook T, Ouyang J, Zimmer C, Orlandi C. Efficacy of Vasopressin Antagonism in Heart Failure Outcome Study with Tolvaptan (EVEREST) Investigators. Effects of oral tolvaptan in patients hospitalized for worsening heart failure: the EVEREST outcome trial. JAMA. 2007;297(12):1319–31.
23. Felker GM, Mentz RJ, Cole RT, Adams KF, Egnaczyk GF, Fiuzat M, et al. Efficacy and safety of tolvaptan in patients hospitalized with acute heart failure. J Am Coll Cardiol. 2017;69(11):1399–406.

24. Konstam MA, Kiernan M, Chandler A, Dhingra R, Mody FV, Eisen H, Haught WH, Wagoner L, Gupta D, Patten R, Gordon P, Korr K, Fileccia R, Pressler SJ, Gregory D, Wedge P, Dowling D, Romeling M, Konstam JM, Massaro JM, Udelson JE, SECRET of CHF Investigators, Coordinators, and Committee Members. Short-term effects of tolvaptan in patients with acute heart failure and volume overload. J Am Coll Cardiol. 2017;69(11):1409–19.
25. Bart BA, Goldsmith SR, Lee KL, Givertz MM, O'Connor CM, Bull DA, et al. Ultrafiltration in decompensated heart failure with cardiorenal syndrome. N Engl J Med. 2012;367(24):2296–304.
26. Dauw J, Charaya K, Lelonek M, Zegri-Reiriz I, Nasr S, Paredes-Paucar CP, Borbély A, Erdal F, Benkouar R, Cobo-Marcos M, Barge-Caballero G, George V, Zara C, Ross NT, Barker D, Lekhakul A, Frea S, Ghazi AM, Knappe D, Doghmi N, Klincheva M, Fialho I, Bovolo V, Findeisen H, Alhaddad IA, Galluzzo A, de la Espriella R, Tabbalat R, Miró Ò, Singh JS, Nijst P, Dupont M, Martens P, Mullens W. Protocolized natriuresis-guided decongestion improves diuretic response: the multicenter ENACT-HF study. Circ Heart Fail. 2024;17(1):e011105.
27. Ter Maaten JM, Beldhuis IE, van der Meer P, Krikken JA, Coster JE, Nieuwland W, van Veldhuisen DJ, Voors AA, Damman K. Natriuresis-guided therapy in acute heart failure: rationale and design of the Pragmatic Urinary Sodium-based treatment algoritHm in Acute Heart Failure (PUSH-AHF) trial. Eur J Heart Fail. 2022;24(2):385–92.
28. Ter Maaten JM, Beldhuis IE, van der Meer P, Krikken JA, Postmus D, Coster JE, Nieuwland W, van Veldhuisen DJ, Voors AA, Damman K. Natriuresis-guided diuretic therapy in acute heart failure: a pragmatic randomized trial. Nat Med. 2023;29(10):2625–32.
29. Damman K, Beldhuis IE, van der Meer P, Krikken JA, Coster JE, Nieuwland W, et al. Renal function and natriuresis-guided diuretic therapy—a pre-specified analysis from the PUSH-AHF trial. Eur J Heart Fail. 2024;26(6):1347–57.
30. Kidney Disease: Improving Global Outcomes (KDIGO) CKD Work Group. KDIGO 2024 Clinical Practice Guideline for the Evaluation and Management of Chronic Kidney Disease. Kidney Int. 2024;105(4S):S117–314.
31. Brenner BM, Cooper ME, de Zeeuw D, Keane WF, Mitch WE, Parving HH, Remuzzi G, Snapinn SM, Zhang Z, Shahinfar S, RENAAL Study Investigators. Effects of losartan on renal and cardiovascular outcomes in patients with type 2 diabetes and nephropathy. N Engl J Med. 2001;345(12):861–9.
32. Bakris GL, Agarwal R, Anker SD, Pitt B, Ruilope LM, Rossing P, et al. Effect of finerenone on chronic kidney disease outcomes in type 2 diabetes. N Engl J Med. 2020;383(23):2219–29.
33. Perkovic V, Tuttle KR, Rossing P, Mahaffey KW, Mann JFE, Bakris G, et al. Effects of semaglutide on chronic kidney disease in patients with type 2 diabetes. N Engl J Med. 2024;391(2):109–21.
34. Heerspink HJL, Agarwal R, Bakris GL, Cherney DZI, Lam CSP, Neuen BL, Sarafidis PA, Tuttle KR, Wanner C, Brinker MD, Dizayee S, Kolkhof P, Schloemer P, Vesterinen P, Perkovic V, FIND-CKD investigators. Design and baseline characteristics of the Finerenone, in addition to standard of care, on the progression of kidney disease in patients with Non-Diabetic Chronic Kidney Disease (FIND-CKD) randomized trial. Nephrol Dial Transplant. 2025;40(2):308–19.
35. Rossing P, Anker SD, Filippatos G, Pitt B, Ruilope LM, Birkenfeld AL, et al. Finerenone in patients with chronic kidney disease and Type 2 diabetes by sodium–glucose cotransporter 2 inhibitor treatment: the FIDELITY analysis. Diabetes Care. 2022;45(12):2991–8.
36. Sarafidis P. Use of ACEi/ARBs, SGLT2 inhibitors and MRAs can help us reach the therapeutic ceiling in CKD. Clin Kidney J. 2024;17(2):sfae014.
37. Agarwal R, Green JB, Heerspink HJL, Mann JFE, McGill JB, Mottl AK, Rosenstock J, Rossing P, Vaduganathan M, Brinker M, Edfors R, Li N, Scheerer MF, Scott C, Nangaku M, CONFIDENCE Investigators. Finerenone with empagliflozin in chronic kidney disease and type 2 diabetes. N Engl J Med. 2025;393(6):533–43.
38. Mebazaa A, Davison B, Chioncel O, Cohen-Solal A, Diaz R, Filippatos G, et al. Safety, tolerability and efficacy of up-titration of guideline-directed medical therapies for acute

heart failure (STRONG-HF): a multinational, open-label, randomised, trial. Lancet. 2022;400(10367):1938–52.

39. Juurlink DN, Mamdani MM, Lee DS, Kopp A, Austin PC, Laupacis A, et al. Rates of hyperkalemia after publication of the randomized aldactone evaluation study. N Engl J Med. 2004;351(6):543–51.
40. Pitt B, Zannad F, Remme WJ, Cody R, Castaigne A, Perez A, et al. The effect of spironolactone on morbidity and mortality in patients with severe heart failure. N Engl J Med. 1999;341(10):709–17.
41. Epstein M, Reaven NL, Funk SE, McGaughey KJ, Oestreicher N, Knispel J. Evaluation of the treatment gap between clinical guidelines and the utilization of renin-angiotensin-aldosterone system inhibitors. Am J Manag Care. 2015;21(11 Suppl):S212–20.
42. Neuen BL, Oshima M, Agarwal R, Arnott C, Cherney DZ, Edwards R, et al. Sodium-glucose cotransporter 2 inhibitors and risk of hyperkalemia in people with type 2 diabetes: a meta-analysis of individual participant data from randomized, controlled trials. Circulation. 2022;145(19):1460–70.
43. Neuen BL, Heerspink HJL, Vart P, Claggett BL, Fletcher RA, Arnott C, et al. Estimated lifetime cardiovascular, kidney, and mortality benefits of combination treatment with SGLT2 inhibitors, GLP-1 receptor agonists, and nonsteroidal MRA compared with conventional care in patients with Type 2 diabetes and albuminuria. Circulation. 2024;149(6):450–62.
44. Minutolo R, Ruotolo C, Conte G, Borrelli S. SGLT2 inhibitors in hemodialysis or peritoneal dialysis patients: rationale and state-of-the art. Clin Kidney J. 2025;19(1):sfaf350.
45. Heerspink HJL, Sjöström CD, Jongs N, Chertow GM, Kosiborod M, Hou FF, et al. Effects of dapagliflozin on mortality in patients with chronic kidney disease: a pre-specified analysis from the DAPA-CKD randomized controlled trial. Eur Heart J. 2021;42(13):1216–27.
46. Agarwal R, Sinha AD, Pappas MK, Abraham TN, Tegegne GG. Hypertension in hemodialysis patients treated with atenolol or lisinopril: a randomized controlled trial. Nephrol Dial Transplant. 2014;29(3):672–81.
47. Tieu A, Velenosi TJ, Kucey AS, Weir MA, Urquhart BL. β-blocker dialyzability in maintenance hemodialysis patients a randomized clinical trial. Clin J Am Soc Nephrol. 2018;13(4):604–11.
48. Charytan DM, Himmelfarb J, Ikizler TA, Raj DS, Hsu JY, Landis JR, et al. Safety and cardiovascular efficacy of spironolactone in dialysis-dependent ESRD (SPin-D): a randomized, placebo-controlled, multiple dosage trial. Kidney Int. 2019;95(4):973–82.
49. Rossignol P, Zannad F, Massy Z, Azizi M, Chorfa F, Coadic J, et al. Spironolactone in patients on chronic haemodialysis at high risk of adverse cardiovascular outcomes (ALCHEMIST): a multicentre, double-blind, randomised, placebo-controlled trial and updated meta-analysis. Lancet. 2025;406(10504):705–18.
50. Walsh M, Collister D, Gallagher M, Mark PB, de Zoysa JR, Tyrwhitt J, et al. Spironolactone versus placebo in patients undergoing maintenance dialysis (ACHIEVE): an international, parallel-group, randomised controlled trial. Lancet. 2025;406(10504):695–704.
51. Matsumoto Y, Mori Y, Kageyama S, Arihara K, Sugiyama T, Ohmura H, et al. Spironolactone reduces cardiovascular and cerebrovascular morbidity and mortality in hemodialysis patients. J Am Coll Cardiol. 2014;63(6):528–36.
52. The EMPA-KIDNEY Collaborative Group, Herrington WG, Staplin N, Wanner C, Green JB, Hauske SJ, Emberson JR, Preiss D, Judge P, Mayne KJ, Ng SYA, Sammons E, Zhu D, Hill M, Stevens W, Wallendszus K, Brenner S, Cheung AK, Liu ZH, Li J, Hooi LS, Liu W, Kadowaki T, Nangaku M, Levin A, Cherney D, Maggioni AP, Pontremoli R, Deo R, Goto S, Rossello X, Tuttle KR, Steubl D, Petrini M, Massey D, Eilbracht J, Brueckmann M, Landray MJ, Baigent C, Haynes R. Empagliflozin in patients with chronic kidney Disease. N Engl J Med. 2023;388(2):117–27.
53. McMurray JJV, Wheeler DC, Stefánsson BV, Jongs N, Postmus D, Correa-Rotter R, et al. Effects of dapagliflozin in patients with kidney disease, with and without heart failure. JACC Heart Fail. 2021;9(11):807–20.

54. Sarraju A, Li J, Cannon CP, Chang TI, Agarwal R, Bakris G, Charytan DM, de Zeeuw D, Greene T, Heerspink HJL, Levin A, Neal B, Pollock C, Wheeler DC, Yavin Y, Zhang H, Zinman B, Perkovic V, Jardine M, Mahaffey KW. Effects of canagliflozin on cardiovascular, renal, and safety outcomes in participants with type 2 diabetes and chronic kidney disease according to history of heart failure: results from the CREDENCE trial. Am Heart J. 2021;233:141–8.
55. Filippatos G, Pitt B, Agarwal R, Farmakis D, Ruilope LM, Rossing P, et al. Finerenone in patients with chronic kidney disease and type 2 diabetes with and without heart failure: a prespecified subgroup analysis of the FIDELIO-DKD trial. Eur J Heart Fail. 2022;24(6):996–1005.
56. Filippatos G, Anker SD, Agarwal R, Ruilope LM, Rossing P, Bakris GL, et al. Finerenone reduces risk of incident heart failure in patients with chronic kidney disease and type 2 diabetes: analyses from the FIGARO-DKD trial. Circulation. 2022;145(6):437–47.
57. Ruilope LM, Pitt B, Anker SD, Rossing P, Kovesdy CP, Pecoits-Filho R, et al. Kidney outcomes with finerenone: an analysis from the FIGARO-DKD study. Nephrol Dial Transplant. 2023;38(2):372–83.
58. Vaduganathan M, Filippatos G, Claggett BL, Desai AS, Jhund PS, Henderson A, et al. Finerenone in heart failure and chronic kidney disease with type 2 diabetes: FINE-HEART pooled analysis of cardiovascular, kidney and mortality outcomes. Nat Med. 2024;30(12):3758–64.
59. Pratley RE, Tuttle KR, Rossing P, Rasmussen S, Perkovic V, Nielsen OW, et al. Effects of semaglutide on heart failure outcomes in diabetes and chronic kidney disease in the FLOW trial. J Am Coll Cardiol. 2024;84(17):1615–28.
60. Bowling CB, Sanders PW, Allman RM, Rogers WJ, Patel K, Aban IB, et al. Effects of enalapril in systolic heart failure patients with and without chronic kidney disease: insights from the SOLVD treatment trial. Int J Cardiol. 2013;167(1):151–6.
61. McCallum W, Tighiouart H, Ku E, Salem D, Sarnak MJ. Trends in kidney function outcomes following RAAS inhibition in patients with heart failure with reduced ejection fraction. Am J Kidney Dis. 2020;75(1):21–9.
62. Lesogor A, Cohn JN, Latini R, Tognoni G, Krum H, Massie B, et al. Interaction between baseline and early worsening of renal function and efficacy of renin-angiotensin-aldosterone systemblockade in patients with heart failure: insights from the Val-HeFT study. Eur J Heart Fail. 2013;15(11):1236–44.
63. Tokmakova MP, Skali H, Kenchaiah S, Braunwald E, Rouleau JL, Packer M, et al. Chronic kidney disease, cardiovascular risk, and response to angiotensin-converting enzyme inhibition after myocardial infarction: the Survival and Ventricular Enlargement (SAVE) study. Circulation. 2004;110(24):3667–73.
64. Konstam MA, Neaton JD, Dickstein K, Drexler H, Komajda M, Martinez FA, Riegger GA, Malbecq W, Smith RD, Guptha S, Poole-Wilson PA, HEAAL Investigators. Effects of high-dose versus low-dose losartan on clinical outcomes in patients with heart failure (HEAAL study): a randomised, double-blind trial. Lancet. 2009;374(9704):1840–8.
65. Kiernan MS, Gregory D, Sarnak MJ, Rossignol P, Massaro J, Kociol R, Zannad F, Konstam MA. Early and late effects of high- versus low-dose angiotensin receptor blockade on renal function and outcomes in patients with chronic heart failure. JACC Heart Fail. 2015;3(3):214–23.
66. Ghali JK, Wikstrand J, Van Veldhuisen DJ, Fagerberg B, Goldstein S, Hjalmarson Å, et al. The influence of renal function on clinical outcome and response to β-blockade in systolic heart failure: insights from metoprolol CR/XL randomized intervention trial in chronic HF (MERIT-HF). J Card Fail. 2009;15(4):310–8.
67. Castagno D, Jhund PS, McMurray JJV, Lewsey JD, Erdmann E, Zannad F, et al. Improved survival with bisoprolol in patients with heart failure and renal impairment: an analysis of the cardiac insufficiency bisoprolol study II (CIBIS-II) trial. Eur J Heart Fail. 2010;12(6):607–16.
68. Wali RK, Iyengar M, Beck GJ, Chartyan DM, Chonchol M, Ann Lukas M, et al. Efficacy and safety of carvedilol in treatment of heart failure with chronic kidney disease: a meta-analysis of randomized trials. Circ Heart Fail. 2011;4(1):18–26.

69. Cohen-Solal A, Kotecha D, Van Veldhuisen DJ, Babalis D, Böhm M, Coats AJ, et al. Efficacy and safety of nebivolol in elderly heart failure patients with impaired renal function: insights from the SENIORS trial. Eur J Heart Fail. 2009;11(9):872–80.
70. Anker SD, Butler J, Filippatos G, Ferreira JP, Bocchi E, Böhm M, et al. Empagliflozin in heart failure with a preserved ejection fraction. N Engl J Med. 2021;385(16):1451–61.
71. Sharma A, Ferreira JP, Zannad F, Pocock SJ, Filippatos G, Pfarr E, et al. Cardiac and kidney benefits of empagliflozin in heart failure across the spectrum of kidney function: insights from the EMPEROR-preserved trial. Eur J Heart Fail. 2023;25(8):1337–48.
72. Packer M, Anker SD, Butler J, Filippatos G, Pocock SJ, Carson P, et al. Cardiovascular and renal outcomes with empagliflozin in heart failure. N Engl J Med. 2020;383(15):1413–24.
73. Zannad F, Ferreira JP, Pocock SJ, Zeller C, Anker SD, Butler J, et al. Cardiac and kidney benefits of empagliflozin in heart failure across the Spectrum of kidney function: insights from EMPEROR-reduced. Circulation. 2021;143(4):310–21.
74. McMurray JJV, Solomon SD, Inzucchi SE, Køber L, Kosiborod MN, Martinez FA, et al. Dapagliflozin in patients with heart failure and reduced ejection fraction. N Engl J Med. 2019;381(21):1995–2008.
75. Jhund PS, Solomon SD, Docherty KF, Heerspink HJL, Anand IS, Böhm M, et al. Efficacy of dapagliflozin on renal function and outcomes in patients with heart failure with reduced ejection fraction: results of DAPA-HF. Circulation. 2021;143(4):298–309.
76. Solomon SD, McMurray JJV, Claggett B, de Boer RA, DeMets D, Hernandez AF, et al. Dapagliflozin in heart failure with mildly reduced or preserved ejection fraction. N Engl J Med. 2022;387(12):1089–98.
77. McCausland FR, Claggett BL, Vaduganathan M, Desai AS, Jhund P, de Boer RA, Docherty K, Fang J, Hernandez AF, Inzucchi SE, Kosiborod MN, Lam CSP, Martinez F, Saraiva JFK, McGrath MM, Shah SJ, Verma S, Langkilde AM, Petersson M, McMurray JJV, Solomon SD. Dapagliflozin and kidney outcomes in patients with heart failure with mildly reduced or preserved ejection fraction: a prespecified analysis of the DELIVER randomized clinical trial. JAMA Cardiol. 2023;8(1):56–65.
78. Pitt B, Bhatt DL, Szarek M, Cannon CP, Leiter LA, McGuire DK, et al. Effect of sotagliflozin on early mortality and heart failure-related events: a post hoc analysis of SOLOIST-WHF. JACC Heart Fail. 2023;11(8):879–89.
79. McMurray JJV, Packer M, Desai AS, Gong J, Lefkowitz MP, Rizkala AR, et al. Angiotensin–neprilysin inhibition versus enalapril in heart failure. N Engl J Med. 2014;371(11):993–1004.
80. Damman K, Gori M, Claggett B, Jhund PS, Senni M, Lefkowitz MP, et al. Renal effects and associated outcomes during angiotensin-Neprilysin inhibition in heart failure. JACC Heart Fail. 2018;6(6):489–98.
81. Solomon SD, McMurray JJV, Anand IS, Ge J, Lam CSP, Maggioni AP, et al. Angiotensin–neprilysin inhibition in heart failure with preserved ejection fraction. N Engl J Med. 2019;381(17):1609–20.
82. Mc Causland FR, Lefkowitz MP, Claggett B, Anavekar NS, Senni M, Gori M, et al. Angiotensin-neprilysin inhibition and renal outcomes in heart failure with preserved ejection fraction. Circulation. 2020;142(13):1236–45.
83. Vardeny O, Wu DH, Desai A, Rossignol P, Zannad F, Pitt B, Solomon SD, RALES Investigators. Influence of baseline and worsening renal function on efficacy of spironolactone in patients with severe heart failure: insights from RALES (Randomized Aldactone Evaluation Study). J Am Coll Cardiol. 2012;60(20):2082–9.
84. Pitt B, Pfeffer MA, Assmann SF, Boineau R, Anand IS, Claggett B, et al. Spironolactone for heart failure with preserved ejection fraction. N Engl J Med. 2014;370(15):1383–92.
85. Solomon SD, McMurray JJV, Vaduganathan M, Claggett B, Jhund PS, Desai AS, et al. Finerenone in heart failure with mildly reduced or preserved ejection fraction. N Engl J Med. 2024;391(16):1475–85.

86. Mc Causland FR, Vaduganathan M, Claggett BL, Kulac IJ, Desai AS, Jhund PS, et al. Finerenone and kidney outcomes in patients with heart failure: the FINEARTS-HF trial. J Am Coll Cardiol. 2025;85(2):159–68.
87. Elsayed EF, Tighiouart H, Griffith J, Kurth T, Levey AS, Salem D, Sarnak MJ, Weiner DE. Cardiovascular disease and subsequent kidney disease. Arch Intern Med. 2007;167(11):1130–6.
88. Go AS, Chertow GM, Fan D, McCulloch CE, Hsu CY. Chronic kidney disease and the risks of death, cardiovascular events, and hospitalization. N Engl J Med. 2004;351(13):1296–305.
89. Tonelli M, Muntner P, Lloyd A, Manns BJ, Klarenbach S, Pannu N, et al. Risk of coronary events in people with chronic kidney disease compared with those with diabetes: a population-level cohort study. Lancet. 2012;380(9844):807–14.
90. Li Y, Jiang R, Ouyang C, Wang J, Yu Q, Lu J, Hong W, Liu S, Chen Y, Cai J, Yuan H, Zhang L, Lu Y. Chronic kidney disease is associated with increased risk of sudden cardiac death. Nat Commun. 2025;16(1):9180.
91. Anavekar NS, McMurray JJ, Velazquez EJ, Solomon SD, Kober L, Rouleau JL, White HD, Nordlander R, Maggioni A, Dickstein K, Zelenkofske S, Leimberger JD, Califf RM, Pfeffer MA. Relation between renal dysfunction and cardiovascular outcomes after myocardial infarction. N Engl J Med. 2004;351(13):1285–95.
92. Marx-Schütt K, Cherney DZI, Jankowski J, Matsushita K, Nardone M, Marx N. Cardiovascular disease in chronic kidney disease. Eur Heart J. 2025;46(23):2148–60.
93. Natale P, Palmer SC, Saglimbene VM, Ruospo M, Razavian M, Craig JC, Jardine MJ, Webster AC, Strippoli GF. Antiplatelet agents for chronic kidney disease. Cochrane Database Syst Rev. 2022;2(2):CD008834.
94. Jardine MJ, Ninomiya T, Perkovic V, Cass A, Turnbull F, Gallagher MP, et al. Aspirin is beneficial in hypertensive patients with chronic kidney disease: a post-hoc subgroup analysis of a randomized controlled trial. J Am Coll Cardiol. 2010;56(12):956–65.
95. Baigent C, Landray MJ, Reith C, Emberson J, Wheeler DC, Tomson C, Wanner C, Krane V, Cass A, Craig J, Neal B, Jiang L, Hooi LS, Levin A, Agodoa L, Gaziano M, Kasiske B, Walker R, Massy ZA, Feldt-Rasmussen B, Krairittichai U, Ophascharoensuk V, Fellström B, Holdaas H, Tesar V, Wiecek A, Grobbee D, de Zeeuw D, Grönhagen-Riska C, Dasgupta T, Lewis D, Herrington W, Mafham M, Majoni W, Wallendszus K, Grimm R, Pedersen T, Tobert J, Armitage J, Baxter A, Bray C, Chen Y, Chen Z, Hill M, Knott C, Parish S, Simpson D, Sleight P, Young A, Collins R, Investigators SHARP. The effects of lowering LDL cholesterol with simvastatin plus ezetimibe in patients with chronic kidney disease (Study of Heart and Renal Protection): a randomised placebo-controlled trial. Lancet. 2011;377(9784):2181–92.
96. Wanner C, Krane V, März W, Olschewski M, Mann JFE, Ruf G, et al. Atorvastatin in patients with type 2 diabetes mellitus undergoing hemodialysis. N Engl J Med. 2005;353(3):238–48.
97. Bangalore S, Maron DJ, O'Brien SM, Fleg JL, Kretov EI, Briguori C, et al. Management of coronary disease in patients with advanced kidney disease. N Engl J Med. 2020;382(17):1608–18.
98. Spertus JA, Jones PG, Maron DJ, Mark DB, O'Brien SM, Fleg JL, et al. Health status after invasive or conservative Care in Coronary and Advanced Kidney Disease. N Engl J Med. 2020;382(17):1619–28.

Chapter 5
Hypertension as a Link Between Renal and Cardiac Dysfunction

Feyyaz Hazar Yagmur and Mehmet Kanbay

5.1 Introduction

Hypertension is strongly influenced by environmental and lifestyle-related factors, among which excessive dietary sodium intake and obesity play a crucial role, and in parallel, insufficient dietary potassium intake has emerged as an important contributor to blood pressure (BP) elevation by impairing vascular and renal sodium handling [1]. These modifiable factors are not only closely linked to the development and persistence of hypertension but also exert direct and indirect effects on both cardiac and kidney health [2]. The modern lifestyle, associated with physical inactivity, weight gain, and increased consumption of processed foods rich in sodium and poor in potassium, creates a metabolic and hemodynamic ambience that simultaneously promotes hypertension, cardiac remodeling, and progressive kidney dysfunction. Hypertension represents a central pathophysiological axis through which kidney and cardiac dysfunction converge and amplify one another. Beyond its role as an isolated hemodynamic abnormality, sustained elevation of BP exerts structural, functional, and molecular effects on both the kidney and the heart, positioning these organs in an interdependent relationship [1–3]. The kidney, as the primary regulator of sodium and water balance, extracellular volume and long-term BP control, is particularly vulnerable to hypertensive injury. Conversely, the heart is continuously exposed to increased afterload and sympathetic activation, leading to progressive myocardial remodeling and functional impairment [2–4].

F. H. Yagmur (✉)
Department of Internal Medicine, Koc University Faculty of Medicine, Istanbul, Türkiye
e-mail: fyagmur@kuh.ku.edu.tr

M. Kanbay
Department of Internal Medicine and Nephrology, Koc University, School of Medicine, Istanbul, Türkiye

A. Covic, A. Burlacu (eds.), *Renal Dysfunction in Cardiovascular Pathologies*,
https://doi.org/10.1007/978-3-032-25434-4_5

The close interdependence between kidney and cardiac systems explains why hypertension frequently manifests not as an isolated condition, but as part of a broader cardiorenal sequence [4]. Declining kidney function is associated with a rising prevalence and severity of hypertension, while poorly controlled BP accelerates both chronic kidney disease (CKD) progression and the development of hypertensive heart disease. Importantly, in patients with established CKD, cardiovascular morbidity and mortality often exceed the risk of progression to end-stage kidney disease, emphasizing the dominant clinical impact of cardiorenal interactions [5, 6].

From a mechanistic perspective, hypertension integrates hemodynamic stress with sympathetic activation, endothelial dysfunction, inflammation, and fibrosis. These processes act in parallel within the kidney and the heart, creating a vicious cycle in which kidney dysfunction promotes cardiac injury and vice versa. Understanding hypertension as a unifying link between kidney and cardiac dysfunction is therefore essential for framing both disease pathogenesis and therapeutic strategies [7, 8].

5.2 Epidemiological Overlap Between Kidney and Cardiac Disease

Kidney and cardiac diseases exhibit a marked epidemiological overlap, reflecting shared risk factors and interconnected disease paths. Hypertension is one of the most prevalent and influential contributors to this overlap, functioning as both a primary driver and an amplifier of organ dysfunction in each system. Epidemiological data consistently demonstrate that kidney impairment and cardiovascular disease frequently coexist, particularly in hypertensive populations [9, 10].

The prevalence of hypertension increases progressively with declining kidney function. More than two-thirds of individuals with early-stage CKD are hypertensive, while prevalence rates exceed 90% in patients with advanced-stage CKD. Conversely, markers of kidney damage are highly prevalent among patients with cardiovascular disease. Even modest reductions in estimated glomerular filtration rate (eGFR) or the presence of albuminuria are associated with a substantial increase in the risk of coronary artery disease, congestive heart failure (CHF), and cardiovascular disease-related mortality. Importantly, these associations follow a continuous and graded relationship rather than a clear threshold, indicating that cardiovascular risk rises early in the course of kidney dysfunction [10, 11].

CHF represents a particularly strong point of convergence between renal and cardiac disease. Kidney impairment is present in a significant proportion of patients with CHF, with prevalence estimates ranging from 30% to over 50%, depending on disease severity and diagnostic criteria. This overlap is especially pronounced in heart failure with preserved ejection fraction, a condition frequently associated with long-standing hypertension. Epidemiological studies further demonstrate that declining kidney function is independently associated with worse CHF-related outcomes, including increased hospitalization rates and mortality [9, 10].

From a nephrological perspective, cardiovascular disease remains the leading cause of death across all stages of CKD, far exceeding the risk of progression to end-stage kidney disease in earlier stages. Hypertensive patients with albuminuria or reduced eGFR exhibit a several-fold increases in cardiovascular event rates compared with those without kidney involvement. Albuminuria has been shown to predict cardiovascular outcomes independently of BP levels, underscoring its role as a systemic vascular risk marker rather than an isolated kidney abnormality [10–12].

These epidemiological observations support the concept of a cardiorenal overlap in which hypertension serves as a central and modifiable determinant linking kidney and cardiac disease. Rather than representing different comorbidities, kidney and cardiac dysfunction frequently progress in parallel, driven by sustained BP elevation and shared pathophysiological mechanisms. Recognition of this epidemiological overlap highlights the need for integrated prevention and management strategies targeting both organ systems in patients with hypertension.

5.3 Common Pathophysiological Mechanisms Linking Kidney and Heart

Hypertension is the leading contributor to the development and progression of kidney dysfunction (Fig. 5.1). Chronic elevation of systemic BP increases intraglomerular pressure, promotes glomerular hypertension and endothelial injury. Over time, these changes lead to albuminuria and progressive loss of nephron function, reflected by declining eGFR [12].

Hypertension is closely linked to activation of the renin–angiotensin–aldosterone system (RAAS), which further exacerbates sodium and water retention, inflammation, and fibrotic remodeling within the kidney. These processes accelerate CKD progression and contribute to the maintenance of elevated BP, reinforcing a vicious cycle between hypertension and kidney dysfunction [5, 9, 10].

In the heart, sustained hypertension imposes a chronic pressure overload that drives structural and functional remodeling. Increased afterload promotes left ventricular hypertrophy and concentric remodeling, adaptive responses that initially preserve systolic performance but ultimately impair diastolic function and myocardial compliance. As a result, long-standing hypertension is strongly associated with the development of heart failure [9–11].

Neurohormonal activation and increased sympathetic tone further contribute to hypertensive cardiac injury by increasing myocardial oxygen demand, promoting fibrosis and altering myocardial energy metabolism and efficiency. These changes reduce cardiac reserve and increase vulnerability to ischemia and arrhythmias, linking chronic BP elevation to adverse cardiovascular outcomes [8, 10].

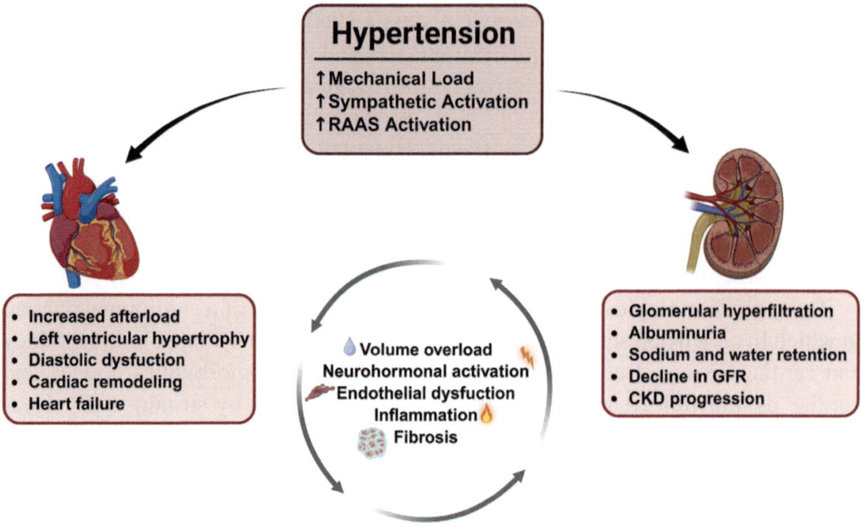

Fig. 5.1 The complex interplay underlying the pathophysiological link between kidney and cardiovascular disorders through high blood pressure. Abbreviations: CKD Chronic kidney disease, GFR Glomerular filtration rate, RAAS Renin-angiotensin-aldosterone system

Hypertension serves as a link between kidney and cardiac dysfunction through a set of shared pathophysiological mechanisms that simultaneously affect both organs. Fundamental to this interaction is persistent activation of the RAAS. Angiotensin II and aldosterone exert parallel harmful effects on the kidney and the heart, promoting vasoconstriction, sodium retention, hypertrophy, inflammation, and fibrosis. These actions not only sustain hypertension but also drive progressive structural damage in both organs [9, 13].

Sympathetic nervous system overactivity represents another critical common pathway. Increased sympathetic tone increases systemic vascular resistance and heart rate while reducing renal blood flow and enhancing renin release. In the kidney, this contributes to sodium retention and ischemic injury; in the heart, it promotes hypertrophy, arrhythmias, and remodeling. Direct measurements of sympathetic activity demonstrate marked elevations in patients with CKD, correlating with left ventricular hypertrophy and increased cardiovascular mortality [7, 8].

Endothelial dysfunction provides an additional mechanistic bridge between kidney and cardiac disease. Impaired nitric oxide bioavailability and increased production of vasoconstrictors such as endothelin lead to increased vascular tone, arterial stiffness, and elevated systolic BP. In the kidney, endothelial dysfunction exacerbates glomerular hypertension and proteinuria, while in the heart it impairs coronary microvascular function and myocardial perfusion [7–9].

Inflammation and fibrosis represent downstream consequences of sustained hypertension and neurohormonal activation. Proinflammatory cytokines and oxidative stress contribute to vascular remodeling, myocardial fibrosis, and tubulointerstitial scarring. These processes reduce organ compliance and functional reserve, further sensitizing both the kidney and the heart to hemodynamic stress [7, 9].

Finally, the mechanical load imposed by hypertension acts directly on both organs. Elevated intraglomerular pressure accelerates nephron loss, while increased ventricular wall stress drives myocardial hypertrophy and remodeling. Through these intertwined mechanisms, hypertension establishes a vicious cycle in which kidney and cardiac dysfunction mutually reinforce each other [10].

5.4 Therapeutic Implications and Cardiorenal Protection

Treatment strategies increasingly emphasize interventions that target shared pathophysiological mechanisms linking cardiac and kidney injury, with particular focus on RAAS blockade and sodium–glucose co-transporter 2 (SGLT2) inhibition (Fig. 5.2).

RAAS blockage remains a fundamental component of hypertension management in patients at risk of cardiac and kidney dysfunction. Angiotensin-converting enzyme inhibitors and angiotensin receptor blockers reduce the adverse effects of chronic RAAS activation by reducing vasoconstriction, sodium retention, and

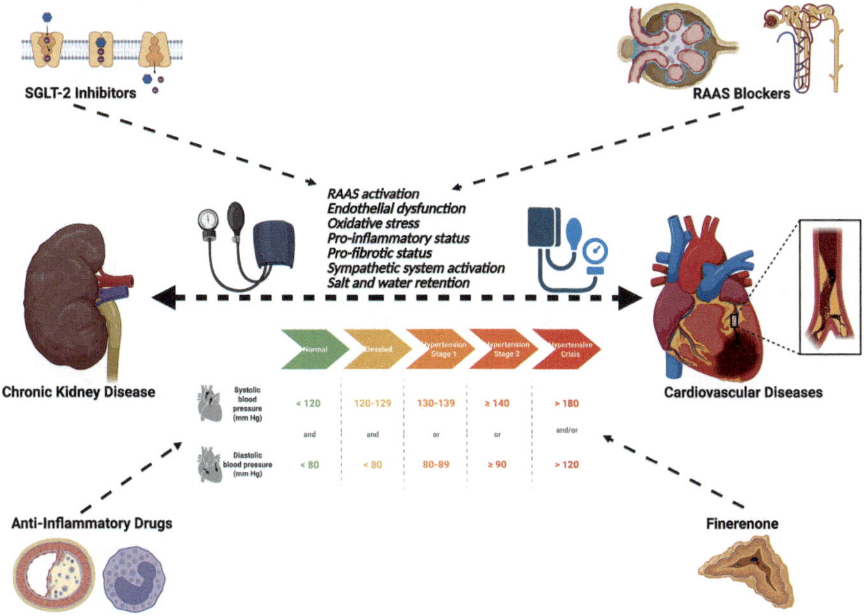

Fig. 5.2 The potential pharmacotherapeutic approaches with kidney and cardiovascular beneficiary effects. Abbreviations: SGLT-2 Sodium-glucose cotransporter-2, RAAS Renin-angiotensin-aldosterone system

intraglomerular hypertension. In the kidney, these agents lower intraglomerular pressure, reduce albuminuria, and slow the progression of CKD. In parallel, RAAS blockade decreases cardiac remodeling by limiting hypertrophy, inflammation and fibrosis. Thereby improving diastolic function and reducing the risk of heart failure development. Beyond hemodynamic effects, RAAS inhibition exerts important anti-fibrotic and anti-inflammatory actions that directly target shared mechanisms of cardiorenal injury [14, 15].

SGLT2 inhibitors have rapidly become a foundational therapy for cardiorenal protection. While originally developed for glycemic control, large-scale randomized clinical trials have consistently shown that SGLT2 inhibitors reduce heart failure hospitalizations and slow kidney function decline across populations with and without diabetes, independent of their glucose-lowering effects. In the DAPA-CKD trial, treatment with dapagliflozin significantly reduced the risk of kidney disease progression, cardiovascular death, and hospitalization for heart failure in patients with CKD, irrespective of diabetes status [16].

Similarly, the EMPA-KIDNEY trial confirmed the broad cardiorenal benefits of SGLT2 inhibition across a wide spectrum of CKD, including patients without diabetes and with lower baseline eGFR. Empagliflozin significantly reduced the risk of kidney disease progression and cardiovascular events, reinforcing the concept that therapies addressing shared kidney and cardiac pathophysiology play a central role in modern cardiorenal protection strategies [17].

Mechanism of effect involves modulation of intrarenal hemodynamics, tubular workload, and systemic metabolic pathways. SGLT2 inhibition reduces intraglomerular pressure and albuminuria, thereby slowing kidney disease progression. Concurrently, these agents promote natriuresis and osmotic diuresis, leading to reductions in plasma volume and preload, which are particularly beneficial in patients with hypertensive heart disease and heart failure [18].

Furthermore, evidence from large randomized clinical trials supports the prognostic importance of intensive BP control in patients at high cardiovascular risk. The Systolic Blood Pressure Intervention Trial (SPRINT) demonstrated that targeting a lower blood pressure (<120 mmHg), compared with standard control (<140 mmHg), significantly reduced major cardiovascular events and all-cause mortality. Importantly, these benefits were observed in a population enriched for hypertension-related target organ damage, including a substantial proportion of patients with CKD. The findings of SPRINT underscore that effective BP lowering not only reduces cardiovascular events but also mitigates the downstream consequences of sustained hemodynamic stress that contribute to integrated cardiorenal dysfunction [19].

Importantly, SGLT2 inhibitors also influence several non-hemodynamic pathways relevant to cardiorenal protection, including reductions in inflammation, oxidative stress, and myocardial fibrosis, as well as improvements in myocardial energy metabolism. These effects translate into consistent reductions in heart failure hospitalization and slowing of kidney function decline observed in large randomized clinical trials [18]. The complementary mechanisms of SGLT2 inhibition and

RAAS blockade provide a strong excuse for their combined use in patients with hypertension-related cardiorenal disease.

In addition to RAAS blockade and SGLT2 inhibition, several emerging therapeutic strategies further target pathways implicated in cardiorenal injury. Dual endothelin receptor antagonists address endothelin-mediated vasoconstriction, sodium retention, and vascular remodeling. Mechanisms that contribute to resistant hypertension and progressive organ damage. By attenuating endothelin-driven glomerular hypertension and systemic vascular stiffness, these agents may offer additive blood pressure reduction and potential renal protection [20].

Nonsteroidal mineralocorticoid receptor antagonists, particularly finerenone, have expanded the therapeutic landscape by selectively modulating aldosterone-mediated inflammation and fibrosis. In large outcome trials involving patients with chronic kidney disease and type 2 diabetes, finerenone significantly reduced renal disease progression and cardiovascular events, supporting the concept that mineralocorticoid receptor overactivation is a central mediator of integrated cardiac and renal injury [21].

Beyond hemodynamic and neurohormonal pathways, inflammation has emerged as a critical contributor to hypertension-associated organ damage. Ziltivekimab, a monoclonal antibody targeting interleukin-6 signaling, has demonstrated substantial reductions in inflammatory biomarkers in patients with chronic kidney disease and elevated cardiovascular risk. Ongoing outcome trials are evaluating whether selective IL-6 inhibition translates into meaningful reductions in cardiovascular and renal events, potentially establishing anti-inflammatory therapy as a complementary strategy in cardiorenal risk modification [22].

Overall, therapeutic strategies targeting both BP control and shared pathophysiological pathways offer the greatest potential to interrupt the vicious cycle linking cardiac and kidney dysfunction. Integration of RAAS blockade and SGLT2 inhibition into hypertension management reflects a shift toward mechanism-based, organ-protective treatment approaches aimed at improving long-term cardiorenal outcomes.

5.5 Future Perspectives

Future research in hypertension-mediated cardiorenal disease is increasingly focused on identifying molecular mechanisms and biomarkers that capture early organ vulnerability and predict disease progression beyond conventional clinical parameters. Omics-based approaches, including genomics, transcriptomics and proteomics, have emerged as promising tools to explain the complex biological networks underlying the interaction between the heart and the kidney. These technologies offer the potential to move from population-based risk assessment toward individualized characterization of cardiorenal risk [23, 24].

Genetic studies have identified variants associated with BP regulation, renal sodium handling, and myocardial remodeling, providing insights into individual susceptibility to hypertensive organ damage. Proteomic and metabolomic profiling has revealed distinct molecular signatures associated with inflammation, oxidative stress, extracellular matrix turnover, and fibrosis, the processes central to both cardiac and kidney dysfunction. Circulating biomarkers reflecting these pathways, such as markers of collagen synthesis and degradation, endothelial dysfunction, and tubular injury, are currently being evaluated for their ability to improve early detection and prognostic stratification in hypertensive populations [25].

In parallel, novel biomarkers are gaining attention as indicators of cardiorenal stress. Fibroblast growth factor 23, soluble urokinase plasminogen activator receptor, and growth differentiation factor-15 have been linked to both cardiovascular and kidney outcomes and may represent upstream mediators rather than downstream consequences of organ damage. Advances in high-sensitivity assays further allow detection of low-grade myocardial injury and subclinical volume overload, refining risk assessment in patients with hypertension and early CKD [26–28].

Finally, the integration of multi-omics data with advanced imaging, longitudinal clinical phenotyping, and machine learning techniques represents a key future direction. Such approaches may enable the construction of predictive models that capture the dynamic evolution of cardiorenal dysfunction in hypertension. By shifting focus toward early molecular alterations and shared pathogenic pathways, future research holds promise for more precise prevention and treatment of hypertension-related cardiac and kidney disease.

5.6 Conclusion

Hypertension represents a central and modifiable driver of both cardiac and kidney dysfunction, linking these two organ systems through shared hemodynamic, neurohormonal, vascular, and inflammatory pathways. Instead of being an isolated risk factor, chronic BP elevation promotes a progressive cardiorenal disease process, leading to parallel structural and functional impairment of both the heart and the kidney.

Recognition of this interaction has important clinical implications. Early identification of subclinical cardiac and kidney involvement offers the opportunity to interrupt disease progression before irreversible organ damage occurs. Current guideline-directed therapies, particularly RAAS blockade and SGLT2 inhibition, support this strategy by addressing shared disease mechanisms and offering effective protection for both the heart and the kidney. Ultimately, approaching hypertension from a cardiorenal perspective supports a move away from isolated, organ-specific management toward integrated strategies that aim to preserve both cardiac and kidney function. Such an approach is essential to reducing the long-term burden of hypertension-mediated organ damage and improving outcomes across a broad spectrum of patients.

References

1. Cockwell P, Fisher LA. The global burden of chronic kidney disease. Lancet. 2020;395(10225):662–4.
2. Vasan RS, Larson MG, Leip EP, Evans JC, O'Donnell CJ, Kannel WB, et al. Impact of high-normal blood pressure on the risk of cardiovascular disease. N Engl J Med. 2001;345(18):1291–7.
3. MacMahon S, Peto R, Cutler J, Collins R, Sorlie P, Neaton J, et al. Blood pressure, stroke, and coronary heart disease. Part 1, prolonged differences in blood pressure: prospective observational studies corrected for the regression dilution bias. Lancet. 1990;335(8692):765–74.
4. de Mast Q, Beutler JJ. The prevalence of atherosclerotic renal artery stenosis in risk groups: a systematic literature review. J Hypertens. 2009;27(7):1333–40.
5. Smink PA, Lambers Heerspink HJ, Gansevoort RT, de Jong PE, Hillege HL, Bakker SJ, et al. Albuminuria, estimated GFR, traditional risk factors, and incident cardiovascular disease: the PREVEND (Prevention of Renal and Vascular Endstage Disease) study. Am J Kidney Dis. 2012;60(5):804–11.
6. Matsushita K, van der Velde M, Astor BC, Woodward M, Levey AS, de Jong PE, et al. Association of estimated glomerular filtration rate and albuminuria with all-cause and cardiovascular mortality in general population cohorts: a collaborative meta-analysis. Lancet. 2010;375(9731):2073–81.
7. Roumeliotis S, Mallamaci F, Zoccali C. Endothelial dysfunction in chronic kidney disease, from biology to clinical outcomes: a 2020 update. J Clin Med. 2020;9(8).
8. Grassi G, Quarti-Trevano F, Seravalle G, Arenare F, Volpe M, Furiani S, et al. Early sympathetic activation in the initial clinical stages of chronic renal failure. Hypertension. 2011;57(4):846–51.
9. Zoccali C, Mallamaci F, Adamczak M, de Oliveira RB, Massy ZA, Sarafidis P, et al. Cardiovascular complications in chronic kidney disease: a review from the European Renal and Cardiovascular Medicine Working Group of the European Renal Association. Cardiovasc Res. 2023;119(11):2017–32.
10. Botdorf J, Chaudhary K, Whaley-Connell A. Hypertension in cardiovascular and kidney disease. Cardiorenal Med. 2011;1(3):183–92.
11. Burnier M, Damianaki A. Hypertension as cardiovascular risk factor in chronic kidney disease. Circ Res. 2023;132(8):1050–63.
12. De Bhailis ÁM, Kalra PA. Hypertension and the kidneys. Br J Hosp Med (Lond). 2022;83(5):1–11.
13. Chue CD, Townend JN, Steeds RP, Ferro CJ. Arterial stiffness in chronic kidney disease: causes and consequences. Heart. 2010;96(11):817–23.
14. Brenner BM, Cooper ME, de Zeeuw D, Keane WF, Mitch WE, Parving HH, et al. Effects of losartan on renal and cardiovascular outcomes in patients with type 2 diabetes and nephropathy. N Engl J Med. 2001;345(12):861–9.
15. McEvoy JW, McCarthy CP, Bruno RM, Brouwers S, Canavan MD, Ceconi C, et al. ESC guidelines for the management of elevated blood pressure and hypertension. Eur Heart J. 2024;45(38):3912–4018.
16. Mark PB, Sarafidis P, Ekart R, Ferro CJ, Balafa O, Fernandez-Fernandez B, et al. SGLT2i for evidence-based cardiorenal protection in diabetic and non-diabetic chronic kidney disease: a comprehensive review by EURECA-m and ERBP working groups of ERA. Nephrol Dial Transplant. 2023;38(11):2444–55.
17. Herrington WG, Staplin N, Wanner C, Green JB, Hauske SJ, Emberson JR, et al. Empagliflozin in patients with chronic kidney disease. N Engl J Med. 2023;388(2):117–27.
18. Heerspink HJL, Stefánsson BV, Correa-Rotter R, Chertow GM, Greene T, Hou FF, et al. Dapagliflozin in patients with chronic kidney disease. N Engl J Med. 2020;383(15):1436–46.
19. Wright JT Jr, Williamson JD, Whelton PK, Snyder JK, Sink KM, Rocco MV, et al. A randomized trial of intensive versus standard blood-pressure control. N Engl J Med. 2015;373(22):2103–16.

20. Schlaich MP, Bellet M, Weber MA, Danaietash P, Bakris GL, Flack JM, et al. Dual endothelin antagonist aprocitentan for resistant hypertension (PRECISION): a multicentre, blinded, randomised, parallel-group, phase 3 trial. Lancet. 2022;400(10367):1927–37.
21. Filippatos G, Anker SD, Agarwal R, Ruilope LM, Rossing P, Bakris GL, et al. Finerenone reduces risk of incident heart failure in patients with chronic kidney disease and type 2 diabetes: analyses from the FIGARO-DKD trial. Circulation. 2022;145(6):437–47.
22. Wada Y, Jensen C, Meyer ASP, Zonoozi AAM, Honda H. Efficacy and safety of interleukin-6 inhibition with ziltivekimab in patients at high risk of atherosclerotic events in Japan (RESCUE-2): a randomized, double-blind, placebo-controlled, phase 2 trial. J Cardiol. 2023;82(4):279–85.
23. Provenzano M, Serra R, Garofalo C, Michael A, Crugliano G, Battaglia Y, et al. OMICS in chronic kidney disease: focus on prognosis and prediction. Int J Mol Sci. 2021;23(1).
24. Virzì GM, Clementi A, Battaglia GG, Ronco C. Multi-omics approach: new potential key mechanisms implicated in cardiorenal syndromes. Cardiorenal Med. 2019;9(4):201–11.
25. He T, Zhang Z, Staessen JA, Mischak H, Latosinska A, Beige J. Proteomic biomarkers in the cardiorenal syndrome: toward deciphering molecular pathophysiology. Am J Hypertens. 2021;34(7):669–79.
26. Tuegel C, Katz R, Alam M, Bhat Z, Bellovich K, de Boer I, et al. GDF-15, galectin 3, soluble ST2, and risk of mortality and cardiovascular events in CKD. Am J Kidney Dis. 2018;72(4):519–28.
27. Marthi A, Donovan K, Haynes R, Wheeler DC, Baigent C, Rooney CM, et al. Fibroblast growth factor-23 and risks of cardiovascular and noncardiovascular diseases: a meta-analysis. J Am Soc Nephrol. 2018;29(7):2015–27.
28. Rotbain Curovic V, Theilade S, Winther SA, Tofte N, Eugen-Olsen J, Persson F, et al. Soluble urokinase plasminogen activator receptor predicts cardiovascular events, kidney function decline, and mortality in patients with type 1 diabetes. Diabetes Care. 2019;42(6):1112–9.

Chapter 6
Vascular Calcification in Advanced Chronic Kidney Disease: Epidemiology, Pathophysiology, and Treatment

Rodolfo Fernando Rivera, Maria Teresa Sciarrone Alibrandi, Nadia Edvige Foligno, Lorenza Magagnoli, Paola Ciceri, and Mario Cozzolino

Abbreviations

AAC	Abdominal Aortic Calcification
ALP	Alkaline Phosphatase
AMPK	AMP-Activated Protein Kinase
ATF4	Activating Transcription Factor 4
BMP	Bone Morphogenetic Protein
BMP7	Bone Morphogenetic Protein 7
CAC	Coronary Artery Calcification
CaSR	Calcium-Sensing Receptor
Ca–Pi	Calcium–Phosphate
CVC	Cardiac Valvular Calcification
CKD	Chronic Kidney Disease
CKD-MBD	Chronic Kidney Disease–Mineral and Bone Disorder
CPPs	Calciprotein Particles
dp-ucMGP	Dephosphorylated–Uncarboxylated Matrix Gla Protein
eGFR	Estimated Glomerular Filtration Rate
ENPP1	Ectonucleotide Pyrophosphatase/Phosphodiesterase 1
ER	Endoplasmic Reticulum
ESRD	End-Stage Renal Disease

R. F. Rivera
Nephrology and Dialysis Unit, Pio XI Hospital, ASST Brianza, Desio, Italy

M. T. S. Alibrandi · N. E. Foligno
Nephrology and Dialysis Unit, IRCCS San Raffaele Scientific Institute, Milan, Italy

L. Magagnoli · P. Ciceri · M. Cozzolino (✉)
Nephrology and Dialysis, ASST Santi Paolo E Carlo, Department of Health Sciences, University of Milan, Milan, Italy
e-mail: mario.cozzolino@unimi.it

A. Covic, A. Burlacu (eds.), *Renal Dysfunction in Cardiovascular Pathologies*,
https://doi.org/10.1007/978-3-032-25434-4_6

EVs	Extracellular Vesicles
FGF23	Fibroblast Growth Factor 23
FGFR	Fibroblast Growth Factor Receptor
FoxO	Forkhead Box O
GFR	Glomerular Filtration Rate
GRP	Gla-Rich Protein
HIF-PHDi	HIF-prolyl hydroxylase inhibitors
IL	Interleukin
IL-17A	Interleukin-17A
IL-6	Interleukin-6
Klotho	Klotho Protein (α-Klotho)
lncRNA	Long Non-Coding RNA
MAPK	Mitogen-Activated Protein Kinase
MGP	Matrix Gla Protein
mTORC1	Mechanistic Target of Rapamycin Complex 1
NF-κB	Nuclear Factor Kappa B
NO	Nitric Oxide
OPG	Osteoprotegerin
OPN	Osteopontin
PTH	Parathyroid Hormone
Pi	Inorganic Phosphate
PiT1/PiT2	Type III Sodium-Dependent Phosphate Transporters
PKC	Protein Kinase C
PPi	Inorganic Pyrophosphate
RAAS	Renin–Angiotensin–Aldosterone System
ROS	Reactive Oxygen Species
Runx2	Runt-Related Transcription Factor 2
SIRT1	Sirtuin 1
SIRT3	Sirtuin 3
sHPT	Secondary Hyperparathyroidism
SOD	Superoxide Dismutase
TNAP	Tissue-Nonspecific Alkaline Phosphatase
TNF-α	Tumour Necrosis Factor Alpha
UPR	Unfolded Protein Response
VC	Vascular Calcification
VDR	Vitamin D Receptor
VSMC	Vascular Smooth Muscle Cell

6.1 Introduction

6.1.1 *Definition of Vascular Calcification in Advanced Chronic Kidney Disease*

Vascular calcification (VC) represents one of the most relevant and complex complications of chronic kidney disease (CKD), with both incidence and severity increasing in parallel with the decline in renal function. Although it may already be present in the early stages of the disease, its prevalence rises sharply in advanced stages—particularly in stages 4 and 5D, collectively referred to as end-stage renal disease (ESRD) [1].

Today, VC is recognised as an active, regulated, and potentially reversible process characterised by the deposition of calcium–phosphate (Ca–Pi) hydroxyapatite crystals within the vascular wall and, at times, in cardiac valves. While it shares common risk factors with ageing, diabetes, and dyslipidaemia, in CKD it develops earlier and progresses more aggressively, thereby contributing substantially to the markedly increased cardiovascular risk that typifies this patient population [2].

From a morphological perspective, two principal forms can be distinguished: intimal calcification, which is associated with atherosclerotic plaques in large elastic arteries, and medial calcification (Mönckeberg's sclerosis), characterised by concentric thickening of the medial layer in the absence of lipid deposition—the predominant form observed in the advanced stages of CKD [3, 4]. This distinction is not merely descriptive but carries important clinical and prognostic implications: each type affects vascular function in a distinct manner and requires targeted therapeutic approaches, while both contribute to increased arterial stiffness, left ventricular overload, and a heightened risk of cardiovascular events and mortality [5].

VC arises from the interplay between osteogenic transformation of Vascular Smooth Muscle Cell (VSMCs), disturbances in mineral metabolism, and uraemic toxins, all of which promote the formation of microcalcifications and the progressive stiffening of the vascular wall [6].

These processes fall within the broader framework of CKD–mineral and bone disorder (CKD-MBD), defined by *Moe* et al. in 2005 [7], which encompasses abnormalities in calcium (Ca), phosphate (Pi), parathyroid hormone (PTH), vitamin D, and Fibroblast Growth Factor 23 (FGF23) metabolism. The consequences range from renal osteodystrophy to the progression of VC, contributing to cardiovascular risk even before conventional biochemical markers become abnormal [8]. A deeper understanding of these mechanisms has profoundly influenced the clinical management of CKD, guiding monitoring and therapeutic strategies towards the prevention of cardiovascular morbidity and mortality.

6.1.2 Differences Between Vascular and Valvular Calcification

VC and cardiac valvular calcification (CVC) share a common pathophysiological substrate—encompassing disturbances in mineral metabolism, chronic inflammation, and osteogenic trans-differentiation of resident cells—yet they differ in localisation, haemodynamic impact, and clinical significance.

VC primarily involves the arterial media and intima, leading to vascular stiffness, increased pulse pressure, and left ventricular overload. Its consequences manifest as left ventricular hypertrophy, arrhythmias, and heart failure, conditions particularly prevalent among patients with advanced CKD and ESRD [9].

CVC, by contrast, predominantly affects the aortic and mitral valves. Progressive Ca deposition leads to valvular stenosis or regurgitation, with a markedly higher incidence and faster progression than in the general population. CVC represents one of the leading causes of cardiovascular morbidity in patients undergoing dialysis [10].

From a functional standpoint, VC acts as a diffuse haemodynamic load, impairing vascular compliance and coronary perfusion, whereas CVC produces a focal mechanical injury, resulting in severe valvular stenosis or regurgitation. Understanding these distinctions is essential for accurate risk stratification and the selection of targeted therapeutic strategies.

As CKD progresses (stages 4–5D), the calcific burden tends to increase in parallel within both the vascular wall and the valvular leaflets. The progression of CVC correlates with declining renal function and rising levels of Pi, PTH and FGF23, suggesting a bidirectional relationship between renal dysfunction and valvular remodelling [11]. Likewise, multiple longitudinal studies have linked the expansion of VC with increased arterial stiffness and cardiovascular mortality [12].

Recent reviews identify CKD-MBD as the common matrix underlying both processes, emphasising the efficacy of anti-crystallisation therapies such as SNF472 in slowing calcific progression in haemodialysis patients [13]. Moreover, meta-analyses and systematic reviews confirm that CVC is highly prevalent and predictive of adverse cardiovascular outcomes, underscoring the importance of parallel monitoring of VC and CVC in clinical practice [14].

To aid comprehension, Table 6.1 compares the key pathophysiological, clinical, and prognostic aspects, highlighting how VC and CVC, while interrelated, demand distinct management approaches.

Overall, VC and CVC represent two interconnected manifestations of a shared pathophysiological continuum. The former leads to a diffuse loss of arterial elasticity and a global haemodynamic overload, whereas the latter causes a focal yet clinically dramatic impairment of valvular function. Recognising this functional and prognostic duality is crucial to guiding monitoring and treatment strategies aimed at reducing cardiovascular risk and improving the quality of life in patients with advanced CKD.

Table 6.1 Vascular and cardiac valve calcification: comparative overview in advanced CKD

Parameter	Vascular calcification (VC)	Cardiac valve calcification (CVC)	Clinical notes/ comments
Main site	Involves primarily the intima and media of elastic and muscular arteries, with diffuse hydroxyapatite deposition [5]	Affects cardiac valves, mainly aortic and mitral, leading to leaflet thickening and stiffness [11]	VC is diffuse along the arterial tree; CVC is localized but with significant hemodynamic impact
Type	Intimal (atherosclerotic) and medial (Mönckeberg) calcification. Medial type predominates in advanced CKD and dialysis [1]	Progressive valvular calcification with nodular mineralization and matrix ossification [13]	The distinction is clinically relevant for prognosis and therapeutic strategies
Main mechanisms	Mineral metabolism imbalance (Ca, P, PTH, FGF23, Vit D), VSMC osteogenic switch, chronic inflammation, uremic toxins [15]	Osteogenic transformation of valvular cells, mineral imbalance, inflammation, local mechanical stress [10]	Both share CKD–MBD as a common pathophysiologic substrate
Evolution pattern	Progressive with CKD stage, correlating with arterial stiffness and CV mortality [16]	Progressive in CKD, leading to valvular stenosis or regurgitation; often parallels VC but with different rates and patterns [11]	CKD progression drives both VC and CVC, though with distinct clinical manifestations
Hemodynamic consequences	Left ventricular overload, increased pulse pressure, arterial stiffness, reduced coronary perfusion [1]	Valvular stenosis or regurgitation, localized pressure gradient, risk of acute heart failure [13]	VC: Diffuse "load"; CVC: Localized "critical point" with severe functional impact
Cardiovascular risk	Higher rates of hypertension, arrhythmia, heart failure, myocardial infarction, and overall CV mortality [5]	Associated with valvular dysfunction, HF, ischemic events, and CV mortality [11]	Both substantially contribute to CV morbidity and mortality in ESRD
Assessment methods	Coronary/aortic CT, X-ray, calcification scoring, vascular ultrasound [10]	Echocardiography, valvular CT, 3D imaging, pressure gradient assessment [11]	Imaging should be site-specific; combined VC/CVC assessment is often needed
Therapeutic options	CKD–MBD management, SNF472, phosphate/Ca/PTH control, optimized dialysis, experimental anti-crystallization agents [13]	CKD–MBD management, anti-crystallization drugs, valve replacement when indicated, emerging pharmacologic options [10]	Pharmacologic strategies still evolving; integrated VC/CVC monitoring is essential

(continued)

Table 6.1 (continued)

Parameter	Vascular calcification (VC)	Cardiac valve calcification (CVC)	Clinical notes/ comments
Prevalence	High in advanced CKD and ESRD; often detectable early in disease [5]	Common in ESRD, with faster progression than in general population [11]	Longitudinal studies confirm parallel progression with renal decline
Prognosis	Strongly linked to arterial stiffness, CV events, and mortality [16]	Powerful predictor of adverse CV outcomes, progressive stenosis, and heart failure [13]	Both require close clinical evaluation and longitudinal follow-up

6.1.3 Epidemiology, Clinical Relevance and Prognostic Impact

VC is an extremely common and progressive complication in patients with CKD, exerting a direct impact on cardiovascular mortality. Its prevalence rises in parallel with declining renal function and may reach up to 90% in patients with ESRD [17]. The most frequently affected sites are the Coronary Artery Calcification (CAC), Abdominal Aortic Calcification (AAC), and CVC [18], with their extent closely correlated to the severity of CKD [19].

The main risk factors include advanced age, hyperphosphatemia, secondary hyperparathyroidism, chronic use of calcium-based binders, and poor control of the Ca-Pi balance. Recent studies have also identified elevated FGF23 levels as a strong predictor of VC progression [20].

The presence and progression of VC are associated with a significant increase in cardiovascular risk, independent of traditional risk factors [21–23], and exhibit a clear dose–response relationship with the decline in glomerular filtration rate (GFR) [24–26].

The CRIC Study by *Tian* et al. [27] confirmed that in patients with CKD stages 2–5, the progression of CAC is strongly associated with major cardiovascular events and all-cause mortality, consolidating the central role of CKD-MBD in the pathogenesis of VC. This dynamic process, linked not only to CKD progression but also to biochemical parameters such as PTH and FGF23, further underscores the pivotal contribution of mineral–bone disorder to vascular damage. *Zhang* et al. [18] also demonstrated that patients with rapid CAC progression exhibit a substantially higher risk profile compared with those with stable calcifications, highlighting the importance of serial monitoring as a key prognostic tool.

Although computed tomography (CT) remains the gold standard for quantifying VC [28], the assessment of AAC using lateral radiography has emerged as a valuable alternative prognostic marker, particularly useful in CKD [25] and ESRD [26], demonstrating a dose–response relationship with the decline in estimated eGFR [24]. Bellasi et al. [29] reported a strong correlation between AAC scores and cardiovascular calcification indices, with a sensitivity of 67% and specificity of 91%, further supported by evidence linking AAC severity to that of CAC [30]. Meta-analyses by Leow et al. [31] and Yao et al. [32] confirmed that both the presence and progression of AAC are strongly associated with cardiovascular and all-cause mortality.

Finally, CVC represents another powerful negative prognostic marker. Prospective studies have shown that their presence in dialysis patients is associated with increased overall [33, 34] and cardiovascular mortality [35, 36], serving as a true pathological hallmark of advanced CKD. Bellasi et al. [37] and Brandenburg et al. [36] describe CVC as a distinctive manifestation of CKD progression, driven by metabolic derangements, chronic inflammation, and disturbances of mineral metabolism within the CKD–MBD framework. The progression of CVC is a robust predictor of adverse outcomes, underscoring the importance of systematic valvular monitoring.

Taken together, these data highlight that integrated assessment of VC, CAC, and CVC is crucial for accurate risk stratification and early identification of targeted preventive and therapeutic strategies, ultimately aiming to reduce cardiovascular morbidity and mortality in advanced CKD.

6.2 Pathophysiological Mechanisms

Initially, VC was regarded as a passive, degenerative process; however, it is now recognised as an active, cell-mediated phenomenon governed by complex molecular and regulatory mechanisms. VC may occur within the intimal layer, where it is typically associated with atherosclerosis and inflammation, or within the medial layer (*Mönckeberg's sclerosis*), a condition particularly common among patients with CKD [3, 4]. Both forms may coexist within the same vessel, exerting synergistic effects that contribute to disease progression and poorer prognosis [38].

The mechanisms underlying accelerated VC in CKD are not yet fully understood. Both traditional risk factors—such as advanced age, hypertension, diabetes, and dyslipidaemia—and non-traditional CKD-specific factors have been identified. The latter include disturbances of mineral metabolism, abnormal PTH levels, and Ca-Pi overload, chronic inflammation, malnutrition, and oxidative stress, all of which contribute to the initiation and progression of VC in this high-risk population.

Far from being a mere passive precipitation of Ca–Pi salts, VC represents an active phenotypic transformation of VSMCs into an osteochondrogenic lineage. This process is driven by the loss of physiological inhibitors and the activation of pro-mineralisation signalling pathways, ultimately leading to the deposition of hydroxyapatite within the vascular wall.

The following sections describe the key molecular mechanisms involved in the initiation and progression of VC, organised according to their pathophysiological roles (see Fig. 6.1).

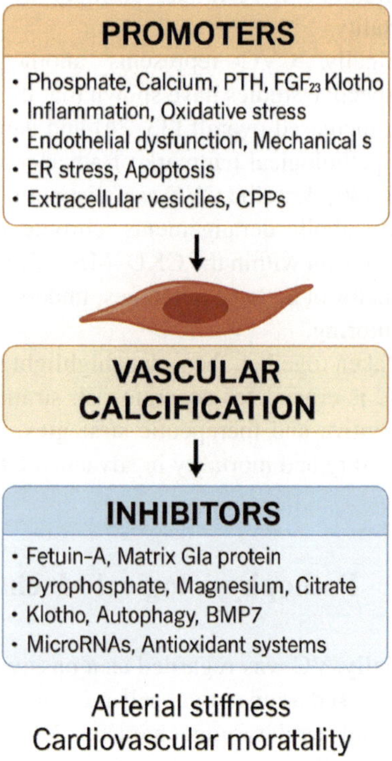

Fig. 6.1 Integrated schematic of vascular calcification mechanisms in CKD. Simplified vertical schematic illustrating the integrated balance between promoters and inhibitors of vascular calcification in CKD. The central vascular smooth muscle cell (VSMC) integrates pro-calcific stimuli (phosphate, calcium, inflammation, oxidative stress) and anti-calcific defences (Fetuin-A, MGP, pyrophosphate, magnesium, Klotho, protective microRNAs). The downstream clinical outcomes—arterial stiffness, endothelial dysfunction, and cardiovascular mortality—reflect the net imbalance of these opposing pathways

6.2.1 *Promoters of Vascular Calcification*

6.2.1.1 Calcium–Phosphate Imbalance and Osteogenic Signalling

Hyperphosphatemia, a hallmark of CKD–MBD, represents one of the primary drivers of vascular mineralization by promoting local supersaturation and nucleation of Ca–Pi crystals within the extracellular matrix [39]. Elevated extracellular Pi concentrations alter osteoblastic gene expression through the type III sodium-dependent Pi co-transporters PiT1 and PiT2 [40]. The increased intracellular influx of Pi triggers a cascade of signalling pathways that culminates in the transcriptional reprogramming of VSMCs, which progressively lose their contractile phenotype and acquire an osteo-chondrogenic profile.

At the core of this process lies the activation of the transcription factor Runx2/Cbfa1, regarded as the *master regulator* of osteoblastic differentiation. Runx2 promotes the expression of bone-related genes such as osteocalcin, Alkaline Phosphatase (ALP), osteopontin (OPN), and type I collagen, while repressing smooth-muscle markers including SM22α and SM–MHC, thus leading to a true *phenotypic conversion* of VSMCs [41].

Upstream of Runx2, a pivotal role is played by Msx2 (muscle segment homeobox 2), a transcription factor induced by BMP-2/BMP-4 signalling and oxidative stress. Msx2 directly activates Runx2 transcription and stimulates the Wnt/β-catenin pathway, amplifying the osteogenic response and enhancing the synthesis of endogenous Bone Morphogenetic Proteins (BMP) [42]. The subsequent induction of Osterix (Sp7), a downstream effector of Runx2, promotes the final maturation of the osteoblastic phenotype with the synthesis of collagen I, osteonectin, and ALP, which are essential for hydroxyapatite crystal nucleation [43].

In parallel, excess extracellular Ca amplifies the effects of Pi by stabilizing Ca–Pi complexes and promoting the nucleation of hydroxyapatite ($Ca_{10}(PO_4)_6(OH)_2$) within EVs of endosomal or apoptotic origin.

These vesicles contain annexins, ALP, sialoproteins, and matrix fragments that act as micro-scaffolds for crystal growth [42].

The accumulation of Ca–Pi complexes further enhances mitochondrial oxidative stress and induces VSMCs apoptosis, leading to the release of apoptotic bodies that serve as additional nucleation sites for mineral deposition [44]. Interaction between Ca– Pi crystals and the cell membrane also activates ion-sensing receptors, including the calcium-sensing receptor (CaSR), which triggers additional pro-calcific signalling cascades [45].

At the systemic level of CKD, Pi retention is accompanied by Klotho Protein (α-Klotho) deficiency and elevated FGF23, which exacerbate endothelial dysfunction and destabilize mineral metabolism, fuelling a self-perpetuating cycle of hyperphosphatemia and progressive VC [46].

In summary, the combined excess of Pi and Ca does not merely produce a passive chemical precipitation but acts as a potent active pathogenic signal capable of reprogramming the vascular genome.

The Msx2 → Runx2 → Osterix transcriptional cascade, together with stimuli mediated by BMPs, Wnt/β-catenin, and reactive oxygen species (ROS), constitutes the molecular core of vascular osteoblastic trans-differentiation, which characterizes advanced-stage CKD calcification.

6.2.1.2 PTH, FGF23 and Klotho

In advanced CKD, progressive Pi retention and reduced calcitriol synthesis trigger a complex hormonal response involving PTH, FGF23, and its co-receptor Klotho—key regulators of the bone–kidney–vascular axis. This network, which physiologically maintains mineral homeostasis, becomes dysregulated in CKD, transforming into a potent driver of VC and endothelial injury [39, 45].

Secondary Hyperparathyroidism (sHPT) initially arises as an adaptive mechanism to early hypocalcaemia and Pi retention, but as CKD progresses, it evolves into a maladaptive state. Chronic PTH excess promotes the mobilization of Ca and Pi from bone, leading to post-resorptive hypercalcemia and systemic mineral overload.

At the vascular level, PTH exerts pleiotropic pro-calcific effects: it induces oxidative stress, enhances ALP activity, and upregulates osteogenic factors in VSMCs, thereby promoting the transition to an osteoblastic phenotype [39, 40]. Moreover, PTH increases intracellular Ca through L-type Ca channels and activates the PKC/MAPK signalling pathway, which in turn amplifies Runx2 and osteocalcin transcription, reinforcing the osteogenic switch [39, 45, 46].

In parallel, elevated FGF23, secreted by osteocytes in response to Pi retention, represents a compensatory attempt to reduce serum phosphate. However, in the uremic milieu, its action becomes pathologically dissociated from normal renal Pi regulation. FGFR1c/3c receptors expressed on endothelial and VSMCs become hyperresponsive, and in the absence of Klotho, they mediate toxic, phosphate-independent signalling [47]. FGF23 activates intracellular cascades such as ERK1/2 and PLCγ, leading to myocardial hypertrophy, oxidative stress, and endothelial dysfunction; within vascular tissues, these pathways enhance ALP expression and suppress anti-calcific mediators such as Klotho and Fetuin-A [45, 46].

Recent evidence has also revealed a close interaction between FGF23 and iron metabolism. Iron deficiency has been shown to upregulate FGF23 synthesis through stabilization of HIF-1α and activation of the proprotein convertase *furin*, leading to increased cleavage of intact FGF23 (iFGF23) into C-terminal fragments (cFGF23) [48–50]. In CKD, this mechanism contributes to elevated circulating FGF23 levels independently of phosphate load or inflammation [48–50].

Importantly, excessive FGF23 can in turn suppress erythropoiesis and promote renal anaemia, establishing a pathogenic loop linking iron deficiency, hypoxia, and mineral dysregulation [50]. Correction of iron deficiency—particularly with oral iron formulations—has been shown to reduce FGF23 overproduction and may thus represent a therapeutic opportunity to modulate the phosphate–FGF23–Klotho axis.

Klotho, a transmembrane protein primarily expressed in the renal distal tubule, functions as an obligatory co-receptor for FGF23 and a pleiotropic regulator of mineral metabolism, redox balance, and vascular aging [51]. In CKD, both renal and vascular Klotho expression are markedly reduced even in early stages, converting FGF23 signalling from a physiological regulator into a pathological driver of vascular injury.

Klotho deficiency leads to multiple pro-calcific alterations: impaired cellular Ca extrusion, increased Pi influx into VSMCs, and suppression of antioxidant pathways such as FoxO/SOD2.

Moreover, loss of Klotho attenuates autophagy and accelerates endothelial senescence, thereby enhancing the vascular inflammatory response and predisposing to accelerated calcification [51].

In the current integrated model, the PTH–FGF23–Klotho axis represents a maladaptive circuit that amplifies VC.

- Elevation of PTH and FGF23 promotes the mobilization and precipitation of Ca and phosphate.
- Reduction of Klotho abolishes its antioxidant and anti-inflammatory protective signals.

- VSMCs, exposed to this altered microenvironment, activate Runx2 and ALP expression and release calcifying EVs.

The result is a pathogenic triad in which PTH, FGF23, and Klotho act synergistically to drive vascular mineralization and arterial stiffness.

Understanding this hormonal network not only clarifies the pathogenesis of calcification, but also provides the rationale for therapeutic strategies aimed at modulating the phosphate–FGF23–Klotho axis and restoring a more physiological mineral balance within the vasculature.

6.2.1.3 Vitamin D and Mineral Metabolism

Vitamin D exerts a complex and ambivalent role in mineral metabolism and in the pathophysiology of VC. Under physiological conditions, it supports cardiovascular health by maintaining Ca– Pi homeostasis, limiting parathyroid activation, and modulating inflammatory responses. However, in CKD this delicate balance is rapidly disrupted [52, 53].

Already in the early stages of CKD, serum 25(OH)-vitamin D levels are significantly reduced due to multiple factors: impaired cutaneous synthesis, altered hepatic metabolism, urinary loss of binding proteins, and—most critically—decreased renal conversion to $1{,}25(OH)_2$-vitamin D (calcitriol) caused by reduced 1α-hydroxylase activity. The resulting vitamin D deficiency contributes to sHPT, Pi retention, and overactivation of the renin–angiotensin–aldosterone system (RAAS), promoting arterial stiffness and endothelial dysfunction [54, 55].

Several studies have demonstrated that vitamin D deficiency is associated with an increased incidence of cardiovascular events and progression of VC, through the upregulation of PTH, activation of inflammatory pathways (notably NF-κB), and accumulation of oxidative stress mediators [55].

Moreover, low vitamin D levels correlate with a pro-inflammatory profile, characterized by elevated TNF-α and decreased IL-10, contributing to the establishment of a pro-calcific endothelial state [56, 57].

On the opposite side, excess active vitamin D (calcitriol or its analogy) may promote vascular mineralization, particularly in uremic patients with hypercalcemia or hyperphosphatemia.

Activation of the vitamin D receptor (VDR) in VSMCs induces the transcription of osteogenic genes such as Runx2, osteocalcin, and ALP, acting synergistically with hypercalcemia to Favor hydroxyapatite deposition within the vascular matrix [45].

The Biphasic Role of Vitamin D in VC:

- Protective, under conditions of sufficiency, where it contributes to mineral homeostasis, limits PTH secretion, and reduces inflammation.
- Potentially harmful, in uremic settings or under high pharmacological dosing, where VDR activation in vascular cells may facilitate osteogenic transdifferentiation and calcific deposition.

This duality underscores the need for a careful therapeutic balance: maintaining an adequate vitamin D status to prevent SHPT and endothelial dysfunction, while avoiding excessive VDR stimulation in the presence of hypercalcemia or hyperphosphatemia.

6.2.1.4 Inflammation and Oxidative Stress

CKD is a state of chronic systemic inflammation, which serves as a powerful promoter of VC. The accumulation of uremic toxins, gut dysbiosis, and hyperphosphatemia stimulates the production of pro-inflammatory cytokines (IL-1β, IL-6, TNF-α) and ROS, which act synergistically to promote the osteogenic trans-differentiation of VSMCs [58, 59].

Inflammatory cytokines activate the NF-κB and NLRP3 inflammasome pathways, leading to increased expression of ALP, Runx2, and OPN, while also promoting cellular apoptosis [45]. Dead or injured vascular cells release apoptotic bodies and calcifying microvesicles enriched in ALP and membrane fragments, which act as nucleation foci for Ca–Pi complex formation [44].

Mitochondrial oxidative stress, amplified by reduced antioxidant activity (superoxide dismutase, catalase, glutathione peroxidase) and Klotho deficiency, intensifies ROS production and compromises cellular integrity. This establishes a self-perpetuating pro-calcific environment, in which inflammation and mineralization mutually reinforce each other, driving the progression of vascular damage in CKD [60].

In summary, chronic inflammation and oxidative stress form a bidirectional pathogenic circuit that converts inflammatory stimuli into structural calcification, thereby driving the progression of arterial stiffness and increasing cardiovascular risk in patients with CKD.

6.2.1.5 Endothelial Dysfunction and Mechanical Stress

In CKD, the vascular endothelium is continuously exposed to a uremic, pro-oxidant, and pro-inflammatory milieu that profoundly impairs its function. The reduced bioavailability of nitric oxide (NO)—resulting from decreased endothelial nitric oxide synthase (eNOS) expression and increased ROS production—disrupts vascular tone regulation and promotes leukocyte adhesion and local inflammation [45, 59].

Senescent or injured endothelial cells release microvesicles enriched in ALP, BMP-2, and annexins, which act as vectors of osteogenic signals toward underlying VSMCs [58, 60]. These vesicles, together with the loss of endothelial anti-calcific factors such as Klotho and Fetuin-A, contribute to the formation of initial mineralization foci within the vascular wall.

Moreover, chronic mechanical stress—arising from hypertension, increased arterial stiffness, and disturbed flow—enhances ROS generation and activates pro-calcific signalling pathways such as TGF-β/Smad and MAPK, establishing a vicious cycle linking endothelial dysfunction, inflammation, and calcification [61].

Altogether, endothelial dysfunction represents one of the earliest and most pivotal events in the pathogenesis of VC in CKD, predisposing the arterial wall to progressive mineralization and stiffness.

Intracellular Alterations: Mitochondria, ER Stress, and Autophagy

Within the uremic microenvironment, VSMCs undergo profound disturbances in the intracellular mechanisms responsible for maintaining energy and redox homeostasis. Mitochondrial injury, triggered by Pi overload, uremic toxins, and oxidative stress, results in ATP depletion and accumulation of ROS, which amplify inflammatory signalling and drive osteogenic trans-differentiation [58].

Concomitantly, endoplasmic reticulum (ER) stress represents an additional pro-calcific stimulus. The accumulation of misfolded proteins within the ER activates the unfolded protein response (UPR) through the PERK → eIF2α → ATF4 pathway, inducing the transcription factor CHOP. This signalling axis is known to mediate apoptosis under chronic stress conditions and, in vascular cell models, has been associated with the upregulation of osteogenic genes such as Runx2 and with enhanced mineral deposition [62]. These processes promote the release of EVs enriched in Ca and ALP, which act as nucleation sites for hydroxyapatite formation [59].

In parallel, reduced autophagy, documented in experimental models of CKD, impairs the clearance of damaged mitochondria and calcifying vesicles. The autophagic deficit disrupts the delicate balance between cellular survival and programmed death, leading to the accumulation of mineralizable material within the extracellular matrix [44].

Altogether, the combination of mitochondrial dysfunction, ER stress, and impaired autophagy defines a metabolic vulnerability that transforms VSMCs from a contractile to an osteogenic phenotype—representing a critical nodal point in the pathophysiology of VC in CKD.

Extracellular Vesicles and Calciprotein Particles (CPPs)

VSMCs and macrophages are the principal sources of EVs in the uremic milieu. These microvesicles, typically 100–300 nm in diameter, are released in response to apoptosis or cellular stress and contain ALP, annexins (II, V), sialoproteins, and nanocrystals of hydroxyapatite, which act as primary nucleation foci for mineral deposition [58, 59].

Under physiological conditions, EVs are neutralized by circulating calcification inhibitors such as Fetuin-A, inorganic pyrophosphate (PPi), and matrix Gla protein (MGP), which prevent crystal growth. However, in advanced CKD, the reduction of these protective factors Favors the transformation of EVs into CPPs—colloidal complexes that transport Ca^{2+}/Pi–Fetuin-A aggregates within the plasma [44].

Type II CPPs, which are denser and richer in hydroxyapatite, lose their inhibitory properties and acquire pro-inflammatory and pro-calcific potential. They induce endothelial dysfunction and stimulate the production of cytokines such as IL-6 and TNF-α, amplifying systemic inflammation and accelerating both VC and arterial stiffness [63].

Overall, EVs and CPPs represent a critical interface between mineral metabolism, inflammation, and innate immunity, acting both as early biomarkers of cardiovascular risk and as active mediators of pathological mineralization in CKD.

6.2.1.6 Immunity and Cellular Cross-Talk

In the context of VC, immune cells play an active and regulatory role, rather than serving as passive bystanders. M1 macrophages (classically polarized) release pro-inflammatory cytokines such as TNF-α, IL-1β, and IL-6, which stimulate the osteogenic trans-differentiation of VSMCs by activating Runx2 and enhancing ALP activity [64]. In contrast, M2 macrophages (alternatively polarized) exhibit a more repair-oriented phenotype, promoting inflammation resolution and secreting anti-inflammatory mediators, which in some experimental models appear to attenuate VC [65].

T cells, particularly the Th17 subset, also contribute to VC. IL-17A, produced by activated T lymphocytes, has been shown both in vitro and ex vivo to promote VC by inducing endothelial senescence, stimulating pro-calcific factor synthesis, and driving the proliferation of vascular mesenchymal cells [66]. Furthermore, IL-17 signalling has been linked to fibroblast proliferation and vascular dysfunction in cardiovascular disease models [67].

This immune–vascular cross-talk establishes a pro-calcific microenvironment, where inflammatory signalling promotes VSMCs transdifferentiation, the release of calcifying vesicles, and the loss of mineralization inhibitors. Conversely, transformed VSMCs can secrete cytokines and growth factors that recruit and further polarize macrophages and lymphocytes, sustaining a self-amplifying inflammatory–calcific loop.

6.2.2 Physiological Inhibitors of Vascular Calcification

VC represents a dynamic process regulated by a continuous balance between pro-calcific and anti-calcific factors. Under physiological conditions, an integrated network of circulating, metabolic, cellular, and genetic molecules tightly controls mineral deposition, preventing the transformation of the vascular wall into an ectopic bone-like tissue. In CKD, however, the quantitative and functional loss of these endogenous inhibitors disrupts this equilibrium and accelerates the deposition of Ca–Pi crystals.

Based on the main mechanisms previously described by other authors [44, 58–60, 63, 68], it is possible to propose an original and innovative classification of the physiological inhibitors of VC.

This framework, which distinguishes five major categories, provides a clearer conceptual structure and ensures didactic continuity with the pathophysiological mechanisms outlined earlier.

6.2.2.1 Classical Circulating Inhibitors

Systemic circulating inhibitors represent the first line of defence against ectopic mineralization.

Fetuin-A, a liver-derived glycoprotein, binds Ca–Pi complexes to form soluble CPPs, thereby preventing crystal growth and precipitation [44, 60]. Serum Fetuin-A levels are markedly reduced in CKD and in chronic inflammatory states, showing an inverse correlation with the severity of VC and cardiovascular mortality [69].

A second key regulator is MGP, a vitamin K–dependent protein synthesized by VSMCs and endothelial cells, which inhibits BMP-2 activity and hydroxyapatite nucleation. Only the γ-carboxylated form of MGP is biologically active; hence, vitamin K deficiency or the use of vitamin K antagonists impairs its protective function [68].

Gla-Rich Protein (GRP), recently identified as a potent negative modulator of vascular and cartilage calcification, acts synergistically with MGP to reinforce the anti-mineralization barrier [55].

Among the matrix-associated inhibitors, OPN and Osteoprotegerin (OPG) play additional roles. OPN, a phosphorylated glycoprotein, binds to hydroxyapatite crystals, slowing their growth and modulating macrophage responses; OPG, acting as a soluble decoy receptor for RANKL, attenuates the osteogenic trans-differentiation of vascular cells [58].

6.2.2.2 Mineral and Metabolic Inhibitors

Among soluble inhibitors, PPi is one of the most potent and evolutionarily conserved regulators of mineralization. PPi prevents the nucleation and growth of hydroxyapatite crystals and is generated extracellularly through ATP hydrolysis mediated by ecto-nucleotide pyrophosphatase/phosphodiesterase-1 (ENPP1). Mutations or down-regulation of ENPP1, ANK, or ABCC6 lead to a marked reduction in PPi availability and result in widespread ectopic calcification [68].

In CKD, the concomitant activation of tissue-nonspecific alkaline phosphatase (TNAP) further accelerates PPi degradation, thereby amplifying the risk of vascular mineralization.

Magnesium (Mg^{2+}) is another key inhibitory ion, acting as a competitive antagonist of Ca at nucleation sites and stabilizing the amorphous phases of Pi salts, thus delaying their transformation into crystalline hydroxyapatite [70]. Both experimental and clinical studies have shown that magnesium supplementation exerts a significant anti-calcific effect, even under hyperphosphatemic conditions.

Finally, citrate, though often underestimated, plays a protective role by chelating ionized Ca and reducing crystal aggregation. Its decline in CKD contributes to microenvironmental instability and the progression of VC [44].

6.2.2.3 Cellular and Endogenous Mechanisms

At the cellular level, autophagy represents a fundamental defense mechanism. By removing damaged mitochondria and pro-calcific vesicles, autophagy helps preserve the contractile phenotype of VSMCs. Its activation, mediated through the AMP-Activated Protein Kinase (AMPK/m)TORC1 pathway, counteracts osteogenic trans-differentiation and limits the accumulation of mineralizing vesicles [58, 59].

The redox balance plays an equally crucial role. Endogenous antioxidant enzymes such as SOD, catalase, and glutathione peroxidase reduce intracellular oxidative stress, thereby suppressing NF-κB activation and downstream pro-calcific signalling pathways [59].

Among systemic regulators, Klotho exerts an indirect anti-calcific action by modulating Pi metabolism through FGF23 and inhibiting the Wnt/β-catenin pathway. Similarly, BMP7 acts as a physiological antagonist of BMP2/4, preventing osteoblastic trans-differentiation of VSMCs and preserving vascular integrity [45].

6.2.2.4 Emerging Molecular and Epigenetic Regulators

Among emerging epigenetic regulators of VC, long non-coding RNAs (lncRNAs) have gained increasing prominence. For instance, lncRNA-ANCR (Anti-Differentiation Non-Coding RNA) has been identified in vitro and in murine models as a protective modulator of VC. Its overexpression in VSMCs reduces Runx2 and BMP-2 expression, attenuates the formation of mineralized nodules, and promotes autophagy as a cytoprotective mechanism [71].

Conversely, lncRNA-H19 has been implicated as a pro-calcific factor in response to hyperphosphatemic stimuli. Recent studies have shown that H19 modulates the miR-138/TLR3 axis, enhancing osteogenic differentiation in phosphate-overloaded VSMCs [72]. Moreover, aldosterone-induced upregulation of H19 accelerates the expression of osteogenic markers in vascular cells [73].

Other recently characterized lncRNAs include SENCR, whose modulation mitigates VC by reducing ER stress through the miR-4731-5p/ER stress signalling axis [74].

Updated reviews on the epigenetic regulation of VC further highlight that restoring anti-calcific lncRNAs (e.g., ANCR, GAS5) may limit vascular mineralization by activating PTEN signalling and promoting autophagic pathways [75].

In parallel, microRNAs (miRNAs) remain among the most consistently validated molecular modulators. For example, miR-204-5p and miR-133a suppress Runx2 and BMP2 expression, exerting a potent anti-calcific effect in VSMCs models [75].

Additional emerging mechanisms include the modulatory role of complement proteins (C1q, C3a), which regulate sterile inflammation and vascular immune responses, and the sirtuins (SIRT1 and SIRT3), which preserve mitochondrial integrity and reduce oxidative stress within vascular cells [44].

6.2.2.5 Pharmacologically Induced or "Functional" Inhibitors

Beyond endogenous mechanisms, several pharmacological compounds have been developed to mimic or potentiate physiological inhibitors of VC. Representative examples include SNF472, a derivative of *myo*-inositol hexaphosphate capable of binding hydroxyapatite crystals and preventing their growth, and vitamin K_2 (menaquinone-7), which restores the anti-calcific activity of MGP through γ-carboxylation [63]. Although these agents are not physiological inhibitors in the strict sense, they reflect an attempt to reactivate the body's natural protective systems and will be discussed in greater detail in the subsequent section dedicated to therapeutic strategies (Table 6.2).

The combination of these mechanisms outlines a complex and dynamic regulatory network in which the interplay between mineral metabolism, oxidative stress, immunity, autophagy, and epigenetic regulation determines whether the vascular wall follows a calcifying or protective trajectory.

Understanding, preserving, and enhancing these physiological inhibitors of calcification currently represents one of the most promising research avenues for the prevention and treatment of VC in CKD.

6.2.3 Integration of Mechanisms

VC in CKD represents the convergence of interdependent promotive and inhibitory processes operating at molecular, cellular, and systemic levels. Hyperphosphatemia, oxidative stress, and chronic inflammation trigger the osteogenic trans-differentiation of VSMCs, while the progressive loss of physiological inhibitors—such as Fetuin-A, MGP, pyrophosphate, and Klotho—undermines the intrinsic capacity of the vascular system to resist mineral deposition.

These mechanisms mutually amplify one another: apoptosis and the release of calcifying microvesicles provide the initial nucleation sites for mineral deposition; endothelial dysfunction and mechanical stress enhance the generation of ROS; and

Table 6.2 Promoters and inhibitors of vascular calcification in CKD: a dynamic balance between metabolic, cellular, and molecular mechanisms

Category	Promoters of calcification	Physiological inhibitors of calcification	Main mechanism or target	Key Ref.
Mineral metabolism	Inorganic phosphate ↑, calcium ↑, TNAP activation	Pyrophosphate (PPi), ENPP1/ANK/ ABCC6, magnesium, citrate	Regulate hydroxyapatite crystal nucleation and growth	[44, 45, 68]
Hormonal and systemic regulators	PTH ↑, FGF23 ↑, Klotho deficiency, vitamin D deficiency	Klotho, BMP7, physiological vitamin D	Phosphate–calcium homeostasis, modulation of Wnt/β-catenin signalling	[58]
Inflammation and oxidative stress	TNF-α, IL-1β, IL-6, ROS, NF-κB, NLRP3	SOD, catalase, glutathione peroxidase, autophagy	Redox regulation and local immune response	[58, 59]
Cellular and structural factors	Apoptosis, necroptosis, calcifying microvesicles, type II CPPs	Autophagy, Fetuin-A, osteopontin (OPN), osteoprotegerin (OPG)	Control of vesicle release and extracellular matrix stability	[60, 63]
Endothelial and mechanical factors	Endothelial dysfunction, hypertension, altered shear stress	Nitric oxide (NO), Klotho, Gla-rich protein (GRP)	Vascular barrier integrity and paracrine signalling	[55]
Epigenetic and molecular regulators	Runx2, Msx2, Osterix, miR-223, H19 (pro-calcific)	miR-30b, miR-125b, miR-143/145, miR-204, lncRNA-ANCR, GAS5	Transcriptional and post-transcriptional regulation of osteogenic transdifferentiation	[58, 59, 75]
Systemic and circulating factors	Uremia, hyperuricemia, metabolic acidosis, chronic infections	Fetuin-A, matrix Gla protein (MGP), GRP, OPG	Control of solubility and transport of Ca–P complexes	[60, 63]
Pharmacological and nutritional (overview)	Vitamin K antagonists, excess calcitriol	SNF472, vitamin K_2, magnesium supplementation	Mimic or potentiate natural anti-calcifying mechanisms	[63]

the activation of epigenetic pathways involving microRNAs and lncRNAs consolidates the osteoblastic phenotype.

The result is a self-reinforcing pathogenic loop in which the accumulation of promoters and the loss of inhibitors drive arterial stiffness, microvascular dysfunction, and the progression of cardiovascular and renal injury [58–60].

A deeper understanding of this integrated regulatory network provides the pathophysiological rationale for developing targeted therapeutic strategies—pharmacological, nutritional, and cellular—aimed not only at reducing calcification promoters but also at restoring or enhancing physiological inhibitors. This integrated approach defines the new frontier of *Therapeutic Strategies* and *Future Perspectives* in CKD-related VC.

6.3 Therapeutics Strategies

6.3.1 General Rationale

The management of VC in CKD requires a multidimensional and integrated approach (see Table 6.3).

Since VC arises from a disequilibrium between promotors and physiological inhibitors of mineral metabolism, each therapeutic strategy must aim to restore this balance by acting simultaneously on systemic metabolism, molecular signalling pathways, and cellular responses.

The overarching therapeutic goal is to shift the vascular phenotype from pro-calcific to protective, through integrated, personalized, and mechanism-oriented interventions tailored to the patient's specific pathophysiological profile (see Fig. 6.2) [13, 60, 76].

Table 6.3 Pharmacologic and molecular strategies for vascular calcification in CKD: mechanisms and level of evidence

Therapeutic class	Mechanistic target	Representative agent(s)	Evidence level	Notes
Phosphate binders	↓ Pi absorption	Sevelamer, lanthanum	Phase III, established	Standard of care
Vitamin D analogs	↓ PTH, VDR modulation	Paricalcitol	Phase III	Risk of hypercalcemia
Calcimimetics	CaSR activation	Cinacalcet, etelcalcetide	Phase III	Reduces Ca × P product
TNAP inhibitors	↓ Hydrolysis of Ppi	SBI-425	Preclinical	Prevents plaque mineralization
Iron citrate	Induces autophagy	Ferric citrate	Phase II	Antioxidant & antiapoptotic
SNF472	Blocks hydroxyapatite growth	SNF472	Phase III	Reduces coronary Ca progression
ENPP1 (INZ-701)	↑ Extracellular Ppi	INZ-701	Phase II (ongoing)	Genetic/uremic calcification
Vitamin K_2	γ-carboxylation of MGP	MK-7	Phase II–III	Safe, low cost
SIRT/AMPK activators	Mitochondrial function, redox	Metformin, resveratrol	Preclinical–translational	Anti-inflammatory

This table summarizes the principal therapeutic classes currently used or under investigation for vascular calcification in chronic kidney disease, highlighting their primary molecular targets, representative agents, and stage of clinical development. The evidence level ranges from established clinical practice to emerging preclinical interventions

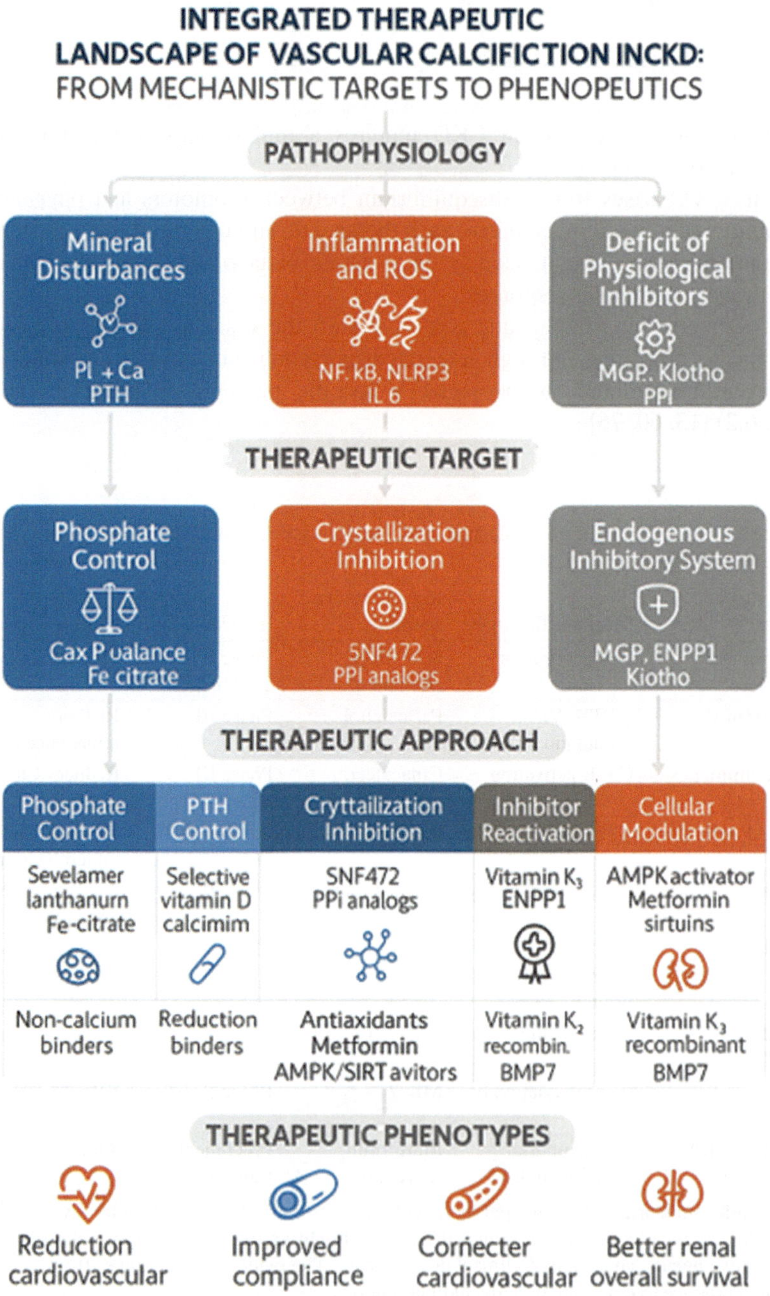

Fig. 6.2 Integrated therapeutic landscape of vascular calcification in chronic kidney disease. *Integrated therapeutic phenotypes in vascular calcification and CKD.* This infographic illustrates the three major therapeutic phenotypes underlying vascular calcification in chronic kidney disease:

6.3.2 Interventions on Mineral Metabolism

Phosphate control remains the cornerstone of VC prevention. Non-calcium-based phosphate binders—including sevelamer, lanthanum, and magnesium oxide or carbonate—reduce the Ca-Pi product saturation and attenuate osteogenic stimulation of VSMCs [77].

Magnesium plays a dual role: beyond its systemic effect on mineral balance, it acts as a competitive inhibitor of Ca-Pi nucleation, maintaining the amorphous stability of mineral complexes and delaying crystal maturation [70].

Among emerging molecular targets, Tissue-Nonspecific Alkaline Phosphatase (TNAP) has gained particular interest. In ApoE-deficient mice fed an atherogenic diet, pharmacologic inhibition of TNAP with SBI-425 significantly reduced plaque calcification, improved lipid profile, and protected against atherosclerosis, without adverse effects on bone structure [78]. As highlighted by Goettsch et al. [79], TNAP is not only a key enzyme in bone mineralization but also an important vascular modulator of the phosphate–pyrophosphate equilibrium. Therefore, TNAP modulation represents a critical therapeutic node to halt VC progression.

Another innovative approach involves ferric citrate, a compound traditionally used as a Pi binder but now recognized for its direct anti-calcific effects. In vitro studies on calcified VSMCs have demonstrated that ferric citrate halts Ca deposition, reduces apoptosis, and stimulates autophagy. The ferrous chromate complex further attenuates osteo-chondrogenic transformation of the extracellular matrix [80]. In complementary models, ferric citrate prevents phosphate-induced calcification by upregulating miR-30c and modifying extracellular matrix composition [81].

Together, these findings support TNAP inhibition and ferric citrate therapy as promising emerging options in VC management. However, their application requires careful calibration: TNAP modulation must preserve the bone–vascular balance, and iron-based interventions must be evaluated for potential redox toxicity and bioavailability concerns.

Beyond their phosphate-binding and direct anti-calcific actions, iron-based therapies have shown additional benefits in modulating the FGF23–erythropoietin axis. Iron deficiency is a potent stimulator of FGF23 transcription and cleavage, leading to elevated circulating levels of both intact (iFGF23) and C-terminal (cFGF23) fragments, which contribute to disordered mineral metabolism and renal anaemia.

Fig. 6.2 (continued) *hyperphosphatemic*, *inflammatory/oxidative*, and *inhibitor-deficiency* profiles. Each phenotype is linked to its dominant pathophysiologic mechanisms, corresponding molecular targets, and specific therapeutic strategies. The vertical flow highlights the transition from systemic metabolic imbalance to targeted interventions—such as phosphate control, antioxidant activation, and restoration of endogenous inhibitors—culminating in improved vascular compliance, reduced arterial stiffness, and enhanced cardio-renal outcomes

Treatments with iron-based phosphate binders—such as sucroferric oxyhydroxide and ferric citrate—have been shown to significantly reduce serum FGF23 levels in haemodialysis patients, while improving phosphate control and iron parameters [82, 83].

Similarly, oral iron supplementation has been associated with lower FGF23 concentrations in patients with iron-deficiency anaemia or autosomal dominant hypophosphatemic rickets (ADHR), whereas certain intravenous preparations, such as ferric carboxymaltose, may transiently increase iFGF23 levels [84, 85].

Experimental studies in CKD models further demonstrate that optimizing iron utilization with erythropoietin or HIF-prolyl hydroxylase inhibitors (HIF-PHDi) reduces iFGF23 expression and ameliorates mineral metabolism abnormalities [86].

These findings reinforce the dual benefit of iron-based interventions in CKD—combining phosphate control with restoration of iron homeostasis and attenuation of FGF23-driven hormonal dysregulation.

6.3.2.1 Vitamin D and Selective Analogues

Vitamin D and its selective VDR analogues remain a cornerstone in the management of sHPT. Agents such as paricalcitol and doxercalciferol allow for more targeted suppression of PTH while reducing the risk of hypercalcemia and hyperphosphatemia compared with native calcitriol [39, 46]. Maintaining adequate 25(OH)D levels is associated with lower arterial stiffness and reduced expression of osteogenic markers in VSMCs. However, excessive doses of active vitamin D or highly calcaemic analogues can promote VC, particularly in the presence of latent hypercalcemia or elevated Pi levels [58]. For this reason, the use of selective VDR activators—characterized by a balanced receptor activity and lower impact on the Ca × P product—represents a preferred therapeutic strategy for achieving safe and physiologic PTH control in advanced CKD.

6.3.2.2 Calcimimetics

Calcimimetics, such as cinacalcet and etelcalcetide, act as allosteric activators of the CaSR on parathyroid cells, thereby reducing PTH secretion and improving overall mineral metabolism control.

Beyond PTH suppression, these agents help lower serum Ca levels and reduce the Ca × P product, indirectly mitigating the progression of VC [13].

Post-hoc analyses from the EVOLVE and PARADIGM trials have shown a lower incidence of cardiovascular events and a stabilization of valvular calcification in patients treated with cinacalcet, although the impact on overall mortality remains a subject of debate.

The combined use of calcimimetics and vitamin D analogues provides synergistic PTH control, minimizing the risk of hypercalcemia and excess Pi burden—two of the main pro-calcific triggers in CKD.

6.3.3 Inhibitors of Mineral Crystallization and Growth

Among innovative pharmacological approaches aimed at blocking mineralization, the most extensively studied agent is SNF472, a derivative of *myo*-inositol hexaphosphate (phytate) that binds to the surface of hydroxyapatite crystals, inhibiting their growth and maturation.

The CaLIPSO trial [87]—a multicentre, randomized, double-blind, placebo-controlled study—evaluated the efficacy of SNF472 in haemodialysis patients with cardiovascular calcifications.

Clinical results, later reported by Raggi et al. [88, 89], demonstrated that SNF472 significantly slows the progression of coronary and valvular calcification, as measured by CAC scores, compared with placebo, while maintaining a favourable safety profile and no adverse skeletal effects.

A subsequent clinical study, CALCIPHYX [83], confirmed the anti-mineralizing effects of SNF472 in patients with calciphylaxis, showing marked pain reduction and improvement in wound healing.

Collectively, these findings establish SNF472 as the first pharmacologic agent with clinical evidence of efficacy in slowing active VC in patients with advanced CKD, paving the way for therapies that directly target mineral crystallization control.

Other agents, such as non-hydrolysable analogues of PPi—notably bisphosphonates—have demonstrated partial prevention of VC in animal models of ENPP1 or ABCC6 deficiency [76]. However, their clinical translation remains limited due to poor bioavailability, potential skeletal toxicity, and interference with normal bone mineralization [90].

6.3.4 Reactivation of Physiological Inhibitors

Reactivating the body's natural anti-calcifying mechanisms represents one of the most promising—and yet underexplored—therapeutic strategies in VC.

Vitamin K_2 (menaquinone-7) remains the most practical approach currently available to restore the γ-carboxylated form of MGP—its active isoform, which is a potent inhibitor of vascular mineralization.

Vitamin K supplementation has been shown to lower circulating levels of dephosphorylated–uncarboxylated MGP (dp-ucMGP) [63], and meta-analyses have reported an association with slower progression of CAC in patients with CKD [91]. However, most of the clinical evidence remains preliminary and heterogeneous, and the overall benefit should therefore be interpreted with caution [92].

In parallel, the use of recombinant ENPP1 enzyme (INZ-701, ENPP1-Fc) represents a major therapeutic frontier, particularly in cases where VC is associated with defects in the pyrophosphate-generating system.

A recent CKD rat model study demonstrated that administration of INZ-701 significantly reduced vascular and soft tissue calcification and prevented osteoid expansion, a hallmark of CKD–MBD [93]. In genetic models, INZ-701 has been shown to restore circulating PPi levels and prevent systemic calcification in mice with ENPP1 deficiency [94].

Finally, pharmacologic or nutraceutical modulation of Klotho and BMP7 expression may help limit the osteogenic transdifferentiation of VSMCs and support endothelial function.

Although these pathways have been widely discussed in pathophysiological reviews [13, 58], direct clinical evidence of therapeutic benefit remains limited.

6.3.5 Interventi Cellular and Molecular Interventions

The most advanced molecular strategies aim to preserve the vitality and anti-calcific function of vascular cells, counteracting the intracellular processes that drive osteogenic transdifferentiation.

6.3.5.1 Antioxidants and Inflammatory Modulation

The use of antioxidants and the inhibition of NF-κB and NLRP3 pathways represent established approaches to mitigate oxidative stress and sterile inflammation, both of which are central drivers of VC.

In uremic conditions, these pathways are chronically activated, promoting the release of pro-oxidant cytokines and osteogenic factors that accelerate mineral deposition. Recent reviews on CKD-related VC emphasize the phosphate- and uremic toxin–induced activation of NF-κB signalling as a critical step in this process [95].

Dietary antioxidants—including flavonoids, vitamins, and trace minerals—have been shown in both in vitro and in vivo studies to reduce VC, attenuating oxidative injury and preserving VSMCs phenotype [96].

6.3.5.2 Activation of Autophagy (via AMPK/mTORC1)

Autophagy has emerged as a key defensive mechanism against VC. Activation of AMP-activated protein AMPK stimulates autophagy and inhibits mTORC1, promoting the degradation of calcifying vesicles and reducing osteogenic transdifferentiation of VSMCs [97]. In experimental models, canagliflozin has been shown to attenuate VC in rats by enhancing AMPK activity and autophagic flux, leading to a reduction in osteogenic markers such as ALP, Runx2, and BMP-2 [98].

Similarly, other studies have demonstrated that pharmacologic or genetic activation of autophagy significantly reduces Ca deposition in VSMCs exposed to high Pi concentrations, highlighting its potential as a therapeutic target in CKD-related VC [99].

6.3.5.3 Sirtuins (SIRT1/SIRT3) and Mitochondrial Protection

Sirtuins, particularly SIRT1 and SIRT3, play a crucial role in maintaining mitochondrial integrity and modulating redox metabolism, thereby contributing to the inhibition of VC.

- *SIRT1* promotes autophagy activation through the AMPK signalling pathway and suppresses the inflammatory response. Recent studies in renal and vascular models suggest that SIRT1 modulation may delay the progression of kidney disease and, by extension, reduce the associated VC processes [100].
- *SIRT3,* acting primarily at the mitochondrial level, promotes the clearance of damaged mitochondria (mitophagy) and reduces the release of pro-calcific ROS, establishing a positive feedback loop with AMPK/mTORC1 signalling. In renal and cardiovascular contexts, SIRT3 activation has been proposed as a protective strategy against oxidative stress and cellular senescence [101].

6.3.6 Integrated and Personalized Strategies

Because VC in patients with CKD exhibits marked phenotypic heterogeneity—driven by the interplay of genetic, metabolic, and inflammatory factors—future therapeutic approaches must evolve toward personalized medicine.

The goal is to identify the predominant pathophysiological profile of each patient early and tailor therapy toward the dominant mechanisms driving VC progression.

6.3.6.1 Hyperphosphatemic Phenotype

This phenotype is characterized by a high Pi load and relative hypercalcemia, typically observed in advanced CKD stages. In this setting, non–calcium-based Pi binders (such as *sevelamer* or *lanthanum carbonate*) and iron-based binders (e.g., *sodium ferric citrate* or *ferric citrate*) are recommended. These agents not only reduce intestinal Pi absorption but also exert antioxidant and pro-autophagic effects on vascular cells [80]. In patients with active calcification, SNF472 represents an additional therapeutic option, capable of directly inhibiting hydroxyapatite crystal growth, as demonstrated in the CaLIPSO trial [87].

6.3.6.2 Inflammatory/Oxidative Phenotype

This phenotype predominates in patients with heightened immune activation and systemic oxidative stress, such as those with diabetes or advanced uremic syndrome. Therapeutic strategies in this context aim to reduce sterile inflammation and oxidative damage through targeted antioxidants and metabolic modulators such as *metformin*, *resveratrol*, and activators of the AMPK/SIRT1–3 pathways. These interventions enhance autophagy, improve mitochondrial function, and suppress NF-κB and NLRP3 signalling, thereby inhibiting the osteogenic transdifferentiation of VSMCs [58, 59].

6.3.6.3 Phenotype of Physiological Inhibitor Deficiency

This phenotype includes patients in whom VC progression is primarily driven by a reduced expression or functional impairment of endogenous mineralization inhibitors, such as MGP, Klotho, BMP7, and ENPP1. The dysfunction of these mechanisms disrupts the delicate equilibrium between PPi and Pi, thereby reducing the ability of vascular cells to maintain a non-calcifying phenotype.

In such patients, vitamin K_2 (menaquinone-7) represents the most direct therapeutic approach to reactivate the γ-carboxylated form of MGP, partially restoring the vascular anti-calcifying defense [63].

In parallel, experimental therapies based on recombinant ENPP1 (INZ-701) aim to increase plasma PPi levels, thereby counteracting hydroxyapatite crystal nucleation and restoring the inhibitory capacity of the extracellular compartment [58].

Finally, strategies designed to enhance Klotho or BMP7 expression or stability, through pharmacological or nutraceutical interventions, have shown protective effects in CKD models, reducing osteogenic transdifferentiation and improving endothelial function [13, 58].

Overall, these interventions aim to restore the network of physiological inhibitors that maintains the vascular wall in a state of metabolic quiescence and resistance to mineral deposition.

6.4 Future Perspectives: Landscape of Ongoing Trials in VC IN CKD

Research on VC in CKD is undergoing a phase of remarkable expansion, marked by the transition from a purely preventive approach to a form of true vascular interventional medicine. Today, the therapeutic goal is no longer limited to slowing disease progression, but rather to restore a dynamic biological equilibrium between calcification promoters and inhibitors, through the targeted modulation of the cellular, enzymatic, and metabolic processes that govern vascular mineralization (see Fig. 6.3).

Clinical trials currently registered on ClinicalTrials.gov depict an increasingly articulated and promising landscape. Among the most relevant studies, the SNF472 development program *(NCT02966028; NCT04195906)* stands as a milestone in the field. Derived from *myo-inositol hexaphosphate*, SNF472 binds to the surface of hydroxyapatite crystals, preventing their growth and promoting the stabilization of non-pathogenic amorphous forms. In haemodialysis patients, SNF472 has demonstrated a significant reduction in the progression of coronary and valvular calcification, paving the way for a new generation of crystal-targeted therapies.

In parallel, several ongoing trials are exploring the potential of micronutrients and metabolic agents, such as magnesium supplementation *(NCT02542319)*, vitamin K_2 *(NCT04539418)*, and bisphosphonates *(NCT00395382)*, with the goal of restoring mineral balance and enhancing endogenous defences against calcification nucleation. Moreover, dialysate composition adjustments *(NCT07163936)* represent a pragmatic intervention aimed at limiting the vascular Ca and Pi burden directly at the interface between blood and vessel wall.

Alongside these established strategies, even more innovative perspectives are emerging.

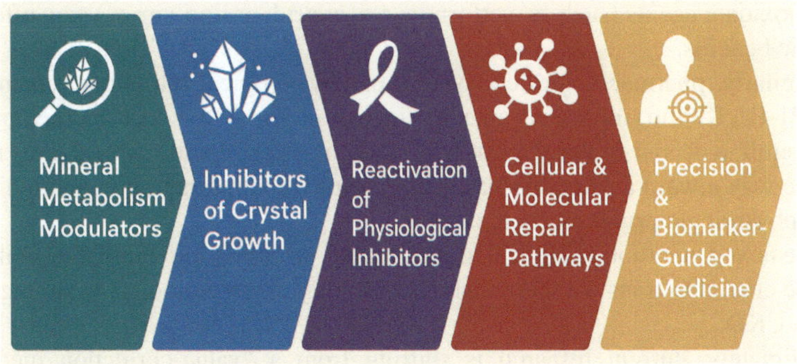

Fig. 6.3 Future therapeutic directions in vascular calcification. This schematic overview summarizes the emerging therapeutic landscape for vascular calcification (VC) in chronic kidney disease (CKD), structured into five interconnected axes reflecting the underlying pathophysiology. The first dimension targets *mineral metabolism modulation*, encompassing phosphate binders, magnesium, and TNAP inhibitors to rebalance the Ca–P product and restore phosphate homeostasis. The second focuses on *crystal-growth inhibition*, with SNF472 and non-hydrolysable pyrophosphate analogues directly preventing hydroxyapatite nucleation. The third axis aims to *reactivate physiological inhibitors* such as MGP, Klotho, and ENPP1, through vitamin K_2 supplementation, recombinant enzymes, and epigenetic modulation. The fourth represents *cellular and molecular repair*, enhancing autophagy, antioxidant defense, and sirtuin signalling to counter oxidative and inflammatory injury. Finally, the fifth embodies the transition toward *precision and biomarker-guided medicine*, integrating patient-specific phenotypes—hyperphosphatemic, inflammatory, or inhibitor-deficient—to achieve personalized therapeutic targeting. Together, these strategies outline a paradigm shift from damage containment to vascular resilience and biological repair

The use of recombinant ENPP1 (INZ-701), developed to increase circulating PPi levels, offers a promising solution for patients with genetic ENPP1 or ABCC6 deficiencies, and potentially an extended therapeutic application in advanced CKD. In parallel, targeted inhibition of TNAP—as demonstrated in preclinical studies with SBI-425—represents a highly appealing frontier to rebalance the PPi/Pi ratio and protect vascular tissues without impairing bone mineralization [78].

Despite these advances, clinical translation remains challenging. Most ongoing trials rely on surrogate endpoints (such as CAC scores or arterial stiffness indices), which, although sensitive, do not always reflect true reductions in cardiovascular risk.

Moreover, the marked phenotypic heterogeneity of CKD—encompassing hyperphosphatemic, inflammatory, and inhibitor-deficient forms—calls for a higher degree of therapeutic personalization.

The bone–vascular balance remains a critical issue, since inhibition of vascular mineralization must not compromise skeletal integrity.

In addition, the lack of standardized biomarkers (such as plasma PPi, dp-ucMGP, or circulating Klotho) limits cross-trial comparability and hinders the definition of precise therapeutic targets.

Looking ahead, the most promising direction lies in the development of combined and modular strategies, capable of acting simultaneously on multiple pathogenic mechanisms.

The association of crystal-growth inhibitors (e.g., SNF472) with pro-autophagic or antioxidant agents (such as metformin, resveratrol, or iron-citrate) may offer synergistic benefits.

Similarly, pharmacologic reactivation of physiological inhibitors (vitamin K_2, ENPP1-Fc, Klotho) represents an emerging paradigm of "vascular biotherapy."

Overall, a deeper molecular understanding, integrated with clinical data, is paving the way toward a precision-based therapeutic model cantered on the individual pathophysiologic profile of each patient.

The next generation of clinical trials—longer, stratified, and biomarker-guided—will be crucial to translate these insights into truly disease-modifying strategies for VC in CKD.

Ultimately, current research is shifting from a "value-correction medicine" toward a "medicine of vascular resilience," grounded in biological intervention and personalized therapy.

6.5 Conclusion

VC in CKD emerges as a dynamic and multifactorial process, shaped by the interplay between metabolic imbalance, inflammation, oxidative stress, and loss of endogenous inhibitors. Recent advances reveal that vascular mineralization is not an irreversible degenerative event but a regulated, targetable phenomenon. The integration of molecular, cellular, and systemic approaches—together with precision strategies tailored to specific CKD phenotypes—offers a realistic opportunity to restore vascular resilience. Future therapeutic success will depend on translating mechanistic insight into individualized, mechanism-based interventions.

Declarations

Competing Interests The author(s) has no competing interests to declare that are relevant to the content of this manuscript.

Ethics Approval The author(s) declares that this manuscript does not include primary research with human participants.

The author(s) declares that this manuscript does not include primary studies involving animals.

References

1. Benz K, Hilgers KF, Daniel C, Amann K. Vascular calcification in chronic kidney disease: the role of inflammation. Int J Nephrol. 2018;2018:4310379.
2. Amann K. Media calcification and intima calcification are distinct entities in chronic kidney disease. Clin J Am Soc Nephrol CJASN. 2008;3(6):1599–605.
3. Shanahan CM, Cary NR, Salisbury JR, Proudfoot D, Weissberg PL, Edmonds ME. Medial localization of mineralization-regulating proteins in association with Mönckeberg's sclerosis: evidence for smooth muscle cell-mediated vascular calcification. Circulation. 1999;100(21):2168–76.
4. Guérin AP, London GM, Marchais SJ, Metivier F. Arterial stiffening and vascular calcifications in end-stage renal disease. Nephrol Dial Transplant. 2000;15(7):1014–21.
5. Kim JS, Hwang HS. Vascular calcification in chronic kidney disease: distinct features of pathogenesis and clinical implication. Korean Circ J. 2021;51(12):961–82.
6. Yang S, Zeng Z, Yuan Q, Chen Q, Wang Z, Xie H, et al. Vascular calcification: from the perspective of crosstalk. Mol Biomed. 2023;4(1):35.
7. Moe S, Drüeke T, Cunningham J, Goodman W, Martin K, Olgaard K, et al. Definition, evaluation, and classification of renal osteodystrophy: a position statement from kidney disease: improving global outcomes (KDIGO). Kidney Int Giugno. 2006;69(11):1945–53.
8. Waziri B, Duarte R, Duarte R, Naicker S. Chronic kidney disease-mineral and bone disorder (CKD-MBD): current perspectives. Int J Nephrol Renov Dis. 2019;12:263–76.
9. London GM, Guérin AP, Marchais SJ, Métivier F, Pannier B, Adda H. Arterial media calcification in end-stage renal disease: impact on all-cause and cardiovascular mortality. Nephrol Dial Transplant. 2003;18(9):1731–40.
10. Raggi P, Boulay A, Chasan-Taber S, Amin N, Dillon M, Burke SK, et al. Cardiac calcification in adult hemodialysis patients. A link between end-stage renal disease and cardiovascular disease? J Am Coll Cardiol. 2002;39(4):695–701.
11. Di Lullo L, Floccari F, Santoboni A, Barbera V, Rivera RF, Granata A, et al. Progression of cardiac valve calcification and decline of renal function in CKD patients. J Nephrol. 2013;26(4):739–44.
12. Sigrist MK, Taal MW, Bungay P, McIntyre CW. Progressive vascular calcification over 2 years is associated with arterial stiffening and increased mortality in patients with stages 4 and 5 chronic kidney disease. Clin J Am Soc Nephrol CJASN. 2007;2(6):1241–8.
13. Cozzolino M, Maffei Faccioli F, Cara A, Boni Brivio G, Rivela F, Ciceri P, et al. Future treatment of vascular calcification in chronic kidney disease. Expert Opin Pharmacother. 2023;24(18):2041–57.

14. Zhang J, Pang Q, Wang S, Wu L, Zhang A. Associated factors of cardiac valve calcification and its prognostic effects among patients with chronic kidney disease: a systematic review and meta-analysis. Front Cardiovasc Med. 2023;10:1120634.
15. Pongsuwan K, Kusirisin P, Narongkiattikhun P, Chattipakorn SC, Chattipakorn N. Mitochondria and vascular calcification in chronic kidney disease: lessons learned from the past to improve future therapy. J Cell Physiol. 2022;237(12):4369–96.
16. Shah A, Hashmi MF, Aeddula NR. Chronic kidney disease-mineral bone disorder (CKD-MBD). In: StatPearls [internet]. Treasure Island: StatPearls Publishing; 2025. http://www.ncbi.nlm.nih.gov/books/NBK560742/.
17. Verma H, Sunder S, Sharma BB, Sharma N, Verma R. Prevalence of vascular calcification in chronic kidney disease stage 4 and 5 patients and its correlation with inflammatory markers of atherosclerosis. Saudi J Kidney Dis Transplant. 2021;32(1):30.
18. Zhang H, Li G, Yu X, Yang J, Jiang A, Cheng H, et al. Progression of vascular calcification and clinical outcomes in patients receiving maintenance dialysis. JAMA Netw Open. 2023;6(5):e2310909.
19. Peeters MJ, van den Brand JA, van Zuilen AD, Koster Y, Bots ML, Vervloet MG, et al. Abdominal aortic calcification in patients with CKD. J Nephrol. 2017;30(1):109–18.
20. Jimbo R, Kawakami-Mori F, Mu S, Hirohama D, Majtan B, Shimizu Y, et al. Fibroblast growth factor 23 accelerates phosphate-induced vascular calcification in the absence of Klotho deficiency. Kidney Int. 2014;85(5):1103–11.
21. Nelson AJ, Raggi P, Wolf M, Gold AM, Chertow GM, Roe MT. Targeting vascular calcification in chronic kidney disease. JACC Basic Transl Sci. 2020;5(4):398–412.
22. Budoff MJ, Hokanson JE, Nasir K, Shaw LJ, Kinney GL, Chow D, et al. Progression of coronary artery calcium predicts all-cause mortality. JACC Cardiovasc Imaging. 2010;3(12):1229–36.
23. Detrano R, Guerci AD, Carr JJ, Bild DE, Burke G, Folsom AR, et al. Coronary calcium as a predictor of coronary events in four racial or ethnic groups. N Engl J Med. 2008;358(13):1336–45.
24. Budoff MJ, Rader DJ, Reilly MP, Mohler ER, Lash J, Yang W, et al. Relationship of estimated GFR and coronary artery calcification in the CRIC (chronic renal insufficiency cohort) study. Am J Kidney Dis. 2011;58(4):519–26.
25. Chen J, Budoff MJ, Reilly MP, Yang W, Rosas SE, Rahman M, et al. Coronary artery calcification and risk of cardiovascular disease and death among patients with chronic kidney disease. JAMA Cardiol. 2017;2(6):635–43.
26. Sarnak MJ, Amann K, Bangalore S, Cavalcante JL, Charytan DM, Craig JC, et al. Chronic kidney disease and coronary artery disease: JACC state-of-the-art review. J Am Coll Cardiol. 2019;74(14):1823–38.
27. Tian L, Jaeger BC, Scialla JJ, Budoff MJ, Mehta RC, Jaar BG, et al. Progression of coronary artery calcification and risk of clinical events in CKD: the chronic renal insufficiency cohort study. Am J Kidney Dis. 2025;85(1):67–77.e1.
28. Agatston AS, Janowitz WR, Hildner FJ, Zusmer NR, Viamonte M, Detrano R. Quantification of coronary artery calcium using ultrafast computed tomography. J Am Coll Cardiol. 1990;15(4):827–32.
29. Bellasi A, Ferramosca E, Muntner P, Ratti C, Wildman RP, Block GA, et al. Correlation of simple imaging tests and coronary artery calcium measured by computed tomography in hemodialysis patients. Kidney Int. 2006;70(9):1623–8.
30. Takayama Y, Yasuda Y, Suzuki S, Shibata Y, Tatami Y, Shibata K, et al. Relationship between abdominal aortic and coronary artery calcification as detected by computed tomography in chronic kidney disease patients. Heart Vessel. 2016;31(7):1030–7.
31. Leow K, Szulc P, Schousboe JT, Kiel DP, Teixeira-Pinto A, Shaikh H, et al. Prognostic value of abdominal aortic calcification: a systematic review and meta-analysis of observational studies. J Am Heart Assoc. 2021;10(2):e017205.

32. Yao Z, Wang C, Zhang Q, Ma S, Gui B, Duan C. Prevalence of abdominal artery calcification in dialysis patients with end-stage renal disease: a systematic review and meta-analysis. Int Urol Nephrol. 2017;49(11):2061–9.
33. Wang AYM, Wang M, Woo J, CWK L, PKT L, Lui SF, et al. Cardiac valve calcification as an important predictor for all-cause mortality and cardiovascular mortality in long-term peritoneal dialysis patients: a prospective study. J Am Soc Nephrol JASN. 2003;14(1):159–68.
34. Raggi P, Bellasi A, Gamboa C, Ferramosca E, Ratti C, Block GA, et al. All-cause mortality in hemodialysis patients with heart valve calcification. Clin J Am Soc Nephrol. 2011;6(8):1990–5.
35. Marwick TH, Amann K, Bangalore S, Cavalcante JL, Charytan DM, Craig JC, et al. Chronic kidney disease and valvular heart disease: conclusions from a kidney disease: improving global outcomes (KDIGO) controversies conference. Kidney Int. 2019;96(4):836–49.
36. Brandenburg VM, Schuh A, Kramann R. Valvular calcification in chronic kidney disease. Adv Chronic Kidney Dis. 2019;26(6):464–71.
37. Bellasi A, Galassi A, Papagni S, Cozzolino M. Cardiac valve calcification: an immutable pathologic finding in chronic kidney disease? J Nephrol. 2013;26(4):606–9.
38. McCullough PA, Agrawal V, Danielewicz E, Abela GS. Accelerated atherosclerotic calcification and Monckeberg's sclerosis: a continuum of advanced vascular pathology in chronic kidney disease. Clin J Am Soc Nephrol. 2008;3(6):1585–98.
39. Cozzolino M, Brancaccio D, Gallieni M, Slatopolsky E. Pathogenesis of vascular calcification in chronic kidney disease. Kidney Int. 2005;68(2):429–36.
40. Jono S, McKee MD, Murry CE, Shioi A, Nishizawa Y, Mori K, et al. Phosphate regulation of vascular smooth muscle cell calcification. Circ Res. 2000;87(7):E10–7.
41. Speer MY, Li X, Hiremath PG, Giachelli CM. Runx2/Cbfa1, but not loss of myocardin, is required for smooth muscle cell lineage reprogramming toward osteochondrogenesis. J Cell Biochem. 2010;110(4):935–47.
42. Shanahan CM, Crouthamel MH, Kapustin A, Giachelli CM. Arterial calcification in chronic kidney disease: key roles for calcium and phosphate. Circ Res. 2011;109(6):697–711.
43. Mizobuchi M, Towler D, Slatopolsky E. Vascular calcification: the killer of patients with chronic kidney disease. J Am Soc Nephrol. 2009;20(7):1453–64.
44. Villa-Bellosta R. Vascular calcification: a passive process that requires active inhibition. Biology. 2024;13(2):111.
45. Yamada S, Giachelli CM. Vascular calcification in CKD-MBD: roles for phosphate, FGF23, and klotho. Bone. 2017;100:87–93.
46. Kanbay M, Copur S, Tanriover C, Yavuz F, Galassi A, Ciceri P, et al. The pathophysiology and management of vascular calcification in chronic kidney disease patients. Expert Rev Cardiovasc Ther. 2023;21(2):75–85.
47. Faul C, Amaral AP, Oskouei B, Hu MC, Sloan A, Isakova T, et al. FGF23 induces left ventricular hypertrophy. J Clin Invest. 2011;121(11):4393–408.
48. Lewerin C, Ljunggren Ö, Nilsson-Ehle H, Karlsson MK, Herlitz H, Lorentzon M, et al. Low serum iron is associated with high serum intact FGF23 in elderly men: the Swedish MrOS study. Bone. 2017;98:1–8.
49. Mehta R, Cai X, Hodakowski A, Lee J, Leonard M, Ricardo A, et al. Fibroblast growth factor 23 and anemia in the chronic renal insufficiency cohort study. Clin J Am Soc Nephrol. 2017;12(11):1795.
50. Eisenga MF, van Londen M, Leaf DE, Nolte IM, Navis G, Bakker SJL, et al. C-terminal fibroblast growth factor 23, iron deficiency, and mortality in renal transplant recipients. J Am Soc Nephrol. 2017;28(12):3639.
51. Kuro-O M. The Klotho proteins in health and disease. Nat Rev Nephrol. 2019;15(1):27–44.
52. Habas E, Eledrisi M, Khan F, Elzouki ANY. Secondary hyperparathyroidism in chronic kidney disease: pathophysiology and management. Cureus. 2021;13(7):e16388.

53. Cozzolino M, Minghetti P, Navarra P. Extended-release calcifediol in stage 3-4 chronic kidney disease: a new therapy for the treatment of secondary hyperparathyroidism associated with hypovitaminosis D. J Nephrol. 2022;35(3):863–73.
54. Khodadadiyan A, Rahmanian M, Shekouh D, Golmohammadi M, Ghaedi A, Bazrgar A, et al. Evaluating the effect of vitamin D supplementation on serum levels of 25-hydroxy vitamin D, 1,25-dihydroxy vitamin D, parathyroid hormone and renin-angiotensin-aldosterone system: a systematic review and meta-analysis of clinical trials. BMC Nutr. 2023;9(1):132.
55. Izzo C, Secondulfo C, Bilancio G, Visco V, Virtuoso N, Migliarino S, et al. Chronic kidney disease with mineral bone disorder and vascular calcification: an overview. Life Basel Switz. 2024;14(3):418.
56. Loh HH, Azizan EA, Sukor N. Connecting the dots: renin-angiotensin-aldosterone system, vitamin D, and hypertension. J Hypertens. 2025;43(7):1136–45.
57. Li YC, Kong J, Wei M, Chen ZF, Liu SQ, Cao LP. 1,25-Dihydroxyvitamin D(3) is a negative endocrine regulator of the renin-angiotensin system. J Clin Invest. 2002;110(2):229–38.
58. Pan W, Jie W, Huang H. Vascular calcification: molecular mechanisms and therapeutic interventions. MedComm. 2023;4(1):e200.
59. Siracusa C, Carabetta N, Morano MB, Manica M, Strangio A, Sabatino J, et al. Understanding vascular calcification in chronic kidney disease: pathogenesis and therapeutic implications. Int J Mol Sci. 2024;25(23):13096.
60. Marreiros C, Viegas C, Simes D. Targeting a silent disease: vascular calcification in chronic kidney disease. Int J Mol Sci. 2022;23(24):16114.
61. Zhang L, Yao J, Yao Y, Boström KI. Contributions of the endothelium to vascular calcification. Front Cell Dev Biol. 2021;9:620882.
62. Rao Z, Zheng Y, Xu L, Wang Z, Zhou Y, Chen M, et al. Endoplasmic reticulum stress and pathogenesis of vascular calcification. Front Cardiovasc Med. 2022;9:918056.
63. Adoberg A, Leis L, Luman M, Uhlin F, Fridolin I, Viigimaa M, et al. Vascular calcification inhibitors in chronic kidney disease. Clin Chim Acta Int J Clin Chem. 2025;572:120271.
64. Wang C, Liang Q, He S, Zhu J, Lin X, Lin G, et al. Role of inflammation and immunity in vascular calcification: a bibliometric and visual analysis, 2000–2022. Front Cardiovasc Med. 2023;10:1258230.
65. Chen R, Zhang H, Tang B, Luo Y, Yang Y, Zhong X, et al. Macrophages in cardiovascular diseases: molecular mechanisms and therapeutic targets. Signal Transduct Target Ther. 2024;9(1):130.
66. Hiramatsu-Asano S, Mukai T, Akagi T, Uchida HA, Fujita S, Nakano K, et al. IL-17A promotes vascular calcification in an ex vivo murine aorta culture. Biochem Biophys Res Commun. 2022;604:83–7.
67. Schüler R, Efentakis P, Wild J, Lagrange J, Garlapati V, Molitor M, et al. T cell-derived IL-17A induces vascular dysfunction via perivascular fibrosis formation and dysregulation of ·NO/cGMP signaling. Oxidative Med Cell Longev. 2019;2019:6721531.
68. Bäck M, Aranyi T, Cancela ML, Carracedo M, Conceição N, Leftheriotis G, et al. Endogenous calcification inhibitors in the prevention of vascular calcification: a consensus statement from the COST action EuroSoftCalcNet. Front Cardiovasc Med. 2018;5:196.
69. Akbari M, Nayeri H, Nasri H. Association of fetuin-A with kidney disease; a review on current concepts and new data. J Nephropharmacol. 2018;8(2):e14.
70. Ter Braake AD, Shanahan CM, de Baaij JHF. Magnesium counteracts vascular calcification: passive interference or active modulation? Arterioscler Thromb Vasc Biol. 2017;37(8):1431–45.
71. Zhang X, Chen J, Meng Q, Li D, Hu FZ, Zhu YQ, et al. The protective effects of long noncoding RNA-ANCR on arterial calcification. J Bone Miner Metab. 2020;38(4):421–31.
72. Liu Q, Qi H, Yao L. A long non-coding RNA H19/microRNA-138/TLR3 network is involved in high phosphorus-mediated vascular calcification and chronic kidney disease. Cell Cycle. 21(16):1667–83.

73. Li XZ, Xiong ZC, Zhang SL, Hao QY, Liu ZY, Zhang HF, et al. Upregulated LncRNA H19 sponges MiR-106a-5p and contributes to aldosterone-induced vascular calcification via activating the Runx2-dependent pathway. Arterioscler Thromb Vasc Biol. 2023;43(9):1684–99.
74. Huang Y, Zhan W, Song C, Tan M, Wu L, Wu S. The lncRNA SENCR knockdown alleviates vascular calcification via miR-4731-5p by suppressing endoplasmic reticulum stress. PLoS One. 2025;20(5):e0323058.
75. Kajuluri LP, Guo YY, Lee S, Christof M, Malhotra R. Epigenetic regulation of human vascular calcification. Genes. 2025;16(5):506.
76. O'Brien K, Husson H, Sabbagh Y. Therapeutic approaches for the treatment of genetic and acquired cardiovascular calcification. Front Cardiovasc Med. 2025;12:1636432.
77. Xu C, Smith ER, Tiong MK, Ruderman I, Toussaint ND. Interventions to attenuate vascular calcification progression in chronic kidney disease: a systematic review of clinical trials. J Am Soc Nephrol. 2022;33(5):1011–32.
78. Bessueille L, Kawtharany L, Quillard T, Goettsch C, Briolay A, Taraconat N, et al. Inhibition of alkaline phosphatase impairs dyslipidemia and protects mice from atherosclerosis. Transl Res J Lab Clin Med. 2023;251:2–13.
79. Goettsch C, Strzelecka-Kiliszek A, Bessueille L, Quillard T, Mechtouff L, Pikula S, et al. TNAP as a therapeutic target for cardiovascular calcification: a discussion of its pleiotropic functions in the body. Cardiovasc Res. 2020;118(1):84–96.
80. Ciceri P, Falleni M, Tosi D, Martinelli C, Cannizzo S, Marchetti G, et al. Therapeutic effect of iron citrate in blocking calcium deposition in high Pi-calcified VSMC: role of autophagy and apoptosis. Int J Mol Sci. 2019;20(23):5925.
81. Ciceri P, Elli F, Braidotti P, Falleni M, Tosi D, Bulfamante G, et al. Iron citrate reduces high phosphate-induced vascular calcification by inhibiting apoptosis. Atherosclerosis. 2016;254:93–101.
82. Maruyama N, Otsuki T, Yoshida Y, Nagura C, Kitai M, Shibahara N, et al. Ferric citrate decreases fibroblast growth factor 23 and improves erythropoietin responsiveness in hemodialysis patients. Am J Nephrol. 2018;47(6):406–14.
83. Sinha S, Gould LJ, Nigwekar SU, Serena TE, Brandenburg V, Moe SM, et al. The CALCIPHYX study: a randomized, double-blind, placebo-controlled, phase 3 clinical trial of SNF472 for the treatment of calciphylaxis. Clin Kidney J. 2022;15(1):136–44.
84. Wolf M, Koch TA, Bregman DB. Effects of iron deficiency anemia and its treatment on fibroblast growth factor 23 and phosphate homeostasis in women. J Bone Miner Res Off J Am Soc Bone Miner Res. 2013;28(8):1793–803.
85. Imel EA, Biggin A, Schindeler A, Munns CF. FGF23, hypophosphatemia, and emerging treatments. JBMR Plus. 2019;3(8):e10190.
86. Noonan ML, Clinkenbeard EL, Ni P, Swallow EA, Tippen SP, Agoro R, et al. Erythropoietin and a hypoxia-inducible factor prolyl hydroxylase inhibitor (HIF-PHDi) lowers FGF23 in a model of chronic kidney disease (CKD). Physiol Rep. 2020;8(11):e14434.
87. Bellasi A, Raggi P, Bover J, Bushinsky DA, Chertow GM, Ketteler M, et al. Trial design and baseline characteristics of CaLIPSO: a randomized, double-blind placebo-controlled trial of SNF472 in patients receiving haemodialysis with cardiovascular calcification. Clin Kidney J. 2021;14(1):366–74.
88. Raggi P, Bellasi A, Bushinsky D, Bover J, Rodriguez M, Ketteler M, et al. Slowing progression of cardiovascular calcification with SNF472 in patients on hemodialysis: results of a randomized phase 2b study. Circulation. 2020;141(9):728–39.
89. Raggi P, Bellasi A, Sinha S, Bover J, Rodriguez M, Ketteler M, et al. Effects of SNF472, a novel inhibitor of hydroxyapatite crystallization in patients receiving hemodialysis — subgroup analyses of the CALIPSO trial. Kidney Int Rep. 2020;5(12):2178–82.
90. Li Q, Kingman J, Sundberg JP, Levine MA, Uitto J. Etidronate prevents, but does not reverse, ectopic mineralization in a mouse model of pseudoxanthoma elasticum (*Abcc6−/−*). Oncotarget. 2018;9(56):30721–30.

91. Li T, Wang Y, Tu W ping. Vitamin K supplementation and vascular calcification: a systematic review and meta-analysis of randomized controlled trials. Front Nutr 2023;10:1115069. doi:https://doi.org/10.3389/fnut.2023.1115069. PMID: 37252246; PMCID: PMC10218696.
92. Neofytou IE, Stamou A, Demopoulos A, Roumeliotis S, Zebekakis P, Liakopoulos V, et al. Vitamin K for vascular calcification in kidney patients: still alive and kicking, but still a lot to learn. Nutrients. 2024;16(12):1798.
93. O'Brien K, Laurion L, Sullivan C, Howe J, Lynch AM, Cheng Z, et al. Recombinant ectonucleotide pyrophosphatase/phosphodiesterase 1 (ENPP1) decreases vascular calcification and prevents osteomalacia in a rat model of chronic kidney disease. JBMR Plus. 2025;9(6):ziaf065.
94. Cheng Z, O'Brien K, Howe J, Sullivan C, Schrier D, Lynch A, et al. INZ-701 prevents ectopic tissue calcification and restores bone architecture and growth in ENPP1-deficient mice. J Bone Miner Res. 2021;36(8):1594–604.
95. Yuan Q, Tang B, Zhang C. Signaling pathways of chronic kidney diseases, implications for therapeutics. Signal Transduct Target Ther. 2022;7(1):182.
96. Lian Y, Li Y, Liu A, Ghosh S, Shi Y, Huang H. Dietary antioxidants and vascular calcification: from pharmacological mechanisms to challenges. Biomed Pharmacother. 2023;168:115693.
97. Lu Y, Yuan T, Min X, Yuan Z, Cai Z. AMPK: potential therapeutic target for vascular calcification. Front Cardiovasc Med. 2021;8 https://doi.org/10.3389/fcvm.2021.670222. PMID: 34046440; PMCID: PMC8144331.
98. Hewedy WA, Abdulmalek SA, Ghareeb DA, Habiba ES. AMPK-mediated autophagy is involved in the protective effect of canagliflozin in the vitamin D3 plus nicotine calcification model in rats. Naunyn Schmiedeberg's Arch Pharmacol. 2024;397(2):873–88.
99. Zhou X, Xu SN, Yuan ST, Lei X, Sun X, Xing L, et al. Multiple functions of autophagy in vascular calcification. Cell Biosci. 2021;11:159.
100. Jin Q, Ma F, Liu T, Yang L, Mao H, Wang Y, et al. Sirtuins in kidney diseases: potential mechanism and therapeutic targets. Cell Commun Signal CCS. 2024;22:114.
101. Peng X, Ni H, Kuang B, Wang Z, Hou S, Gu S, et al. Sirtuin 3 in renal diseases and aging: from mechanisms to potential therapies. Pharmacol Res. 2024;206:107261.

Chapter 7
Advanced Imaging Modalities in Cardio-Renal Syndromes

Adrian Covic and Vlad Vasiliu

7.1 Introduction

The bidirectional interaction between the heart and kidney in CRS is mediated not only by neurohormonal and systemic inflammatory pathways, but also by structural and functional changes in the two organs, which can be evaluated by noninvasive imaging. Structural imaging targets offer a perspective on organ remodeling that can foreshadow overt organ dysfunction [5]. Functional imaging targets in CRS are equally important as structural modifications. These include macro and microvascular perfusion, tissular composition (fibrosis versus edema), venous congestion, renal hemodynamics and ventricular-venous coupling [6].

Cardiac structural targets refer to alterations in the left ventricular geometry and mass, atrial enlargement and myocardial fibrosis. Cardiac functional targets include parameters of left ventricular systolic and diastolic function as well as tissue characterization on MRC. Evaluation of congestion by ultrasound using the inferior vena cava (IVC) diameter is also a functional hemodynamic target linked to renal dysfunction [1, 7, 8].

Renal structural targets include the reduction of renal cortex volume, interstitial fibrosis, vascular modifications (arterial stenosis, venous congestion) and parenchymal alterations such as echogenicity. Renal ultrasound can evaluate kidney size, cortical thickness, Doppler resistivity indices and discontinuity of the intrarenal venous flow, indicators of increased renal venous pressure in heart failure [8, 9]. Renal functional targets include renal perfusion, microvascular flow, oxygenation

A. Covic
University of Medicine and Pharmacy "Grigore T. Popa", Iasi, Romania

Nephrology Clinic, Dialysis and Renal Transplant Center – 'C.I. Parhon' University Hospital, Iasi, Romania

V. Vasiliu (✉)
University of Medicine and Pharmacy "Grigore T. Popa", Iasi, Romania

A. Covic, A. Burlacu (eds.), *Renal Dysfunction in Cardiovascular Pathologies*,
https://doi.org/10.1007/978-3-032-25434-4_7

by blood-oxygen-level-dependent (BOLD) MRI, intrarenal venous flow and renal tubulointerstitial integrity. Advanced imaging such as functional MRI can quantify interstitial water in the renal parenchyma, reflecting congestion or edema [6].

Thus, imaging offers structural and functional targets which can clarify physiopathology, guide risk stratification, and monitor treatment response, creating a comprehensive representation of the problem. By using advanced technology that allows for multi-organ evaluation, clinicians can more precisely characterize CRS, detect preclinical damage earlier, personalize treatment and improve results.

7.2 Echocardiography and Ultrasound

Echocardiography remains an essential tool in the evaluation and longitudinal management of CRS, mainly due to its accessibility, feasibility at the patient's bedside and capacity to characterize hemodynamic and structural cardiac changes relevant to the kidney-heart axis. In CRS patients, echocardiography contributes to multiple levels: quantification of wall thickness, evaluation of systolic and diastolic function, filling pressures and congestion, as well as advanced techniques like speckle-tracking.

Chronic kidney disease (CKD) patients with CRS usually present with left ventricular hypertrophy driven by both pressure and volume overload. In this scenario, echocardiographic measurement of left ventricular mass and relative wall thickness are staple parameters for cardiac remodeling [6]. Ejection fraction (EF) is still universally used for stratification, but in CRS a preserved EF does not exclude subclinical contractile dysfunction. Speckle tracking echocardiography (STE) allows for the measurement of global longitudinal strain (GLS), detecting early myocardial dysfunction before the reduction of EF. CKD patients have reduced left ventricular GLS values. Moreover, impaired left ventricular GLS is associated with adverse outcomes in renal patients [10].

Beyond the left ventricle, the structure and function of the left atrium (LA) offer important information regarding diastolic dysfunction in CRS. LA enlargement and impaired reservoir strain reflect on increased filling pressures and chronic overload and have been associated with worse kidney and cardiovascular outcomes in CKD cohorts [11].

Echocardiography also allows for the indirect evaluation of systemic congestion and right-side pressures by measurement of IVC diameter and collapsibility, tricuspid regurgitation velocity and the estimation of pulmonary artery pressures. In the context of CRS, where venous congestion is a key mediator of insufficient renal perfusion, these measurements are especially valuable. Increased IVC diameter correlates with worse outcomes and can guide decongestive therapy, even though its limitations due to interobserver variability and the influence of intrathoracic pressure must be acknowledged [6].

Noninvasive left ventricular pressure-strain loop, an advanced method that combines strain data with estimated brachial artery blood pressure, has shown promise as a quantitative biomarker of myocardial work. In a small CKD population with preserved EF, this approach has been used for the early detection of myocardial injury, increasing sensitivity beyond standard strain measurements [12].

Point-of-care ultrasonography (POCUS) has emerged as an extension of echocardiography in the management of CRS, offering a bedside dynamic evaluation of cardiac function and systemic congestion. Portable ultrasound machines allow for rapid, repeatable evaluations that can be performed by cardiologists, nephrologists or intensivists, improving real-time decision making in the context of CRS. POCUS includes the assessment of cardiac performance, venous congestion and pulmonary congestion. Focused cardiac ultrasound (FoCUS), a standardized and simplified echocardiography, offers basic and rapid information on ventricular function, pericardial effusion and chamber dilation, while allowing the estimation of filling pressures by Doppler surrogates. Venous congestion can be presently quantified by calculating the venous excess ultrasound score (VExUS), which integrates hepatic, portal and renal venous doppler waves with IVC diameter and collapsibility. High VExUS grades have been associated with worse renal outcomes and have shown predictive value for adverse outcomes in patients with heart failure and CRS [7].

Similarly, lung ultrasound (LUS) detects pulmonary congestion through the presence and distribution of B-lines, also referred to as comet tails—vertical artifacts that extend from the pleural line into the lung, which reflect extravascular fluid. LUS represents a sensitive, radiation-free method for monitoring fluid shifts and guiding decongestive therapy [13].

Recent studies assert that integrating POCUS into clinical management leads to a higher accuracy in assessing volume status and a better adjustment of diuretic or ultrafiltration strategies. Moreover, as portable devices improve in image quality and AI-assisted interpretation, POCUS will increasingly be adopted beyond intensive care units, including nephrology wards and outpatient heart failure clinics [7].

Contrast ultrasonography (CUS), in which ultrasound-enhancing agents (usually microbubbles) are injected to improve visualization, has a well-established role in clinical cardiology. Its applications include the detection with higher accuracy of segmental wall motion abnormalities of the ventricular wall at rest and during stress, as well as better quantification of the EF. The use of contrast agents facilitates the detection of intracavitary thrombi and the characterization of non-thrombotic masses. Additionally, it contributes to the diagnosis of apical hypertrophic cardiomyopathy, the evaluation of eosinophilic and non-compaction cardiomyopathy and the detection of ventricular pseudoaneurysms. It also has a role in the augmentation of Doppler signals and the detection of aortic thrombi and dissections, offering a superior delimitation of the endocardial borders and improving diagnostic confidence. Novel investigational contrast agents, such as nano-emulsion or nanodroplets which are <1 μm have been developed with potential clinical applications including molecular and cellular imaging (risk assessment in atherosclerosis, allograft rejection, myocarditis, recent myocardial ischemia and risk of remodeling), sonothrombolysis for enhanced clot penetration in the treatment of the acute coronary syndrome, vascular or graft thrombosis, stroke or pulmonary embolism or the targeted delivery of drugs, genes or radiosensitizers [14].

More recently, CUS has been used for the assessment of kidney perfusion and the characterization of indeterminate renal masses, due to its increased accuracy, low cost, reproducibility and absence of nephrotoxicity. Doppler ultrasound, the preferred noninvasive method for determining kidney perfusion, cannot estimate microvascular and regional blood flow. CUS has been shown to accurately detect early changes in renal microvascular perfusion, due to the low-diffusibility and similar size and flow of microbubbles as red blood cells; decreased microvascular perfusion using CUS has been shown to be directly related to a drop in estimated glomerular filtration rate (eGFR) [15, 16].

7.3 Computed Tomography

Recent advances in CT have significantly improved its use in the multimodal evaluation of CRS. Among the most relevant innovations are dual-energy CT (DECT) and photon-counting detector CT (PCD-CT), both allowing an improved tissue characterization and spatial resolution, as well as a reduction in contrast and radiation doses. DECT, through material decomposition, opens the possibility of iodine mapping and monochromatic reconstructions, which improve the contrast-to-noise ratio (CNR) and provide a semi-quantitative evaluation of renal and myocardial perfusion. In heart imaging, DECT iodine maps have significantly improved the accuracy of ischemia detection in comparison to conventional CT, while also offering the means to differentiate hyperemia from fibrosis [17].

PCD-CT counts individual photons and distinguishes between them based on energy levels, offering a superior spatial resolution and a reduction in noise compared to conventional CT. This translates into a higher quality representation of vascular calcifications and the possibility to reduce the dose of iodine contrast without a compromise in image quality [18, 19]. Cardiovascular studies show that PCD-CT reduces "blooming" artifacts caused by coronary calcifications and allows for a more precise analysis of stenosis in segments in which conventional CT was not accurate [18].

Low-dose contrast DECT has been utilized in CKD patients undergoing transcatheter aortic valve replacement, with as little as 30 mL of iodine contrast, without a significant rise in creatinine levels at 48–72 h, further proving the feasibility of contrast-sparing CT in high-risk populations [20].

There is also an improved understanding of the safety profile of iodine contrast. Modern data suggests that the real incidence of contrast-associated acute kidney injury (CA-AKI) is lower than was historically presumed, after adjusting for confounders. Recent studies have shown that when modern low-osmolarity agents and adequate prophylaxis are used, the risk of CA-AKI in stable patients is relatively low [21]. The focus has shifted from avoiding contrast to optimization of its usage. The 2024 ACR manual on contrast media recommends an individualized assessment in place of contraindication of contrast, highlighting the role of volume expansion, usage of the minimal effective dose and avoidance of nephrotoxic agents in patients at high risk. Among the practical measures that can be applied are the baseline eGFR and volume status assessment prior to scanning, the utilization of low-kVp and contrast-sparing protocols, the avoidance of repeated exposure (in 24–48 h) unless necessary, tailored hydration strategies according to cardiac and renal function and post-scan monitoring of eGFR for individuals at risk [22].

CT complements ultrasound and MRI in the setting of CRS. Echocardiography and Doppler ultrasound are first-line for cardiac and venous evaluation, while MRI offers a superior tissue characterization. However, CT offers unmatched spatial resolution and a simultaneous evaluation of coronary, renal and systemic vascularization. In this scenario, CT is to be considered the "anatomical backbone" for CRS imaging, with DECT and PCD-CT being the bridge between functional and structural perspectives [1, 6].

While reporting CT in CRS, the interpretation should include kidney function and type and dosage of contrast used, vascular findings, with a focus on coronary, aortic and renal findings (stenosis, calcifications, plaque structure), signs of congestion, as previously mentioned (VCI diameter, ascites, renal tissue heterogenicity), quantitative parameters, where available (iodine concentration, myocardial blood flow, calcium score) as well as mention of contrast-sparing or spectral technique used.

7.3.1 Clinical Applications of CT in CRS

7.3.1.1 Arterial Disease

Arterial disease sits at the center of the CRS physiopathology, affecting coronary, aortic and renal circulation. Coronary CT angiography (CCTA) offers a noninvasive, high-resolution insight into coronary artery disease (CAD), which is disproportionately prevalent in CKD and CRS patients. Extensive coronary calcifications can obstruct the visualization of the vascular lumen on standard CT. PCD-CT mitigates these limitations by reducing blooming artifacts and improving contrast resolution and allowing for a precise characterization of the lumen and plaques even in segments in which there are important calcifications [18, 19].

In advanced CKD patients, combined functional and anatomical CT scanning, like CCTA with myocardial perfusion (CTP) integrations, improves risk stratification. In a recent study with ESRD patients, the combination of obstructive CAD in CCTA with reduced myocardial blood flow shown by dynamic CTP predicted major adverse cardiovascular events (MACE) better than each individual parameter [23].

CT angiography of renal arteries and veins remains the gold standard of noninvasive evaluation of renal artery stenosis, fibromuscular dysplasia, aneurysms or thrombosis, all of which have the potential of exacerbating CRS. Adapted protocols, such as low-kVp or monochromatic imaging with iterative reconstruction, improve vascular visibility as well as renal safety [24].

7.3.1.2 Congestion and Edema

Systemic and renal congestion is acknowledged as one of the main triggers of renal dysfunction in CRS. CT offers cross-sectional markers of congestion across multiple systems: IVC dilation, contrast reflux in hepatic and portal veins, intestinal wall enhancement, ascites, and heterogeneous renal parenchymal enhancement. Recent reviews highlight the diagnostic and prognostic value of integrating these CT findings with echocardiographic and laboratory parameters for guiding decongestive therapy [6].

Within the renal parenchyma, iodine DECT mapping can differentiate perfusion from congestion by measuring cortical and medullary iodine concentrations. Decreased or heterogeneous cortical iodine uptake may reflect renal ischemia, venous hypertension, or microvascular dysfunction—pathophysiologic hallmarks of CRS [1]. While validation in CRS cohorts is ongoing, early studies in abdominal imaging have established the reproducibility and quantitative potential of DECT iodine measurements [25].

Beyond only qualitative imaging, there are potential quantitative biomarkers that emerge.

Iodine Concentration Mapping Derived from DECT, the iodine concentration (mg/mL) serves as a substitute for tissue perfusion. In myocardial studies, iodine maps had successfully differentiated ischemic from healthy tissue [17]. A similar application can be extended to evaluating renal cortical perfusion and to improve congestion scores in CRS [1, 25].

Quantifying Vascular Calcifications Coronary artery calcium score remains an important predictor in CKD, even though important calcifications hinder the measurements. PCD-CT improves spatial resolution and reduces artifacts, refining quantification and allowing a potential longitudinal monitoring of the calcium burden [18, 19].

Congestion Scores Composite markers—VCI diameter, hepatic reflux, renal heterogenicity, could be integrated in congestion scores correlating with diuretic response and renal outcomes [19].

Artificial Intelligence and Deep Learning Artificial intelligence and deep learning. Automated segmentation and pseudo-dual-energy reconstruction using deep learning may expand perfusion mapping to conventional CT systems and facilitate automated quantification of cardiac and renal morphology in CRS [26].

The evolution of CT from a purely anatomical tool to a quantitative multimodal imaging platform is what positions it in the center of future CRS evaluation. Future research priorities include the validation of quantitative biomarkers, correlation of outcomes with iodine-based indices and integration of AI spectral reconstruction techniques for reductions in contrast usage. With the development of PCD-CT, a complete evaluation of the heart-kidney axis using minimal contrast exposure is looking like an attainable goal for CRS patients.

7.4 Magnetic Resonance Imaging

CMR has become an essential tool for the evaluation of the cardiac structure and function, as well as the myocardial tissue composition in patients with CRS. It allows for quantification of fibrosis, edema, perfusion and ventricular function, which are parameters directly involved in the two-way interaction between the heart and kidney.

The uremic cardiomyopathy is often described in ESRD patients, and it is characterized by interstitial diffuse fibrosis, left ventricular hypertrophy and subclinical systolic dysfunction. Non-contrast T1 and T2 mapping techniques are particularly useful in CRS, as they are able to detect fibrosis and diffuse inflammation without the need for gadolinium administration. A prospective study, which included CKD patients stages 1–5, showed that both T1 and T2 values increased progressively with renal function decline, with GLS worsening in parallel [2]. These findings support the idea that myocardial injury in CRS appears before the installation of overt heart failure. A recent meta-analysis has reported significantly elevated native T1 values in CKD and ESRD patients (mean difference of ~1.1 from control groups), suggesting diffuse myocardial fibrosis and extracellular volume overload [27]. Given that myocardial fibrosis is a strong predictor of adverse events (heart failure worsening, arrhythmias, sudden cardiac death) [28], its early detection has major implications in risk stratification in CRS patients. CMR also consistently shows a higher left ventricular mass index and a higher systolic strain impairment with CKD progression [2, 27]. When gadolinium can be administered, late gadolinium enhancement and extracellular volume quantification provide a direct assessment of fibrosis. When contrast is contraindicated, non-contrast mapping (T1/T2 native, strain) remains powerful. Up-to-date guidelines acknowledge that macrocyclic group II gadolinium-based contrast agents (GBCAs) are generally safe even in moderate CKD, though caution persists in stage 5 disease [29].

Perfusion MRI (contrast or stress perfusion) is less commonly used in CKD patients due to limitations related to contrast administration. Nevertheless, it offers important information on microvascular ischemia contributing to neurohormonal activation and renal dysfunction in CRS [30].

Beyond cardiac imaging, MRI has a central role in vascular and renal assessment in CRS. Magnetic resonance angiography (MRA) allows the visualization of renal arteries and veins, as well as systemic vessels, without exposure to ionizing radiation. It is the standard reference for diagnosing renal artery stenosis, fibro-muscular dysplasia and renal vein thrombosis—all being potential contributors to CRS pathophysiology [31].

Multiparametric renal MRI (mpMRI) combines multiple noninvasive parameters of renal function and structure—T1 and T2 mapping for the quantification of fibrosis and edema, diffusion-weighted imaging (DWI) for microstructure, arterial spin labelling (ASL) for renal cortical perfusion, and BOLD-MRI for oxygenation, thus generating reproducible quantitative markers of cortical perfusion, interstitial fibrosis and renal oxygenation without the need of contrast [3]. In CRS, such techniques can differentiate between structural renal dysfunction (fibrosis, ischemia) and hemodynamic dysfunction (reversible congestion). Multicentric validation is needed to acknowledge these as reliable predictors of clinical outcomes, such as heart failure hospitalization, acute kidney injury or mortality.

Combined cardiac–renal MRI—incorporating ventricular function, myocardial tissue mapping, renal morphology, and perfusion—provides a comprehensive view of the heart–kidney axis and may help phenotype CRS into fibrotic, ischemic, or congestive subtypes. These methods, which have been validated as secure and reproducible in CKD cohorts [32, 33], can also be utilized for monitoring of the therapeutic strategies (e.g., decongestion of nephroprotection), supporting MRI's role as a monitoring tool in CRS.

When reporting MRI in CRS, interpretation should be clinically-oriented, integrating cardiac, kidney and vascular information in a holistic functional context. It is essential to reference renal function and the type of contrast administered, including the dose used. The report should specify the sequences and quantitative parameters analyzed, such as native T1 and T2 values, ECV, apparent diffusion coefficient (ADC), and perfusion metrics derived from ASL. Cardiac findings should include ventricular volume and mass, EF, LVMi, myocardial strain and the extent and pattern of fibrosis. For the kidneys, it is recommended to report the morphology and quantitative results, with an emphasis on cortico-medullar differentiation, fibrosis indicators and tissue perfusion. The vascular anatomy must also be reported on, leaning into renal artery stenosis, venous thromboses or systemic atherosclerosis. The report should conclude with a concise clinical interpretation, highlighting the implications of the findings in the management of the patient.

Integrating the cardiac and renal MRI in a single protocol will allow a simultaneous and comprehensive evaluation of the patient. Advancements in artificial intelligence will play a major role, automating tasks such as tissue characterization and quantitative analysis of fibrosis or perfusion. The development of non-contrast MRI protocols will be essential to enable safe and radiation-free evaluation of the heart–kidney axis, especially for patients with advanced renal impairment where gadolinium use is limited.

7.5 Nuclear Imaging

Nuclear imaging offers major advantages in understanding and managing CRS, by enabling direct assessment of perfusion, function and physiopathology of the cardio-renal axis.

Myocardial perfusion scintigraphy (MPS) is an essential tool for risk stratification in CKD and ESRD populations. A recent meta-analysis which included 16 studies and 7834 patients has shown that stress-test MPS anomalies had a hazard ratio (HR) of 2.02 (CI 95% 1.68–2.42) for adverse cardiovascular events; when adjusted for major cardiovascular events only (myocardial infarction, cardiovascular death), the HR climbed to 2.36 (CI 95% 1.77–3.13) [4], which suggests that impaired myocardial perfusion has an independent prognostic value in the setting of kidney disfunction. MPS in ESRD patients who are transplant candidates offers further prognostic value compared to standard clinical and echocardiographic variables, guiding decisions regarding revascularization, the moment of enlisting on the transplant waiting list or the necessity of further cardiovascular investigations. The key limitation is that MPS, in the context of CKD/ESRD, may underestimate diffuse microvascular disease or give false positives in the case of thick myocardium and vascular calcifications, necessitating a specialized context of interpretation [34].

Renal scintigraphy using radiotracers such as ^99mTc-MAG3 and ^99mTc-DTPA offers quantitative and semi-quantitative evaluations of renal perfusion, tubular transit time, excretion and percent differential renal function, parameters often altered in the setting of CRS. This method is preferred where contrast cannot be administered and provides information beyond only anatomy. Comparative studies have shown that MAG3 and DTPA dynamic renography correlate well for relative renal function evaluation, supporting their interchangeability in the clinical setting. In the CRS serial renal scintigraphy can help distinguish pre-renal or tubular dysfunction from obstructive or parenchymal damage, guiding decongestion therapy, fluid resuscitation or urologic referral. In addition, as renal perfusion abnormalities well reflect the hemodynamic burden of heart failure, they can help link the cardiac and renal imaging [35].

PET extends the role of nuclear imaging, allowing precise quantitative data and the possibility of multi-organ simultaneous assessment. A recent feasibility study demonstrated the possibility of quantification of both cardiac and renal perfusion in a single axial ^13N-ammonia PET/CT scan, opening perspectives in discovering therapies with overlapping cardiac and renal benefits [36]. PET allows for the measurement of myocardial flow reserve (MFR), a biomarker of microvascular disease extremely relevant in CKD populations, where epicardial coronary lesions can coexist with diffuse microvascular remodeling. Even though large-scale studies are limited, MFR measured by PET could predict cardiovascular events better than perfusion defects alone [37]. Regarding the kidney, recent literature shows the role of PET in assessing renal perfusion, metabolic activity, inflammation and fibrosis in CKD and transplant populations [38].

PET/MRI is a highly advanced hybrid technique which combines the metabolic and molecular sensitivity of PET with the superior tissular resolution of MRI, offering a comprehensive evaluation of inflammation, perfusion and tissular structure of the heart and kidney. In the setting of CRS, this allows for simultaneous investigation of microvascular and metabolic dysfunctions and fibrosis, without the radiation exposure of the PET/CT. Its clinical applications in cardiology include MPI with the possibility of absolute quantification of the myocardial blood flow, detection of myocardial viability in the setting of repetitive or chronic ischemia and noninvasive quantification of inflammation in disorders such as myocarditis or sarcoidosis, with the potential of presenting a prognostic value for ventricular remodeling in scenarios such as the postischemic myocardial inflammation or after the administration of chemo and radiotherapy in oncologic patients [39].

7.6 Integrating Guidelines

In the contemporary cardiology and nephrology practice, guidelines converge towards a consistent, multimodal imaging strategy in the setting of CRS. However, some variation persists, highlighting the need for local tailoring and the need for a multidisciplinary collaborative interpretation [40–42].

The ESC 2021 Heart Failure guidelines and their 2023 update position transthoracic echocardiography (TTE) as the first line imaging modality in all patients with a diagnosis or suspicion of HF, with clear recommendations for the evaluation of the right and left ventricular size and function, valvular disease, pulmonary pressures and pericardial effusion, as well as for seriated examinations in the context of clinical evolution or before major therapeutic decisions [40]. In parallel, the 2024 KDIGO guidelines for the evaluation and management of CKD highlight the necessity of imaging in the diagnosis and phenotyping of CKD, recommending ultrasound as routine for identifying structural anomalies and early recourse to cardiac imaging for quantification of the burden of left ventricular hypertrophy, systolic and diastolic disfunction or pulmonary hypertension, especially in patients with albuminuria or advanced CKD (G3b-G5) [41]. The ESC 2023 for the management of cardiovascular disease in patients with diabetes, which explicitly integrates CKD in its risk stratification, aligns with KDIGO by recommending systematic cardiovascular imaging in high-risk patients, using TTE for detecting subclinical cardiomyopathy and CCTA or functional stress imaging for detecting silent ischemia when such changes would influence management [42, 43].

In practice, integrating the guidelines in the CRS context begins with echocardiography as common ground—both cardiologists and nephrologists recommend TTE for the initial evaluation of patients with symptomatic heart failure, advanced CKD, kidney and heart transplant, as well as resistant hypertension or unexplained volume overload, with seriated evaluations being based on patient evolution rather than fixed intervals [40–42]. Current ASE and EACVI echocardiography guidelines refine this approach, recommending standardized systolic and diastolic function evaluation, chamber and wall dimensions, and the routine use of two-dimensional speckle-tracking strain when available to expose early myocardial dysfunction—recommendations especially relevant in heart failure with preserved ejection fraction and CKD [44].

ESC HF and CVD-in-diabetes guidelines, together with AHA/ACC chronic coronary disease recommendations, integrate CMR, CCTA and nuclear imaging in decision algorithms, while KDIGO offers the safety frame for their implementation. CMR is recommended by HF guidelines when the TTE images are suboptimal or when there is a suspicion of specific cardiomyopathies such as myocarditis, infiltrative disease, iron overload or non-compaction [40].

KDIGO insists on the careful evaluation of eGFR, cumulative contrast exposure and risk-benefit balance before iodine-contrast CT or gadolinium MRI, without setting absolute eGFR thresholds, proposing instead risk reduction strategies, such as volume expansion, avoidance of nephrotoxics and contrast-sparing protocols where advanced imaging has the potential of influencing prognosis or management [41].

Regarding CAD in CKD or HF patients, ESC and AHA/ACC guidelines encourage the usage of noninvasive imaging, favoring CCTA or functional stress imaging (echocardiography, SPECT/PET or CMR) depending on local experience, patient risk and kidney function, while KDIGO highlights that CKD G3b-G5 patients are at the highest risk and are most likely to benefit from imaging when it guides revascularization or treatment tailoring [42, 43].

Nuclear imaging maintains a defined niche. ESC and AHA/ACC guidelines acknowledge the value of bone-tracer scintigraphy for transthyretin cardiac amyloidosis and myocardial perfusion SPECT or PET for ischemia evaluation. KDIGO warns mainly about radiation exposure in young CKD patients, without major preoccupation concerning the renal safety of radioisotopes [40–42].

Integrating these recommendations is particularly relevant in the diagnostic algorithms of HF in the setting of CKD. ESC HF guidelines mandate ETT for all patients with suspected HF, followed by CMR for tissue characterization and CCTA/nuclear imaging for ischemia evaluation, while KDIGO and ESC CVD-in-diabetes guidelines stratify patients by eGFR and albuminuria for identifying those with the highest risk, which would call for more aggressive imaging for cardiomyopathy or silent ischemia [37–40].

The use of advanced modalities such as strain imaging, 3D echocardiography and right ventricle-focused protocols, even though not imposed in current guidelines, is supported by ASE/EACVI echocardiography guidelines for the refinement of volume status, pulmonary pressures and right ventricle evaluation—pivotal elements in the decision of ultrafiltration initiation moment, dialysis prescription and transplant waiting list enlistment [44].

All the above-cited guidelines consistently warn against the exhaustive, indiscriminate use of imaging. Seriated contrast CT imaging in CKD patients without therapeutic consequence is discouraged, seriated echocardiography is only recommended when it affects clinical and treatment courses, and screening functional stress testing in asymptomatic low-risk patients is not yet supported by evidence [40–42].

The implementation of an integrated imaging strategy in CRS calls for the development of protocols that can unify the step-by-step algorithms found in the ESC and ACC/AHA HF and CVD guidelines with the risk stratification strategies and contrast safety principles proposed by KDIGO, while maintaining conformity to the ASE/EACVI standards to ensure the reproducibility of seriated measurements. Multidisciplinary cardio-renal teams offer a practical way of harmonizing sometimes divergent tones (e.g., the situation where cardiology guidelines support the utilization of contrast CMR for characterization of infiltrative disease, while the nephrology guideline prioritizes renal contrast safety and poor vascular access), integrating guidelines imaging recommendation and steering clinical practice toward a coherent pathway, where TTE remains the first line modality, and each exposure to contrast, ionizing radiation or gadolinium is personalized in the context of the patient's long term evolution rather than viewed in isolation.

Declarations

Competing Interests The author(s) has no competing interests to declare that are relevant to the content of this manuscript.

Ethics Approval The author(s) declares that this manuscript does not include primary research with human participants.

The author(s) declares that this manuscript does not include primary studies involving animals.

References

1. Lin L, Zhou X, Dekkers IA, Lamb HJ. Cardiorenal syndrome: emerging role of medical imaging for clinical diagnosis and management. J Pers Med. 2021;11(8):734.
2. Jia X, Han X, Wang Y, He F, Zhou X, Zheng Y, et al. Cardiac magnetic resonance imaging parameters show association between myocardial abnormalities and severity of chronic kidney disease. Front Cardiovasc Med. 2022;9:1053122. Available from: https://www.frontiersin.org/journals/cardiovascular-medicine/articles/10.3389/fcvm.2022.1053122.
3. Francis ST, Selby NM, Taal MW. Magnetic resonance imaging to evaluate kidney structure, function, and pathology: moving toward clinical application. Am J Kidney Dis. 2023;82(4):491–504.
4. Cantoni V, Green R, Acampa W, Assante R, Zampella E, Nappi C, et al. Prognostic value of myocardial perfusion imaging in patients with chronic kidney disease: a systematic review and meta-analysis. J Nucl Cardiol. 2022;29(1):141–54.
5. Jin L, Zong Y, Pan Y, Hu Y, Xie Q, Wang Z. Application of functional magnetic resonance imaging to evaluate renal structure and function in type 2 cardiorenal syndrome. BMC Cardiovasc Disord. 2024;24(1):637.
6. Ei Khin HH, Cuthbert JJ, Koratala A, Aquaro GD, Pugliese NR, Gargani L, et al. Imaging of congestion in cardio-renal syndrome. Curr Heart Fail Rep. 2025;22(1):10.
7. Argaiz ER, Romero-Gonzalez G, Rola P, Spiegel R, Haycock KH, Koratala A. Bedside ultrasound in the management of cardiorenal syndromes: an updated review. Cardiorenal Med. 2023;13(1):372–84.
8. Mitsas AC, Elzawawi M, Mavrogeni S, Boekels M, Khan A, Eldawy M, et al. Heart failure and Cardiorenal syndrome: a narrative review on pathophysiology, diagnostic and therapeutic regimens—from a cardiologist's view. J Clin Med. 2022;11(23):7041.
9. Grande D, Terlizzese P, Iacoviello M. Role of imaging in the evaluation of renal dysfunction in heart failure patients. World J Nephrol. 2017;6(3):123–31.
10. Mehta R, Buzkova P, Patel H, Cheng J, Kizer JR, Gottdiener JS, et al. Cardiac mechanics and kidney function decline in the cardiovascular health study. Kidney360. 2023;4(5):622–30. Available from: https://journals.lww.com/kidney360/fulltext/2023/05000/cardiac_mechanics_and_kidney_function_decline_in.11.aspx.
11. Ji L, Gao X, Xiao W, Yu S. Assessment of left atrial function provides incremental value: the left atrial volumetric/mechanical coupling index in patients with chronic kidney disease. Front

Cardiovasc Med. 2024;11:1407531. Available from: https://www.frontiersin.org/journals/cardiovascular-medicine/articles/10.3389/fcvm.2024.1407531
12. Wang Q, Wang JP, Li Y, Zhang J, Wang R, Xu HY. Noninvasive left ventricular pressure-strain loop for quantitative assessment of early left ventricular systolic dysfunction in patients with chronic kidney disease. Echocardiography. 2024;41(10):e15941.
13. Platz E, Campbell RT, Claggett B, Lewis EF, Groarke JD, Docherty KF, et al. Lung ultrasound in acute heart failure. JACC Heart Fail. 2019;7(10):849–58.
14. Lindner JR. Contrast echocardiography: current status and future directions. Heart. 2021;107(1):18.
15. Garessus J, Brito W, Loncle N, Vanelli A, Hendriks-Balk M, Wuerzner G, et al. Cortical perfusion as assessed with contrast-enhanced ultrasound is lower in patients with chronic kidney disease than in healthy subjects but increases under low salt conditions. Nephrol Dial Transplant. 2022;37(4):705–12.
16. Velasquez-Botero F, Balasubramanya A, Tang Y, Lu Q, Liu JB, Eisenbrey JR. Renal contrast-enhanced ultrasound: clinical applications and emerging research. Adv Ultrasound Diagn Ther. 2022;6(4):129–46.
17. Dell'Aversana S, Ascione R, De Giorgi M, De Lucia DR, Cuocolo R, Boccalatte M, et al. Dual-energy CT of the heart: a review. J Imaging. 2022;8(9):236.
18. Flohr T, Schmidt B, Ulzheimer S, Alkadhi H. Cardiac imaging with photon counting CT. Br J Radiol. 2023;96(1152):20230407.
19. Shiyovich A, Singh A, Blair CV., Cardoso R, Huck D, Peng G, et al. Photon-counting computed tomography in cardiac imaging. JACC Cardiovasc Imaging. [cited 2025 Nov 16]. 2025. Available from: https://doi.org/10.1016/j.jcmg.2025.07.022.
20. Chang S, Jung JI, Beck KS, Chang K, Kim Y, Han K. Diagnostic efficacy and safety of low-contrast-dose dual-energy CT in patients with renal impairment undergoing transcatheter aortic valve replacement. Korean J Radiol. 2024;25(7):634–43.
21. McDonald JS, McDonald RJ. Risk of acute kidney injury following IV iodinated contrast media exposure: 2023 update, from the AJR special series on contrast media. Am J Roentgenol. 2024;223(1):e2330037.
22. American college of radiology. ACR manual on contrast media. 2025.
23. Araki S, Kitagawa K, Nakamura S, Michallek F, Kokawa T, Takafuji M, et al. Integrating myocardial CT perfusion with coronary CT angiography improves risk stratification in patients with dialysis-dependent end-stage renal disease. Jpn J Radiol. 2025;43(3):402–11.
24. Meng Z, Guo Y, Deng S, Xiang Q, Cao J, Zhang Y, et al. Improving image quality of triple-low-protocol renal artery CT angiography with deep-learning image reconstruction: a comparative study with standard-dose single-energy and dual-energy CT with adaptive statistical iterative reconstruction. Clin Radiol. 2024;79(5):e651–8.
25. Parrott D, Smereka P, Dane B. Dual-energy CT systems: technical aspects and selected clinical applications†. Br J Radiol. 2025;98:tqaf086.
26. Yuasa Y, Shiinoki T, Fujimoto K, Tanaka H. Pseudo dual-energy CT-derived iodine mapping using single-energy CT data based on a convolution neural network. BJR|Open. 2023;5(1):20220059.
27. Chandramohan D, Rajasekaran R, Konda R, et al. Cardiac magnetic resonance imaging findings in patients with chronic kidney disease and end-stage kidney disease: a systematic review and meta-analysis. Cureus. 2024;16(1):e51672. https://doi.org/10.7759/cureus.51672.
28. Nakata K, Joki N. Non-ischemic myocardial fibrosis in end-stage kidney disease patients: a new perspective. Kidney Dial. 2023;3(3):311–21.
29. Wang KC, Lin LC, Pan SY, Huang JW, Chang YC, Chiang JY, et al. Use of iodinated and gadolinium-based contrast media in patients with chronic kidney disease: Consensus statements from nephrologists, cardiologists, and radiologists at National Taiwan University Hospital. J Formos Med Assoc. 2025; Available from: https://www.sciencedirect.com/science/article/pii/S092966462500035X.
30. Wu M, Zhang JL. MR perfusion imaging for kidney disease. MR Perfus. 2024;32(1):161–70.

31. Fu J, Lin Z, Zhang B, Song L, Qin N, Qiu J, et al. Magnetic resonance imaging in atherosclerotic renal artery stenosis: the update and future directions from interventional perspective. Kidney Dis. 2023;10(1):23–31.
32. Liefke J, Steding-Ehrenborg K, Asgeirsson D, Nordlund D, Kopic S, Morsing E, et al. Non-contrast-enhanced magnetic resonance imaging can be used to assess renal cortical and medullary volumes—a validation study. Acta Radiol Open. 2022;11(1):20584601211072281.
33. Tournebize C, Schleef M, De Mul A, Pacaud S, Derain-Dubourg L, Juillard L, et al. Multiparametric MRI: can we assess renal function differently? Clin Kidney J. 2025;18(1):sfae365.
34. Vij A, Doukky R. The prognostic value of MPI in CKD: can we do better? J Nucl Cardiol. 2022;29(1):155–7.
35. Demir F, Demir M. Comparison of 99mTc-DMSA, 99mTc-DTPA and 99mTc-MAG3 renal scintigraphy in the calculation of relative renal function. J Urol Surg. 2020;7(2):130–3. https://doi.org/10.4274/jus.galenos.2019.3107.
36. Brown JM, Park MA, Kijewski MF, Weber BN, Yang Y, Martell L, et al. Feasibility of simultaneous quantification of myocardial and renal perfusion with cardiac positron emission tomography. Circ Cardiovasc Imaging. 2023;16(9):e015324.
37. Dilsizian V, Gewirtz H, Marwick TH, Kwong RY, Raggi P, Al-Mallah MH, et al. Cardiac imaging for coronary heart disease risk stratification in chronic kidney disease. JACC Cardiovasc Imaging. 2021;14(3):669–82.
38. Werner RA, Pomper MG, Buck AK, Rowe SP, Higuchi T. SPECT and PET radiotracers in renal imaging. Semin Nucl Med. 2022;52(4):406–18.
39. Rischpler C, Siebermair J, Kessler L, Quick HH, Umutlu L, Rassaf T, et al. Cardiac PET/MRI: current clinical status and future perspectives. Dev Card Imaging Part 1. 2020;50(3):260–9.
40. McDonagh TA, Metra M, Adamo M, Gardner RS, Baumbach A, Böhm M, et al. 2021 ESC Guidelines for the diagnosis and treatment of acute and chronic heart failure: developed by the task force for the diagnosis and treatment of acute and chronic heart failure of the European Society of Cardiology (ESC) with the special contribution of the Heart Failure Association (HFA) of the ESC. Eur Heart J. 2021;42(36):3599–726.
41. Stevens PE, Ahmed SB, Carrero JJ, Foster B, Francis A, Hall RK, et al. KDIGO 2024 Clinical Practice Guideline for the Evaluation and Management of Chronic Kidney Disease. Kidney Int. 2024;105(4):S117–314.
42. Marx N, Federici M, Schütt K, Müller-Wieland D, Ajjan RA, Antunes MJ, et al. 2023 ESC Guidelines for the management of cardiovascular disease in patients with diabetes: developed by the task force on the management of cardiovascular disease in patients with diabetes of the European Society of Cardiology (ESC). Eur Heart J. 2023;44(39):4043–140.
43. Virani SS, Newby LK, Arnold SV, Bittner V, Brewer LC, Demeter SH, et al. 2023 AHA/ACC/ACCP/ASPC/NLA/PCNA Guideline for the Management of Patients with chronic coronary disease: a report of the American Heart Association/American College of Cardiology Joint Committee on Clinical Practice Guidelines. Circulation. 2023;148(9):e9–119.
44. Taub CC, Stainback RF, Abraham T, Forsha D, Garcia-Sayan E, Hill JC, et al. Guidelines for the standardization of adult echocardiography reporting: recommendations from the American Society of Echocardiography. J Am Soc Echocardiogr. 2025;38(9):735–74.

Chapter 8
Arrhythmias in Patients with Kidney Failure

Simonetta Genovesi

8.1 Atrial Fibrillation in Patients with Kidney Failure

8.1.1 Epidemiology and Pathophysiology of Atrial Fibrillation in Patients with Kidney Failure

Atrial fibrillation (AF) is the most common arrhythmia in the general population. Regardless of severity, chronic kidney disease (CKD) is associated with an increased risk of prevalent and incident AF. The risk increases as CKD worsens [1]. The arrhythmia is particularly prevalent among CKD patients with kidney failure (KF), i.e., CKD in stage G5 or G5D who are undergoing kidney replacement therapy [2, 3]. The prevalence of AF is high in patients with CKD undergoing hemodialysis (HD). The reported prevalence ranges from 7% to 27% [4–6]. The prevalence of AF in patients with KF is likely to be underestimated. Some studies have demonstrated the presence of a significant number of asymptomatic AF episodes, which are often associated with HD sessions [7–9]. It is therefore possible that the diagnostic tools currently used in this population are not sufficiently effective in identifying all AF events.

The prevalence and incidence of AF in patients with CKD has increased over time. The same is true for patients with KF, as demonstrated by data from the United States Renal Data System (USRDS), which shows that the proportion of HD patients with AF increased from 3.5% in the 1990s to 10.7% in the 2000s [5]. The incidence of AF among patients initiating dialysis increased from 1995 to 2007, particularly

S. Genovesi (✉)
School of Medicine and Surgery, University of Milano-Bicocca, Milan, Italy

Istituto Auxologico Italiano, IRCCS, Milan, Italy
e-mail: simonetta.genovesi@unimib.it

A. Covic, A. Burlacu (eds.), *Renal Dysfunction in Cardiovascular Pathologies*,
https://doi.org/10.1007/978-3-032-25434-4_8

in older patients [10]. This data was confirmed by a study conducted in Taiwan among HD patients [11].

Many of the risk factors for AF that are prevalent in the general population are also common in patients with advanced CKD. These include advanced age, hypertension, diabetes mellitus, ischemic heart disease, and left atrial enlargement. Several other factors are more directly associated with CKD itself. The increased risk of developing AF in patients with an estimated glomerular filtration rate (eGFR) of less than 15 ml/min/1.73 m^2 is determined by the accumulation of uremic toxins, electrolyte imbalances, and neurohormonal dysregulation. These factors contribute to systemic and tissue oxidative stress, the activation of the renin–angiotensin–aldosterone system (RAAS) and inflammation [12], which are key mechanisms underlying the development of a pro-arrhythmic substrate. A series of humoral factors, which are pathologically increased in patients with KF, play a fundamental role in exerting a pro-fibrotic action on atrial myocardial tissue. These include angiotensin and TGF-beta [13], TNF-alfa [14] and interleukin 6 [15]. In addition, altered calcium/phosphorus metabolism leads to increased levels of FGF-23, a phosphaturic hormone associated with an increased risk of prevalent and incident AF in patients with CKD [16, 17].

Hemodialysis treatment poses an additional risk. It induces significant volume changes, electrolyte disturbances and pro-inflammatory states, which can cause or exacerbate arrhythmogenic risk acutely. Electrolyte shifts, especially fluctuations in serum potassium, are also implicated in AF risk. Several studies have demonstrated an increased incidence of AF episodes during the dialysis session and on days of dialysis treatment [7, 8]. It has also been demonstrated that electrolyte changes induced by HD sessions are linked to atrial electrophysiology, which could trigger AF episodes [8, 18]. Moreover, lower pre-dialysis serum potassium levels were associated with a higher risk of incident AF [19]. A study examining the impact of ultrafiltration (UF) on the incidence of new-onset AF demonstrated that higher UF rates were associated with a significantly higher risk of AF [20]. These results imply that hemodynamic instability and myocardial stress resulting from aggressive fluid removal could be significant contributors to the development of AF. This hypothesis is supported by observations that patients on peritoneal dialysis (PD) have a lower incidence of arrhythmias than patients undergoing HD, as intravascular volume and electrolyte fluctuations are smaller in PD patients [21]. A cohort study has also shown that improved dialysis adequacy is associated with a lower incidence of AF. This suggests that uremic toxins may increase the risk of AF in patients undergoing maintenance HD [22].

Atrial fibrillation is an indicator of poor prognosis in patients undergoing HD. It has been shown that in HD patients there is an association between AF and increased all-cause and cardiovascular mortality [23, 24]. Atrial fibrillation also increases the risk of ischemic stroke in patients with KF. A large retrospective study showed that patients with AF had a twofold higher thromboembolic risk than patients without AF [25]. Similar conclusions were reached by two other cohort studies, which reported a significantly higher risk of ischemic stroke and associated mortality in HD patients with AF [26, 27].

8.1.2 Prevention of Thromboembolic Risk in Patients with Atrial Fibrillation and Kidney Failure

The main problem for patients with AF is the risk of thromboembolic events. For this reason, cardiology guidelines recommend prescribing oral anticoagulant therapy (OAC) in all patients with documented AF and a thromboembolic score (CHA2DS2-VA score) ≥2. Direct anticoagulants (DOACs) should be preferred over vitamin K antagonists (VKAs) [28]. All randomized controlled trials (RCTs) that led to the recommendation of DOACs in guidelines excluded patients with an eGFR of less than 30 ml/min/1.73 m^2 (25 ml/min/1.73 m^2 for apixaban). For patients with eGFR <50 ml/min/1.73 m^2, a reduced DOAC dosage is recommended. Therefore, the real issue is how to manage patients with CKD stage G5-G5D. Both cardiology and nephrology guidelines are quite vague regarding this group of patients. VKAs, rivaroxaban and apixaban are accepted by the cardiology guidelines ("may be considered"), but are not explicitly recommended [29, 30]. The 2024 Kidney Disease Improving Global Outcomes (KDIGO) clinical practice guideline for the evaluation and management of CKD [31] advises against prescribing dabigatran and edoxaban to patients with an eGFR of less than 15 ml/min/1.73 m^2. It also accepts the use of warfarin (maintaining the international normalized ratio, INR, between 2 and 3) as well as apixaban or rivaroxaban at reduced doses. However, it emphasizes that there is no evidence to support the clinical efficacy of these drugs in this setting. Both cardiology and nephrology guidelines underline the importance of shared decision-making between a multidisciplinary medical team and the patient, taking into account the risks and benefits of therapy. The European Medicines Agency (EMA) advises against the use of all DOACs in patients with KF, while the US Food and Drug Administration (FDA) accepts apixaban, with the same dosage recommended for patients with normal renal function.

These uncertainties mean that only a minority of patients with both KF and AF receive medication to prevent thromboembolic risk [32]. For decades, the most widely used class of drugs for this purpose has been VKAs, but this practice is not supported by any RCT. Observational studies have failed to demonstrate the effectiveness of VKAs in reducing the incidence of ischemic stroke in patients with CKD stage G5-G5D, and there are numerous concerns about their safety. Numerous studies have shown an increased risk of bleeding, particularly intracranial bleeding [33, 34]. It is particularly difficult to maintain the INR within the therapeutic range in these patients, which exposes them to a high risk of bleeding [35, 36]. Furthermore, due to its antagonistic action against vitamin K, warfarin is associated with an increased risk of vascular calcification in both patients with normal renal function and in those with CKD [37, 38]. Finally, warfarin-related nephropathy remains a potential cause of acute kidney injury in patients taking VKAs [39]. It should be noted that a similar issue has also been reported for DOACs [40].

Four major CRTs have demonstrated that in cardiac patients with relatively preserved renal function (eGFR >30–25 ml/min/1.73 m^2), DOACs are at least as effective as VKAs and equally or more safe [41–44]. A patient-level meta-analysis using the COMBINE AF (A Collaboration Between Multiple Institutions to Better Investigate the Use of Non-Vitamin K Antagonist Oral Anticoagulants in Atrial Fibrillation) database suggests that DOACs are safer and more effective than warfarin down to an eGFR of at least 25 mL/min [45]. Unfortunately, the results are less encouraging for RCTs conducted in patients with KF. Four RCTs compared the efficacy and safety of DOACs and VKAs in HD patients [46–49]. Two of these trials were discontinued before the specified sample size was reached [47, 48]. Overall, the number of patients included in the four studies is too small to determine whether VKAs or DOACs are better for patients with KF and AF. Two meta-analyses that incorporated the four RCTs failed to demonstrate a superiority of either drug in terms of efficacy or safety [50, 51]. Other RCTs comparing DOACs with VKAs and with no OAC are currently underway (VISIONAIRE, NCT06402851; SACK, NCT05679024).

Evidence from observational studies comparing DOACs and VKAs in patients with KF and AF is inconsistent. Chan et al. reported an increased risk of major bleeding and mortality associated with two DOACs, dabigatran and rivaroxaban, compared with VKAs [52]. In contrast, Siontis et al. described a reduction in deaths without an increase in bleeding among dialysis patients taking apixaban compared to those taking warfarin [53]. It has been demonstrated that rivaroxaban exhibits a superior safety profile to warfarin in patients with AF and KF [54] and that, in a French patient cohort, DOAC off-label use was associated with a reduced thromboembolic risk despite a comparable bleeding risk to that observed with VKAs [55]. However, a recent meta-analysis, which included both RCTs and observational studies, concluded that the risk of ischemic stroke, bleeding and all-cause mortality was similar in HD patients with AF who were treated with DOACs or VKAs [56].

Data relating to the progression of kidney failure in patients taking DOACs compared to VKAs is more encouraging. A meta-analysis of 285,201 patients showed that DOAC treatment was associated with a lower risk of acute kidney injury and progression to kidney failure than warfarin treatment [57]. Data from the Xareno study confirms this finding [58].

However, the real problem with thromboembolic prophylaxis for patients with KF and AF is that it has yet to be demonstrated that prescribing OAC is more beneficial than not prescribing any therapy for this population. Two meta-analyses, which included a very large number of studies and patients, showed that OAC (both VKAs and DOACs) would not reduce thromboembolism, but would increase bleeding events [59, 60]. In a recent comprehensive analysis of 33 studies involving a total of 137,574 patients, Du et al. showed an equal incidence of stroke between OAC and no therapy. The risk of bleeding was increased with dabigatran and phenprocoumon compared to no therapy [61]. Two other studies [62, 63], too recent to be included in the cited meta-analyses, provided results conflicting with each other. Both are registry studies derived from the administrative databases of Korean HD patients with AF. The two populations had similar clinical characteristics, and the percentage of patients taking OAC was comparable and low in both studies (9.8% vs. 8.5%). Nevertheless, Kim et al. reported a significant reduction in ischemic strokes and mortality without an increase in bleeding in patients taking OAC compared to those not taking anticoagulants [62]. In contrast, Park et al. described an association between warfarin and an increased risk of thromboembolic events compared to no OAC therapy. Direct oral anticoagulants did not appear to be related to an increase or reduction in thromboembolic events compared with no therapy. Moreover, Warfarin and DOACs were both associated with a significant increase in mortality compared to no OAC therapy [63]. These data highlight the ongoing debate surrounding this topic.

The left atrial appendage (LAA) is the primary site for the generation of atrial thrombi in patients with AF [64]. Consequently, left atrial appendage closure (LAAC) has been suggested as an OAC for preventing thromboembolic events in patients with AF. A recent meta-analysis of all available RCTs comparing LAAC with OAC (both VKAs and DOACs) showed that LAAC was associated with significantly lower risk of all-cause and cardiovascular death, hemorrhagic stroke, and clinically relevant non-procedural bleeding, compared to OAC. Furthermore, LAAC was not associated with an increased risk of thromboembolic events or major bleeding [65]. However, the RCTs included in the meta-analysis compared groups of patients with no contraindications to taking anticoagulant drugs. This excluded precisely those patients who could benefit most from the procedure, including those with CKD. For this reason, cardiology guidelines only weakly recommend LAAC as an alternative to OAC in patients with AF and contraindications for long-term anticoagulant treatment to prevent ischemic stroke and thromboembolism (lass IIb, level C) [28]. Recently, an international consensus document emphasized the importance of specialists managing populations of AF patients at high risk of bleeding considering LAAC, including patients with KF [66].

Two RCTs that had the primary outcome of comparing the safety of LAAC to VKAs in patients with an eGFR of less than 30 ml/min/1.73 m^2 (stage CKD G4, G5 and G5D) were discontinued due to a lack of recruitment (Watch-AFIB, NCT02039167 and STOP-ARM, NCT02885545). A third trial with a composite outcome of first stroke, systemic embolism, cardiovascular or unexplained death, or major bleeding is currently ongoing (the LAA-Kidney study, NCT05204212). This trial only includes patients with stage G5-G5D CKD and compares LAAC with all other types of medical therapy.

Although RCTs are lacking, a series of observational studies performed on groups of patients with CKD and AF who underwent the procedure are available. A meta-analysis [67] included 12 studies comparing short-term outcomes associated with LAAC in patients with AF without KF showed a higher in-hospital mortality rate and peri-procedural complication rate in patients with KF. Another meta-analysis, which included 17 studies, confirmed the data relating to an increased risk of short-term complications in patients with CKD G5-G5D compared to patients without KF [68]. However, no significant difference in long-term stroke risk was found, although the incidence of major bleeding events was significantly higher in patients with KF.

Very few studies have compared the efficacy and safety of LAAC and OAC in dialysis patients. Two studies, both derived from a retrospective analysis of the USRDS, provided data favoring LAAC over OAC. The first study demonstrated a lower risk of bleeding and mortality in patients undergoing the procedure, with no advantage in terms of thromboembolic events [69]. The second study showed a lower incidence of the composite endpoint of thromboembolic events, bleeding events and mortality in patients treated with LAAC compared to those taking warfarin or apixaban [70]. Only one study prospectively compared the efficacy and safety of LAAC with both warfarin and no OAC, demonstrating a significant reduction in thromboembolism in the LAAC cohort compared to the other two cohorts. There was a significant reduction in bleeding in the LAAC group compared to patients taking warfarin. There was also a significant reduction in cardiovascular events and mortality in the LAAC group compared to the other two groups [71].

8.1.3 Catheter Ablation in Patients with Kidney Failure

Chronic kidney disease patients are significantly more likely to have AF recurrence after single catheter ablation (CA) therapy [72, 73]. It is unclear whether this is also true for patients with KF and AF undergoing CA, because the current evidence is sparse and consists mainly of heterogeneous observational studies with short follow-up periods. A meta-analysis was conducted on three studies and revealed that dialysis patients had a higher incidence of AF recurrence after CA compared to the control population [74], while another meta-analysis described a non-significant increase in AF recurrence in patients with KF compared to those without [73]. A recent Chinese study of a small group of HD patients suggested that the recurrence rate of AF was higher after a single ablation procedure than in the general population. However, multiple ablation procedures seemed to improve outcomes [75]. Catheter ablation is a potentially effective and safe treatment for AF in patients with heart disease. However, RCTs or even observational studies with suitable follow-up times to compare the efficacy of catheter ablation therapy with antiarrhythmic drugs and anticoagulation in this patient group are lacking.

8.2 Ventricular Arrhythmia and Sudden Cardiac Death in Patients with Kidney Failure

For many years, it has been known that dialysis sessions are an arrhythmogenic factor for patients with KF. The first studies on this topic date back to the late 1980s. These studies used Holter ECG recordings to show that the frequency of ventricular arrhythmias increased significantly during the third hour of HD, and that this effect lasted for several hours after dialysis [76]. However, after a 4-year follow-up, ventricular ectopias were not associated with increased mortality, while age and ischemic heart disease were found to correlate independently with lower survival [77].

Subsequent studies have better characterized the factors associated with the excess arrhythmic death observed in patients with KF.

8.2.1 Epidemiology and Pathophysiology of Sudden Cardiac Death in Patients with Kidney Failure

Sudden cardiac death (SCD) is a common cause of death among patients with kidney failure undergoing dialysis. According to the USRDS, approximately 45% of HD patients died from "arrhythmia/cardiac arrest" [2]. This definition is rather general and suggests that it encompasses patients with various clinical characteristics. In particular, no distinction is made between cardiac arrest due to asystole and ventricular fibrillation, or between events occurring during HD sessions and those occurring outside of sessions. Patients with KF undergoing kidney replacement therapy have a high prevalence of ischemic heart disease and heart failure, which are two factors strongly associated with SCD in the general population. This puts the KF population at risk of SCD beyond the specific risk factors associated with uremic disease. However, there are a number of specific SCD risk factors associated with KF, particularly in HD patients [78].

In patients undergoing HD, sudden cardiac arrest (SCA) may occur during the HD session. However, these patients may also experience SCD outside of the dialysis session. The relationship between HD session and SCD in patients undergoing kidney replacement therapy is complex. Intra-dialytic SCA is a rare event with a poor prognosis. There are fewer than 10 events per 100,000 treatments [79, 80], and only 50% of patients survive resuscitation attempts [80, 81]. Studies disagree on which rhythm is responsible for the final event. Davis et al. report that the majority of cases (approximately 70%) involve ventricular tachyarrhythmias and the minority (approximately 30%) involve bradyarrhythmias. Conversely, Pun et al. [82] report a higher prevalence of non-defibrillable rhythms (almost 70%). Although the underlying rhythm of intra-dialytic SCA is not always shock-treatable, patients resuscitated by medical staff within the dialysis unit have a three times higher survival rate than those resuscitated by emergency medical services [82].

The relationship between electrolyte concentration in the dialysis bath and SCA is significant. Indeed, an association has been described between intra-dialytic SCA and HD bath composition. A doubling of the risk of intradialytic SCA has been observed with potassium concentrations in the dialysate of less than 2 mmol/L [79], and a significant increase in SCA incidence has been reported for dialysis patients with low concentrations of ionized calcium in the dialysis bath (i.e., 1.25 mmol/L) [83]. Regarding the timing of SCA, the event appears to be more frequent during the first HD session of the week. Contrary to what might be expected, no association has been described between traditional cardiovascular risk factors, such as coronary artery disease or heart failure with reduced ejection fraction, and intra-dialytic SCA [79, 80].

Hemodialysis sessions are associated with changes in myocardial repolarization, as represented by the QT interval on an electrocardiogram. These changes are related to the concentration of some electrolytes in the dialysis solution, particularly potassium and ionized calcium. Another factor affecting ventricular repolarization is the gradient between the serum concentrations of the two electrolytes at the start and end of the HD session. The potassium concentration in the dialysis bath can vary, typically ranging from 2 to 4 mmol/L. A low concentration of potassium in the dialysate is more readily associated with a higher pre- and post-dialysis serum electrolyte gradient, particularly in patients who arrive at their dialysis session with hyperkalemia. A similar argument can be made for calcium, the concentration of which in dialysate varies from 1.25 to 1.75 mmol/L. An inverse correlation has been described between the change in serum potassium and ionized calcium levels from the start to the end of the HD session, and prolongation of the QT interval [84, 85]. The greater the gradient, the greater the prolongation of repolarization time, a phenomenon which is particularly evident when dialysis baths with low concentrations of both potassium (e.g., 2 mmol/L) and ionized calcium (e.g., 1.25 mmol/L) are used.

Pathological prolongation of ventricular repolarization can trigger potentially fatal tachyarrhythmias, which can occur during and outside dialysis sessions. Ter Meulen et al. compared the incidence of SCD in dialysis patients with a concentration of 1.25 mmol/L of ionized calcium to that in patients with a concentration of 1.50 mmol/L. They demonstrated an excess of SCD when the calcium concentration was lower (HR 0.81, 95% CI 0.67–0.97) [86].

Data from the Dialysis Outcomes and Practice Patterns Study registry showed that, in a large population of hemodialysis patients, the risk of SCD was 40% higher (Hazard ratio, HR 1.39, 95% confidence interval, CI 1.12–1.74) when a dialysis bath with potassium concentrations of less than 1.5 mmol/L was used compared to concentrations of 3 mmol/L. Furthermore, the risk of SCD increased by around 20% for every 1 mmol/L reduction in potassium in the dialysate [87].

The concentration of bicarbonate in the dialysis bath can also affect the duration of the QT interval. The transition from an acidic to a more alkaline plasma pH, which occurs during HD, induces a shift of potassium ions from the extracellular to the intracellular compartment. If acidosis is corrected too quickly, serum potassium levels may drop, causing hypokalemia [88]. Therefore, the use of high concentrations of bicarbonate in the dialysate is not recommended, particularly if low concentrations of potassium and ionized calcium are maintained [89]. Particular attention should be paid to patients with a prolonged baseline QT interval, a condition not uncommon in patients with KF [90, 91]. As with the general population, the presence of long QT syndrome is associated with an increased risk of total and sudden mortality in patients undergoing HD [91, 92]. Several drugs used to treat various conditions can cause the QT interval to lengthen, which can lead to life-threatening arrhythmias. This has also been observed in HD patients. These drugs include certain antiemetics (e.g., ondansetron), antibiotics (e.g., quinolones) and antidepressants (e.g., selective serotonin reuptake inhibitors) [93–95]. Therefore, careful electrocardiographic monitoring should be performed in patients with KF who are taking these classes of drugs.

When talking about SCD, magnesium is an electrolyte that is often overlooked. A Japanese study of almost 150,000 HD patients revealed a J-shaped curve relating to magnesium concentrations and cardiovascular and all-cause mortality [96]. Furthermore, an inverse association was observed between magnesium concentrations and all-cause mortality, cardiovascular mortality and SCD in a population of European HD patients [97].

The volume of fluid removed from patients during HD may also be a risk factor for SCD. An ultrafiltration volume of more than 5.7% of body weight has been found to increase the risk of SCD by 13% (HR 1.13; 95% CI 1.00–1.27) [87]. Pun et al. demonstrated a significant association between intra-dialysis SCA and increased ultrafiltration volumes [79].

Although most SCDs occur outside dialysis hours, a link has been described between the timing of HD sessions and when SCDs occur. In fact, two peaks in the incidence of SCDs have been identified in dialysis patients: the first occurs immediately after the first HD session of the week (i.e., during the initial short interdialytic interval), and the second occurs immediately before the first session of the week (i.e., at the end of the extended interdialytic interval) [98, 99]. Furthermore, it has been demonstrated that patients arriving at dialysis with high potassium levels have a higher incidence of SCD [100]. While it is known that the majority of SCDs in the general population are due to ventricular tachyarrhythmias, this does not seem to be the case with regard to sudden mortality in HD patients. Indeed, although data derived from Implantable Cardioverter Defibrillator (ICD) interrogation in patients with KF who have the device suggests that ventricular fibrillation is the arrhythmia responsible for death [101], more recent evidence obtained from loop recorder recordings seems to indicate that brady-arrhythmic phenomena may be the main cause of SCD in dialysis patients [102–104]. Most brady-arrhythmias occur during the long interdialytic interval [103]. This data suggests that the pathogenesis of SCD in patients with KF may differ somewhat from that in the general population. The fatal arrhythmias that lead to SCD in patients with KF are likely to be non-uniform, depending partly on the presence of underlying heart disease; however, in other cases, they may be due to electrolyte imbalances that lead to life-threatening arrhythmias. The interdialytic interval is often characterized by severe hyperkalemia, which may be due to the brady-arrhythmias recorded at that time. Conversely, severe pre-dialysis hyperkalemia often prompts the nephrologist to use a dialysis bath with a low potassium concentration to correct the electrolyte imbalance quickly. However, too rapid a correction may lead to electrical instability of the myocardium and possibly trigger lethal ventricular tachyarrhythmias immediately following the session [85]. A recently published study seems to support these hypotheses. In HD patients for whom continuous arrhythmia monitoring was possible using a loop recorder, a dialysate potassium concentration of 3 mmol/L, combined with potassium binding to prevent hyperkemia, was associated with a lower incidence of clinically significant arrhythmias (such as ventricular tachycardia, bradycardia, and asystole) than dialysis baths with a potassium concentration of 2 mmol/L [105]. In light of this evidence, we can hypothesize that eliminating the long interdialytic interval could reduce the risk of SCD in HD patients. However, to date, there are no solid data to support this hypothesis.

Beyond electrolyte imbalances, cardiovascular comorbidities, highly prevalent in CKD patients undergoing HD, particularly heart failure with reduced ejection fraction and coronary artery disease, contribute to an increased SCD incidence [78]. Moreover, some evidence showed an association between AF and increased SCD in patients with KF [101], a finding that is also evident in the general population [106, 107]. Finally, the presence of inflammation/malnutrition syndrome has been suggested as a contributor to the excess of SCD in the KF population [108].

Compared with HD, peritoneal dialysis (PD) is associated with a lower incidence of electrolyte imbalances and should ensure greater hemodynamic stability [109]. However, large registries report a high prevalence of SCD in patients undergoing PD [2], which is not significantly different from that found in HD patients. In PD patients, it is likely that cardiac comorbidities are an important risk factor for SCD. This is suggested by a study that showed a significant association between higher plasma pro-BNP and troponin levels and SCD in a PD population [110]. This observation is supported by a study comparing the incidence of SCD in HD and PD patients. The study demonstrated that there was no significant difference and that factors associated with SCD in peritoneal dialysis patients included reduced left ventricular ejection fraction, previous stroke and ischemic heart disease [111]. These results suggest that the high incidence of SCD in PD patients is primarily due to the high prevalence of heart disease, meaning that the causes of SCD may differ between the two dialysis modalities.

In vitro models of cardiomyocytes have demonstrated that uremic toxins can alter certain ion channels. These toxins reduce IKr, IK and L-type calcium currents in myocardial cells, resulting in altered ventricular repolarization. In vivo animal models with advanced renal failure have demonstrated that uremic toxins can slow conduction velocity and prolong action potential and ventricular repolarization times. Ventricular tachyarrhythmias and SCD have also been observed in animal models in which uremia was induced [112]. These experimental observations suggest that advanced renal failure is a condition with arrhythmogenic potential, putting patients at risk to life.

8.2.2 Role of Cardiac Devices in the Prevention of Sudden Cardiac Death in Patients with Kidney Failure

For patients with an ICD due to a cardiologic indication, the presence of advanced kidney disease is a significant predictor of mortality [113]. A meta-analysis combining data from the MADIT-I, MADIT-II and SCD-HFT studies showed that patients with preserved renal function had improved survival, whereas those with an eGFR of less than 60 ml/min/1.73 m^2 had less improvement [114]. This finding has been confirmed by other observational studies [115–117].

This result is particularly evident among HD patients. In a population of patients with ICDs in primary prevention, the risk of death was 5 times higher (HR 4.80, 95% CI 4.46–5.17) [116]. These data have also been confirmed in a series of other studies [118, 119]. This raises the question of whether the indications in the cardiology guidelines regarding the use of ICDs for the prevention of SCD can be transferred to and applied to patients with KF.

One thing we can expect is that patients with severe CKD will have a higher mortality rate than those without it. However, the real question is whether ICD implantation can lead to an improvement in total and sudden mortality within populations with KF. Several studies comparing HD patients with an indication for ICD implantation for primary or secondary prevention of SCD, who have or have not received the device, are available. Unfortunately, there are no randomized studies on this topic. The only RCT available compared the usefulness of ICD implantation for SCD prevention in two groups of HD patients, neither of which had a cardiologic indication for device implantation. Therefore, this study has special features and will be discussed separately [120].

Some studies recruiting HD patients for whom primary prevention ICD implantation was indicated failed to demonstrate improved survival in patients who received the device compared to those who did not [121, 122]. However, there is also evidence of the benefits of an ICD for the primary prevention of SCD in patients with KF [123].

More encouraging and consistent data exist for patients with KF who underwent ICD implantation for secondary prevention. In a large population of patients who had undergone resuscitation following cardiac arrest, receiving an ICD was associated with improved survival. However, it should be noted that fewer than 10% of patients had undergone implantation, clearly demonstrating how rarely cardiological indications are considered in this population [124]. A recent Japanese study has confirmed the underuse of ICDs in secondary prevention in HD patients. The study showed that, of a large population of cardiac arrest survivors, 27% of HD patients received ICDs, which is a significantly lower percentage than that of non-HD patients (44%) [125]. These data should give us pause for thought, especially in light of the reported findings by Charytan et al., who demonstrated that patients with AF who had received an ICD for secondary prevention were at significantly lower risk of mortality than a population with similar clinical characteristics who had not had the device implanted [126]. These findings were confirmed by a more recent retrospective study using data from the USRDS registry, which demonstrated that ICD implantation doubled 2-year survival in patients who had survived resuscitated cardiac arrest (53% vs 27%, HR 0.54; 95% CI 0.53–0.54), compared to patients who had not received the device [127].

The incidence of SCD has been reported to be high in patients with KF and a cardiological indication for device implantation. However, it is also high in patients without an indication for implantation [128]. Therefore, it appears that the presence of KF itself constitutes a risk factor for SCD. This assumption formed the basis of the only RCT designed and performed on HD patients, which aimed to assess whether primary prevention ICD implantation could protect this population from the onset of SCD [120]. The study excluded patients with a cardiological indication for ICD implantation and therefore included only patients with a left ventricular ejection fraction ≥35%. It did not demonstrate a difference in the cumulative incidence of SCD after 5 years between patients who had received an ICD and those who had not (HR 1.32, 95% CI 0.53–3.29). Five-year mortality was also similar in the two groups (HR 1.02, 95% CI 0.69–1.52; $P = 0.92$). Patients who underwent implantation experienced a higher incidence of device-related adverse events, including inappropriate shocks, subclavian vein stenosis and explantation due to bacteremia.

8.2.3 Role of Drug Therapy in the Prevention of Sudden Cardiac Death in Patients with Kidney Failure

To date, no data have demonstrated a reduction in the risk of SCD in dialysis patients taking a renin-angiotensin-aldosterone system inhibitor. The same applies to the combination of sartans and neprolisin. All of these drugs should be used with caution in patients with KF, as they can cause an increase in serum potassium levels. Indeed, studies have shown that hyperkalemia, particularly pre-dialysis hyperkalemia, is associated with increased all-cause and sudden mortality in this population [99, 100].

The evidence regarding beta-blockers appears to be more robust. Although their use was not associated with a reduction in the incidence of SCD in the total population examined, data from the HEMO study show that beta-blockers were nevertheless associated with a greater protective effect in patients with coronary artery disease than in those without (HR, 0.65; 95% CI 0.42–1.01 vs. HR, 1.61; 95% CI 0.92–2.80; interaction $P = 0.03$) [129]. The protective effect of beta-blockers on the risk of SCD has been demonstrated in HD patients [130]. In particular, data from the DOPPS registry in a large HD population show a 12% reduction in the risk of SCD (HR, 0.88; 95% CI, 0.78–0.99) for patients taking beta-blockers compared to those not taking them [87]. Furthermore, it appears that this class of drugs can reduce short- and medium-term mortality after intradialytic SCA [131].

Declarations

Competing Interests The author(s) has no competing interests to declare that are relevant to the content of this manuscript.

Ethics Approval The author(s) declares that this manuscript does not include primary research with human participants.

The author(s) declares that this manuscript does not include primary studies involving animals.

References

1. Kim S, Jeong Y, Kim YL, Kang M, Kang E, Ryu H, et al. Association of chronic kidney disease with atrial fibrillation in the general adult population: a Nationwide Population-Based Study. J Am Heart Assoc. 2023;12:e028496. https://doi.org/10.1161/JAHA.122.028496.
2. Johansen KL, Chertow GM, Foley RN, Gilbertson DT, Herzog CA, Ishani A, et al. US Renal Data System 2020 Annual Data Report: epidemiology of kidney disease in the United States. Am J Kidney Dis. 2021;77(4):Svii–Sviii, S1–S597.
3. Genovesi S, Camm AJ, Covic A, Bulracu A, Meijers B, Franssen C, et al. Treatment strategies of the thromboembolic risk in kidney failure patients with atrial fibrillation. Nephrol Dial Transplant. 2024;39(8):1248–57. https://doi.org/10.1093/ndt/gfae121.
4. Genovesi S, Pogliani D, Faini A, Valsecchi MG, Riva A, Stefani F, et al. Prevalence of atrial fibrillation and associated factors in a population of long-term hemodialysis patients. Am J Kidney Dis. 2005;46:897–902. https://doi.org/10.1053/j.ajkd.2005.07.044.
5. Winkelmayer WC, Patrick AR, Liu J, Brookhart MA, Setoguchi S. The increasing prevalence of atrial fibrillation among hemodialysis patients. J Am Soc Nephrol. 2011;22(2):349–57. https://doi.org/10.1681/ASN.2010050459.
6. Zimmerman D, Sood MM, Rigatto C, Holden RM, Hiremath S, Clase CM. Systematic review and meta-analysis of the incidence, prevalence and outcomes of atrial fibrillation in patients on dialysis. Nephrol Dial Transplant. 2012;27(10):3816–22. https://doi.org/10.1093/ndt/gfs416.
7. Buiten MS, de Bie MK, Rotmans JI, Gabreëls BA, van Dorp W, Wolterbeek R, et al. The dialysis procedure as a trigger for atrial fibrillation: new insights into the development of atrial fibrillation in dialysis patients. Heart. 2014;100(9):685–90. https://doi.org/10.1136/heartjnl-2013-305417.
8. Vincenti A, Passini E, Fabbrini P, Luise MC, Severi S, Genovesi S. Recurrent intradialytic paroxysmal atrial fibrillation: hypotheses on onset mechanisms based on clinical data and computational analysis. Europace. 2014;16(3):396–404. https://doi.org/10.1093/europace/eut346.
9. Koplan BA, Winkelmayer WC, Costea AI, Roy-Chaudhury P, Tumlin JA, Kher V, et al. Implantable loop recorder monitoring and the incidence of previously unrecognised atrial fibrillation in patients on haemodialysis. Kidney Int Rep. 2021;7(2):189–99. https://doi.org/10.1016/j.ekir.2021.10.001.
10. Goldstein BA, Arce CM, Hlatky MA, Turakhia M, Setoguchi S, Winkelmayer WC. Trends in the incidence of atrial fibrillation in older patients initiating dialysis in the United States. Circulation. 2012;126(19):2293–301. https://doi.org/10.1161/CIRCULATIONAHA.112.099606.
11. Hung TW, Huang JY, Jong GP. Long-term outcomes of dialysis in patients with chronic kidney disease and new-onset atrial fibrillation: a population-based cohort study. PLoS One. 2019;14(9):e0222656. https://doi.org/10.1371/journal.pone.0222656.
12. Hatamizadeh P, Fonarow GC, Budoff MJ, Darabian S, Kovesdy CP, Kalantar-Zadeh K. Cardiorenal syndrome: pathophysiology and potential targets for clinical management. Nat Rev Nephrol. 2013;9:99–111. https://doi.org/10.1038/nrneph.2012.279.
13. Liu Y, Lv H, Tan R, An X, Niu XH, Liu YJ, et al. Platelets promote Ang II (angiotensin II)-induced atrial fibrillation by releasing TGF-beta1 (transforming growth factor-beta1) and interacting with fibroblasts. Hypertension. 2020;76(6):1856–67. https://doi.org/10.1161/HYPERTENSIONAHA.120.15016.
14. Liew R, Khairunnisa K, Gu Y, Tee N, Yin O, Naylynn TM, Moe KT. Role of tumor necrosis factor-alpha in the pathogenesis of atrial fibrosis and development of an arrhythmogenic substrate. Circ J. 2013;77(5):1171–9. https://doi.org/10.1253/circj.cj-12-1155.
15. Sano M, Fukuda K, Kodama H, Pan J, Saito M, Matsuzaki J, et al. Interleukin-6 family of cytokines mediate angiotensin II-induced cardiac hypertrophy in rodent cardiomyocytes. J Biol Chem. 2000;275(38):29717–23. https://doi.org/10.1074/jbc.M003128200.

16. Mehta R, Cai X, Lee J, Scialla JJ, Bansal N, Sondheimer JH, et al. Chronic renal insufficiency cohort study, association of fibroblast growth factor 23 with atrial fibrillation in chronic kidney disease, from the chronic renal insufficiency cohort study. JAMA Cardiol. 2016;1(5):548–56. https://doi.org/10.1001/jamacardio.2016.1445.
17. Mathew JS, Sachs MC, Katz R, Patton KK, Heckbert SR, Hoofnagle AN, Alonso A, Chonchol M, Deo R, Ix JH, Siscovick DS, Kestenbaum B, de Boer IH. Fibroblast growth factor-23 and incident atrial fibrillation: the multi-ethnic study of atherosclerosis (MESA) and the cardiovascular health study (CHS). Circulation. 2014;130(4):298–307. https://doi.org/10.1161/CIRCULATIONAHA.113.005499.
18. Severi S, Pogliani D, Fantini G, Fabbrini P, Viganò MR, Galbiati E, et al. Alterations of atrial electrophysiology induced by electrolyte variations: combined computational and P-wave analysis. Europace. 2010;12(6):842–9. https://doi.org/10.1093/europace/euq042.
19. Hu A, Liu S, Montez–Rath ME, Khairallah P, Niu J, Turakhia MP, et al. Associations of serum and dialysate potassium concentrations with incident atrial fibrillation in a cohort study of older US persons initiating hemodialysis for kidney failure. Kidney Int Rep. 2022;8(2):305–16. https://doi.org/10.1016/j.ekir.2022.11.003.
20. Flythe JE, Liu S, Montez-Rath ME, Winkelmayer WC, Tara I, Chang TI. Ultrafiltration rate and atrial fibrillation risk among older patients receiving hemodialysis. Nephrol Dial Transplant. 2021;36(11):2084–93. https://doi.org/10.1093/ndt/gfaa332.
21. Niu J, Shah MK, Perez JJ, Airy M, Navaneethan SD, Turakhia MP, et al. Dialysis modality and incident atrial fibrillation in older patients with ESRD. Am J Kidney Dis. 2019;73(3):324–31. https://doi.org/10.1053/j.ajkd.2018.09.011.
22. Heo GY, Park JT, Kim HJ, Kim KW, Kwon YU, Kim SH, et al. Adequacy of dialysis and incidence of atrial fibrillation in patients undergoing hemodialysis. Circ Cardiovasc Qual Outcomes. 2024;17(8):e010595. https://doi.org/10.1161/CIRCOUTCOMES.123.010595.
23. Genovesi S, Vincenti A, Rossi E, Pogliani D, Acquistapace I, Stella A, et al. Atrial fibrillation and morbidity and mortality in a cohort of long-term hemodialysis patients. Am J Kidney Dis. 2008;51(2):255–62. https://doi.org/10.1053/j.ajkd.2007.10.034.
24. Hsieh HL, Hsu SC, Cheng HS, et al. The influence of atrial fibrillation on the mortality of incident ESRD patients undergoing maintenance hemodialysis. PLoS One. 2020;15(1):e0228405. https://doi.org/10.1371/journal.pone.0228405.
25. Kimura A, Tanaka M, Moniwa M, Osanami A, Abe K, Myamori D, et al. Atrial fibrillation as a risk factor for ischemic stroke in dialysis patients: results from a Japanese multicenter registry. Clin Exp Nephrol. 2021;25(3):297–304. https://doi.org/10.1007/s10157-020-01991-9.
26. Joki N, Toida T, Nakata K, Abe M, Hanafusa N, Kurita N. Effect of atherosclerosis on the relationship between atrial fibrillation and ischemic stroke incidence among patients on hemodialysis. Sci Rep. 2024;14(1):1330. https://doi.org/10.1038/s41598-024-51439-3.
27. Findlay M, MacIsaac R, MacLeod MJ, Metcalfe W, Sood MM, Traynor JP, et al. The Association of Atrial Fibrillation and Ischemic Stroke in patients on hemodialysis: a competing risk analysis. Can J Kidney Health Dis. 2019;27(6):2054358119878719. https://doi.org/10.1177/2054358119878719.
28. Van Gelder IC, Rienstra M, Bunting KV, Casado-Arroyo R, Caso V, Crijns HJGM, et al. 2024 ESC guidelines for the management of atrial fibrillation developed in collaboration with the European Association for Cardio-Thoracic Surgery (EACTS). Eur Heart J. 2024;45(36):3314–414. https://doi.org/10.1093/eurheartj/ehae176.
29. Joglar JA, Chung MK, Armbruster AL, Benjamin EJ, Chyou JY, Cronin EM, et al. 2023 ACC/AHA/ACCP/HRS guideline for the diagnosis and management of atrial fibrillation: a report of the American College of Cardiology/American Heart Association Joint Committee on Clinical Practice Guidelines. Circulation. 2024;149(1):e1–e156. https://doi.org/10.1161/CIR.0000000000001193.
30. Hindricks G, Potpara T, Dagres N, Arbelo E, Bax JJ, Blomstrom-Lundqvist C, et al. 2020 ESC guidelines for the diagnosis and management of atrial fibrillation developed in collaboration with the European Association for Cardio-Thoracic Surgery (EACTS): the task force

for the diagnosis and management of atrial fibrillation of the European Society of Cardiology (ESC) developed with the special contribution of the European Heart Rhythm Association (EHRA) of the ESC. Eur Heart J. 2021;42(5):373–498. https://doi.org/10.1093/eurheartj/ehaa612.
31. Kidney Disease: Improving Global Outcomes (KDIGO) CKD Work Group. KDIGO 2024 Clinical Practice Guideline for the Evaluation and Management of Chronic Kidney Disease. Kidney Int. 2024 Apr;105(4S):S117–314. https://doi.org/10.1016/j.kint.2023.10.018.
32. Hu A, Niu J, Winkelmayer WC. Oral anticoagulation in patients with end-stage kidney disease on dialysis and atrial fibrillation. Semin Nephrol. 2018;38(6):618–28. https://doi.org/10.1016/j.semnephrol.2018.08.006.
33. Dahal K, Kunwar S, Rijal J, Schulman P, Lee J. Stroke. Major bleeding and mortality outcomes in warfarin users with atrial fibrillation and chronic kidney disease: a meta-analysis of observational studies. Chest. 2016;149(4):951–9. https://doi.org/10.1378/chest.15-1719.
34. Randhawa MS, Vishwanath R, Rai MP, Wang L, Randhawa AK, Abela G, et al. Association between use of warfarin for atrial fibrillation and outcomes among patients with end-stage renal disease: a systematic review and meta-analysis. JAMA Netw Open. 2020;3(4):e202175. https://doi.org/10.1001/jamanetworkopen.2020.2175.
35. Szummer K, Gasparini A, Eliasson S, Ärnlöv J, Qureshi AR, Bárány P, et al. Time in therapeutic range and outcomes after warfarin initiation in newly diagnosed atrial fibrillation patients with renal dysfunction. J Am Heart Assoc. 2017;6(3):e004925. https://doi.org/10.1161/JAHA.116.004925.
36. Rebora P, Moia M, Carpenedo M, Valsecchi MG, Genovesi S. Best quality indicator of vitamin K antagonist therapy to predict mortality and bleeding in haemodialysis patients with atrial fibrillation. Blood Transfus. 2021;19(6):487–94. https://doi.org/10.2450/2020.0217-20.
37. Schurgers LJ. Vitamin K: key vitamin in controlling vascular calcification in chronic kidney disease. Kidney Int. 2013;83(5):782–4. https://doi.org/10.1038/ki.2013.26.
38. Weijs B, Blaauw Y, Rennenberg RJMW, Schurgers LJ, Timmermans CCMM, Pison L, et al. Patients using vitamin K antagonists show increased levels of coronary calcification: an observational study in low-risk atrial fibrillation patients. Eur Heart J. 2011;32(20):2555–62. https://doi.org/10.1093/eurheartj/ehr226.
39. Brodsky SV, Nadasdy T, Rovin BH, Satoskar AA, Nadasdy GM, Wu M, et al. Warfarin-related nephropathy occurs in patients with and without chronic kidney disease and is associated with an increased mortality rate. Kidney Int. 2011;80(2):181–9. https://doi.org/10.1038/ki.2011.44.
40. Zakrocka I, Załuska W. Anticoagulant-related nephropathy: focus on novel agents. A review. Adv Clin Exp Med. 2022;31(2):165–73. https://doi.org/10.17219/acem/142657.
41. Connolly SJ, Ezekowitz MD, Yusuf S, Eikelboom J, Oldgren J, Parekh A, et al. Dabigatran versus warfarin in patients with atrial fibrillation. N Engl J Med. 2009;361(12):1139–51. https://doi.org/10.1056/NEJMoa0905561.
42. Patel MR, Mahaffey KW, Garg J, Pan G, Singer DE, Hacke W, et al. Rivaroxaban versus warfarin in nonvalvular atrial fibrillation. N Engl J Med. 2011;365(10):883–91. https://doi.org/10.1056/NEJMoa1009638.
43. Granger CB, Alexander JH, McMurray JJV, Lopes RD, Hylek EM, Hanna M, et al. Apixaban versus warfarin in patients with atrial fibrillation. N Engl J Med. 2011;365(11):981–92. https://doi.org/10.1056/NEJMoa1107039.
44. Giugliano RP, Ruff CT, Braunwald E, Murphy SA, Stephen D, Wiviott SD, Halperin JL, et al. Edoxaban versus warfarin in patients with atrial fibrillation. N Engl J Med. 2013;369(22):2093–104. https://doi.org/10.1056/NEJMoa1310907.
45. Harrington J, Carnicelli AP, Hua K, Wallentin L, Patel MR, Hohnloser SH, et al. Direct oral anticoagulants versus warfarin across the spectrum of kidney function: patient-level network meta-analyses from COMBINE AF. Circulation. 2023;147(23):1748–57. https://doi.org/10.1161/CIRCULATIONAHA.122.062752.

46. De Vriese AS, Caluwé R, Van Der Meersch H, De Boeck K, De Bacquer D. Safety and efficacy of vitamin K antagonists versus rivaroxaban in hemodialysis patients with atrial fibrillation: a multicenter randomized controlled trial. J Am Soc Nephrol. 2021;32(6):1474–83. https://doi.org/10.1681/ASN.2020111566.
47. Pokorney SD, Chertow GM, Al-Khalidi HR, Gallup D, Dignacco P, Mussina K, et al. RENAL-AF Investigators. Apixaban for patients with atrial fibrillation on hemodialysis: a multicenter randomized controlled trial. Circulation. 2022;146(23):1735–45. https://doi.org/10.1161/CIRCULATIONAHA.121.054990.
48. Reinecke H, Engelbertz C, Bauersachs R, Breithardt G, Echterhoff HH, Gerß J, et al. A randomized controlled trial comparing apixaban with the vitamin k antagonist phenprocoumon in patients on chronic hemodialysis: the AXADIA-AFNET 8 study. Circulation. 2023;147(4):296–309. https://doi.org/10.1161/CIRCULATIONAHA.122.062779.
49. Harel Z, Smyth B, Badve SV, Blum D, Beaubien-Souligny W, Silver SA, et al. Anticoagulation for patients with atrial fibrillation receiving dialysis a pilot randomized controlled trial. Am Soc Nephrol. 2025;36(5):901–10. https://doi.org/10.1681/ASN.0000000000000495.
50. Faisaluddin M, Alwifati N, Naeem N, Balasubramanian S, Narasimhan B, Iqbal U, et al. Safety and efficacy of direct oral anticoagulants versus warfarin for atrial fibrillation in end-stage renal disease on hemodialysis: a meta-analysis of randomized control trials. Am J Cardiol. 2023;206:309–11. https://doi.org/10.1016/j.amjcard.2023.08.116.
51. de Lucena LA, Freitas MAA, Souza AKC, Silva CHA, Watanabe JMF, Guedes FL, et al. Direct oral anticoagulants versus vitamin K antagonists in patients with atrial fibrillation and stage 5 chronic kidney disease under dialysis: a systematic review and meta-analysis of randomized controlled trials. J Thromb Thrombolysis. 2024;57(3):381–9. https://doi.org/10.1007/s11239-023-02945-0.
52. Chan KE, Edelman ER, Wenger JB, Thadhani RI, Maddux FW. Dabigatran and rivaroxaban use in atrial fibrillation patients on hemodialysis. Circulation. 2015;131(11):972–9. https://doi.org/10.1161/CIRCULATIONAHA.114.014113.
53. Siontis KC, Zhang X, Eckard A, Bhave N, Schaubel DE, He K, et al. Outcomes associated with apixaban use in patients with end-stage kidney disease and atrial fibrillation in the United States. Circulation. 2018;138(15):1519–29. https://doi.org/10.1161/CIRCULATIONAHA.118.035418.
54. Coleman CI, Kreutz R, Sood NA, Bunz TJ, Eriksson D, Meinecke AK, et al. Rivaroxaban versus warfarin in patients with nonvalvular atrial fibrillation and severe kidney disease or undergoing hemodialysis. Am J Med. 2019 Sep;132(9):1078–83. https://doi.org/10.1016/j.amjmed.2019.04.013.
55. Laville SM, Couchoud C, Bauwens M, Coponat HV, Choukroun G, Liabeuf S, REIN Collaborators. Effectiveness and safety of direct oral anticoagulants versus vitamin K antagonists in patients on chronic dialysis: a nationwide registry study. Nephrol Dial Transplant. 2024;39(10):1662–71. https://doi.org/10.1093/ndt/gfae042.
56. Kyriakoulis I, Adamou A, Stamatiou I, Chlorogiannis DD, Kardoutso I, Koukousaki D, et al. Efficacy and safety of direct oral anticoagulants vs vitamin K antagonists in patients with atrial fibrillation and end-stage renal disease on hemodialysis: a systematic review and meta-analysis. Eur J Intern Med. 2024;119:45–52. https://doi.org/10.1016/j.ejim.2023.08.020.
57. Sitticharoenchai P, Takkavatakarn K, Boonyaratavej S, Praditpornsilpa K, Eiam-Ong S, Susantitaphong P. Non-vitamin K antagonist oral anticoagulants provide less adverse renal outcomes than warfarin in non-valvular atrial fibrillation: a systematic review and metaanalysis. J Am Heart Assoc. 2021;10(7):e019609. https://doi.org/10.1161/JAHA.120.019609.
58. Kreutz R, Deray G, Floege J, Gwechenberger M, Hahn K, Luft AR, et al. XARENO registry rivaroxaban vs vitamin K antagonist in patients with atrial fibrillation and advanced chronic kidney disease anticoagulation in atrial fibrillation and CKD. JACC Adv. 2024;3(2):100813. https://doi.org/10.1016/j.jacadv.2023.100813.

59. Kuno T, Takagi H, Ando T, Sugiyama T, Miyashita S, Valentin N, et al. Oral anticoagulation for patients with atrial fibrillation on long-term hemodialysis. J Am Coll Cardiol. 2020;75(3):273–85. https://doi.org/10.1016/j.jacc.2019.10.059.
60. Kao TW, Chen ZW, Lin YH, Yen-Hung. Anticoagulation for patients with concomitant atrial fibrillation and end-stage renal disease: a systematic review and network meta-analysis. J Am Heart Assoc. 2024;13(8):e034176. https://doi.org/10.1161/JAHA.123.034176.
61. Du Y, Zeng Y, Xu S, Shen Q, Hu J, Lip GYH. Oral anticoagulant therapy for patients with atrial fibrillation on long-term dialysis: a network meta-analysis of 137,574 patients. Eur J Clin Investig. 2025;55(12):e70120. https://doi.org/10.1111/eci.70120.
62. Kim DG, Kim SH, Park SY, Han BG, Kim JS, Yang JW, et al. Anticoagulation in patients with end-stage kidney disease and atrial fibrillation: a national population-based study. Clin Kidney J. 2024;17(2):sfae029. https://doi.org/10.1093/ckj/sfae029.
63. Park SJ, Kim YN, Oh BK, Yu H, Moon S, Lee MY, et al. Efficacy and safety of antithrombotics in patients with atrial fibrillation undergoing hemodialysis: a nationwide cohort study in Korea. J Nephrol. 2025;38(8):2229–37. https://doi.org/10.1007/s40620-025-02340-3.
64. Cresti A, García-Fernández MA, Sievert H, Mazzone P, Baratta P, Solari M, et al. Prevalence of extra-appendage thrombosis in non-valvular atrial fibrillation and atrial flutter in patients undergoing cardioversion: a large transoesophageal echo study. EuroIntervention. 2019;15(3):e225–30. https://doi.org/10.4244/EIJ-D-19-00128.
65. Kaisaier W, Xu Z, Guo L, Dong Y, Chen Y, Lip GYH, et al. Left atrial appendage closure vs oral anticoagulation for stroke prevention in atrial fibrillation: long-term outcomes from 4 randomized trials. Heart Rhythm. 2025;22(11):e1086–96. https://doi.org/10.1016/j.hrthm.2025.07.051.
66. Potpara T, Grygier M, Häusler KG, Nielsen-Kudsk JE, Berti S, Genovesi S, et al. Practical guide on left atrial appendage closure for the non-implanting physician. An international consensus paper. Europace. 2024;26(4):euae035. https://doi.org/10.1093/europace/euae035.
67. Liu C, Han S, Cui K, Wang F. Efficacy and safety of left atrial appendage closure in patients with chronic kidney disease and atrial fibrillation: a systematic review and meta-analysis. PLoS One. 2023;18(10):e0287928. https://doi.org/10.1371/journal.pone.0287928.
68. Rodríguez-Riascos JF, Vemulapalli HS, Akin I, Areiza LA, Della Rocca DG, Eitel I, et al. Left atrial appendage occlusion in patients with end-stage renal disease: An individual patient-level meta-analysis. Europace. 2025;27(10):euaf198. https://doi.org/10.1093/europace/euaf198.
69. Dhar G, Phadnis MA, Hunt SL, Du HE, Ong V, Khandekar N, et al. Left atrial appendage occlusion vs anticoagulants in dialysis with atrial fibrillation. JAMA Netw Open. 2025;8(9):e2530990. https://doi.org/10.1001/jamanetworkopen.2025.30990.
70. Al-Abcha A, Saleh G, Sledge H, Abbasi M, Ismayl M, Killu AM, et al. Outcomes of stroke prevention strategies in patients with atrial fibrillation and end-stage renal disease. JACC Cardiovasc Interv. 2025;18(21):2614–24. https://doi.org/10.1016/j.jcin.2025.07.038.
71. Genovesi S, Porcu L, Rebora P, Slaviero G, Casu G, Bertoli S, et al. Long-term safety and efficacy of left atrial appendage occlusion in dialysis patients with atrial fibrillation: a multi-center, prospective, open label, observational study. Clin Kidney J. 2023;16(12):2683–92. https://doi.org/10.1093/ckj/sfad221.
72. Li M, Liu T, Luo D, Li G. Systematic review and meta-analysis of chronic kidney disease as predictor of atrial fibrillation recurrence following catheter ablation (CA). Cardiol J. 2014;21(1):89–95. https://doi.org/10.5603/CJ.a2013.0116.
73. Chung I, Khan Y, Warrens H, Seshasai RK, Sohal M, Banerjee D. Catheter ablation for atrial fibrillation in patients with chronic kidney disease and on dialysis – a meta-analysis and review. Cardiorenal Med. 2022;12(4):155–72. https://doi.org/10.1159/000525388.
74. Diemberger I, Genovesi S, Massaro G, Reggiani MLB, Frisoni J, Gorlato G, et al. Meta-analysis of clinical outcomes of electrical cardioversion and catheter ablation in patients with atrial fibrillation and chronic kidney disease. Curr Pharm Des. 2018;24(24):2794–801. https://doi.org/10.2174/1381612824666180829112019.

75. Chen L, Gao H, Liang T, Zhao X. Catheter ablation for patients on hemodialysis with symptomatic atrial fibrillation. Ann Palliat Med. 2022;11(9):2862–70. https://doi.org/10.21037/apm-22-410.
76. Multicentre, cross-sectional study of ventricular arrhythmias in chronically haemodialysis patients. Haemodialysis and Cardiovascular Diseases Group. Lancet. 1988;2(8606):305–9.
77. Sforzini S, Latini R, Mingardi G, Vincenti A, Redaelli B. Ventricular arrhythmias and four-year mortality in haemodialysis patients. Hemodialysis and Cardiovascular Diseases Group. Lancet. 1992;339(8787):212–3. https://doi.org/10.1016/0140-6736(92)90008-q.
78. Genovesi S, Lieti G, Camm AJ. Sudden cardiac death in patients with kidney failure on renal replacement therapy: An unsolved problem. Heart Rhythm. 2025;22(8):e380–7. https://doi.org/10.1016/j.hrthm.2025.03.1970.
79. Pun PH, Lehrich RW, Honeycutt EF, Herzog CA, Middleton JP. Modifiable risk factors associated with sudden cardiac arrest within hemodialysis clinics. Kidney Int. 2011;79(2):218–27. https://doi.org/10.1038/ki.2010.3153.
80. Karnik JA, Young BS, Lew NL, Herget M, Dubinsky C, Lazarus JM, et al. Cardiac arrest and sudden death in dialysis units. Kidney Int. 2001;60(1):350–7. https://doi.org/10.1046/j.1523-1755.2001.00806.x.
81. Davis TR, Young BA, Eisenberg MS, Rea TD, Copass MK, Cobb LA. Outcome of cardiac arrests attended by emergency medical services staff at community outpatient dialysis centers. Kidney Int. 2008;73(8):933–9. https://doi.org/10.1038/sj.ki.5002749.
82. Pun PH, Dupre ME, Starks MA, Tyson C, Vellano K, Svetkey LP, et al. Outcomes for hemodialysis patients given cardiopulmonary resuscitation for cardiac arrest at outpatient dialysis clinics. J Am Soc Nephrol. 2019;30(3):461–70. https://doi.org/10.1681/ASN.2018090911.
83. Pun PH, Horton JR, Middleton JP. Dialysate calcium concentration and the risk of sudden cardiac arrest in hemodialysis patients. Clin J Am Soc Nephrol. 2013 May;8(5):797–803. https://doi.org/10.2215/CJN.10000912.
84. Severi S, Grandi E, Pes C, Badiali F, Grandi F, Santoro A. Calcium and potassium changes during haemodialysis alter ventricular repolarization duration: in vivo and in silico analysis. Nephrol Dial Transplant. 2008;23(4):1378–86. https://doi.org/10.1093/ndt/gfm765.
85. Genovesi S, Dossi C, Viganò MR, Galbiati E, Prolo F, Stella A, et al. Electrolyte concentration during haemodialysis and QT interval prolongation in uraemic patients. Europace. 2008;10(6):771–7. https://doi.org/10.1093/europace/eun028.
86. Ter Meulen KJ, Carioni P, Bellocchio F, van der Sande FM, Bouman HJ, Stuard S, et al. The effects of dialysate calcium prescription on mortality outcomes in incident patients on hemodialysis. Clin Kidney J. 2024;17(10):sfae288. https://doi.org/10.1093/ckj/sfae288.
87. Jadoul M, Thumma J, Fuller DS, Tentori F, Li Y, Morgenstern H, et al. Modifiable practices associated with sudden death among hemodialysis patients in the dialysis outcomes and practice patterns study. Clin J Am Soc Nephrol. 2012;7(5):765–74. https://doi.org/10.2215/CJN.08850811.
88. Heguilén RM, Sciurano C, Bellusci AD, Fried P, Mittelman G, Rosa Diez G, et al. The faster potassium-lowering effect of high dialysate bicarbonate concentrations in chronic haemodialysis patients. Nephrol Dial Transplant. 2005;20(3):591–7. https://doi.org/10.1093/ndt/gfh661.
89. Di Iorio B, Torraca S, Piscopo C, Sirico ML, Di Micco L, Pota A, Tartaglia D, Berardino L, et al. Dialysate bath and QTc interval in patients on chronic maintenance hemodialysis: pilot study of single dialysis effects. J Nephrol. 2012;25(5):653–60. https://doi.org/10.5301/jn.5000036.
90. Hage FG, de Mattos AM, Khamash H, Mehta S, Warnock D, Iskandrian AE. QT prolongation is an independent predictor of mortality in end-stage renal disease. Clin Cardiol. 2010;33(6):361–6. https://doi.org/10.1002/clc.20768.
91. Genovesi S, Rossi E, Nava M, Riva H, De Franceschi S, Fabbrini P, et al. A case series of chronic haemodialysis patients: mortality, sudden death, and QT interval. Europace. 2013;15(7):1025–33. https://doi.org/10.1093/europace/eus412.

92. Hiyamuta H, Yamada S, Nakano T, Taniguchi M, Masutani K, Tsuruya K, et al. Impact of electrocardiographic parameters on sudden death in patients receiving maintenance hemodialysis: ten-year outcomes of the Q-cohort study. J Atheroscler Thromb. 2024;31(3):214–31. https://doi.org/10.5551/jat.64255.
93. Ismail S, Funk MJ, Flythe JE. Ondansetron and the risk of sudden cardiac death among individuals receiving maintenance hemodialysis. J Am Soc Nephrol. 2024;35(6):761–71. https://doi.org/10.1681/ASN.0000000000000336.
94. Assimon MM, Pun PH, Wang LC, Al-Khatib SM, Brookhart MA, Weber DJ, et al. Analysis of respiratory fluoroquinolones and the risk of sudden cardiac death among patients receiving hemodialysis. JAMA Cardiol. 2022;7(1):75–83. https://doi.org/10.1001/jamacardio.2021.4234.
95. Assimon MM, Pun PH, Al-Khatib SM, Brookhart MA, Gaynes BN, Winkelmayer WC, et al. The modifying effect of the serum-to-dialysate potassium gradient on the cardiovascular safety of SSRIs in the hemodialysis population: a pharmacoepidemiologic study. Nephrol Dial Transplant. 2022;37(11):2241–52. https://doi.org/10.1093/ndt/gfac214.
96. Sakaguchi Y, Fujii N, Shoji T, Hayashi T, Rakugi H, Isaka Y. Hypomagnesemia is a significant predictor of cardiovascular and non-cardiovascular mortality in patients undergoing hemodialysis. Kidney Int. 2014;85(1):174–81. https://doi.org/10.1038/ki.2013.327.
97. de Roij van Zuijdewijn CL, Grooteman MP, Bots ML, Blankestijn PJ, Steppan S, Büchel J, et al. Serum magnesium and sudden death in European hemodialysis patients. PLoS One. 2015;10(11):e0143104. https://doi.org/10.1371/journal.pone.0143104.
98. Bleyer AJ, Hartman J, Brannon PC, Reeves-Daniel A, Satko SG, Russell G. Characteristics of sudden death in hemodialysis patients. Kidney Int. 2006;69(12):2268–73. https://doi.org/10.1038/sj.ki.5000446.
99. Genovesi S, Valsecchi MG, Rossi E, Pogliani D, Acquistapace I, De Cristofaro V, et al. Sudden death and associated factors in a historical cohort of chronic haemodialysis patients. Nephrol Dial Transplant. 2009;24(8):2529–36. https://doi.org/10.1093/ndt/gfp104.
100. Karaboyas A, Zee J, Brunelli SM, Usvyat LA, Weiner DE, Maddux FW, et al. Dialysate potassium, serum potassium, mortality, and arrhythmia events in hemodialysis: results from the dialysis outcomes and practice patterns study (DOPPS). Am J Kidney Dis. 2017;69(2):266–77. https://doi.org/10.1053/j.ajkd.2016.09.015.
101. Wan C, Herzog CA, Zareba W, Szymkiewicz SJ. Sudden cardiac arrest in hemodialysis patients with wearable cardioverter defibrillator. Ann Noninvasive Electrocardiol. 2014;19(3):247–57. https://doi.org/10.1111/anec.12119.
102. Wong MC, Kalman JM, Pedagogos E, Toussaint N, Vohra JK, Sparks PB, et al. Temporal distribution of arrhythmic events in chronic kidney disease: highest incidence in the long interdialytic period. Heart Rhythm. 2015;12(10):2047–55. https://doi.org/10.1016/j.hrthm.2015.06.033.
103. Sacher F, Jesel L, Borni-Duval C, De Precigout V, Lavainne F, Bourdenx JP, et al. Cardiac rhythm disturbances in hemodialysis patients: early detection using an implantable loop recorder and correlation with biological and dialysis parameters. JACC Clin Electrophysiol. 2018;4(3):397–408. https://doi.org/10.1016/j.jacep.2017.08.002.
104. Roy-Chaudhury P, Tumlin JA, Koplan BA, Costea AI, Kher V, Williamson D, et al. Primary outcomes of the monitoring in dialysis study indicate that clinically significant arrhythmias are common in hemodialysis patients and related to dialytic cycle. Kidney Int. 2018;93(4):941–51. https://doi.org/10.1016/j.kint.2017.11.019.
105. Charytan DM, Winkelmayer WC, Granger CB, Middleton JP, Herzog CA, Chertow GM, et al. Effects of dialysate potassium concentration of 3.0mEq/l with sodium zirconium cyclosilicate on dialysis-free days versus dialysate potassium concentration of 2.0 mEq/l alone on rates of cardiac arrhythmias in hemodialysis patients with hyperkalemia. Kidney Int. 2025;107(1):169–79. https://doi.org/10.1016/j.kint.2024.10.010.

106. Lai Y, Yoshimura H, Zakkak N, Marijon E, Chahal A, Lip GYH, et al. Causes of death in patients with atrial fibrillation in the UK: a nationwide electronic health record study. Eur Heart J Open. 2025;5(1):oeae103. https://doi.org/10.1093/ehjopen/oeae103.
107. Kim YG, Choi YY, Han KD, Min K, Choi HY, Shim J, et al. Atrial fibrillation is associated with increased risk of lethal ventricular arrhythmias. Sci Rep. 2021;11(1):18111. https://doi.org/10.1038/s41598-021-97335-y.
108. Parekh RS, Plantinga LC, Kao WH, Meoni LA, Jaar BG, Fink NE, et al. The association of sudden cardiac death with inflammation and other traditional risk factors. Kidney Int. 2008;74(10):1335–42. https://doi.org/10.1038/ki.2008.449.
109. Genovesi S, Nava E, Bartolucci C, Severi S, Vincenti A, Contaldo G, et al. Acute effect of a peritoneal dialysis exchange on electrolyte concentration and QT interval in uraemic patients. Clin Exp Nephrol. 2019;23(11):1315–22. https://doi.org/10.1007/s10157-019-01773-y.
110. Wang AYM, Lam CWK, Chan IHS, Wang M, Lui SF, Sanderson JE. Sudden cardiac death in end-stage renal disease patients: a 5-year prospective analysis. Hypertension. 2010;56(2):210–6. https://doi.org/10.1161/HYPERTENSIONAHA.110.151167.
111. Genovesi S, Porcu L, Luise MC, Riva H, Nava E, Contaldo G, et al. Sudden death in end stage renal Disease: comparing hemodialysis versus peritoneal dialysis. Blood Purif. 2017;44(1):77–88. https://doi.org/10.1159/000464347.
112. van Ham WB, Cornelissen CM, van Veen TAB. Uremic toxins in chronic kidney disease highlight a fundamental gap in understanding their detrimental effects on cardiac electrophysiology and arrhythmogenesis. Acta Physiol (Oxf). 2022;236(3):e13888. https://doi.org/10.1111/apha.13888.
113. Bilchick KC, Stukenborg GJ, Kamath S, Cheng A. Prediction of mortality in clinical practice for medicare patients undergoing defibrillator implantation for primary prevention of sudden cardiac death. J Am Coll Cardiol. 2012;60(17):1647–55. https://doi.org/10.1016/j.jacc.2012.07.028.
114. Pun PH, Al-Khatib SM, Han JY, Edwards R, Bardy GH, Bigger JT, et al. Implantable cardioverter-defibrillators for primary prevention of sudden cardiac death in CKD: a meta-analysis of patient-level data from 3 randomized trials. Am J Kidney Dis. 2014;64(1):32–9. https://doi.org/10.1053/j.ajkd.2013.12.009.
115. Schefer T, Wolber T, Binggeli C, Holzmeister J, Brunckhorst C, Duru F. Long-term predictors of mortality in ICD patients with non-ischaemic cardiac disease: impact of renal function. Europace. 2008;10(9):1052–9. https://doi.org/10.1093/europace/eun186.
116. Hess PL, Hellkamp AS, Peterson ED, Sanders GD, Al-Khalidi HR, Curtis LH, et al. Survival after primary prevention implantable cardioverter-defibrillator placement among patients with chronic kidney disease. Circ Arrhythm Electrophysiol. 2014;7(5):793–9. https://doi.org/10.1161/CIRCEP.114.001455.
117. Bansal N, Szpiro A, Reynolds K, Smith DH, Magid DJ, Gurwitz JH, et al. Long-term outcomes associated with implantable cardioverter defibrillator in adults with chronic kidney disease. JAMA Intern Med. 2018;178(3):390–8. https://doi.org/10.1001/jamainternmed.2017.8462.
118. Makki N, Swaminathan PD, Hanmer J, Olshansky B. Do implantable cardioverter defibrillators improve survival in patients with chronic kidney disease at high risk of sudden cardiac death? A meta-analysis of observational studies. Europace. 2014;16(1):55–62. https://doi.org/10.1093/europace/eut277.
119. Varga CR, Cleland JGF, Abraham WT, Lip GYH, Leyva F, Hatamizadeh P. Implantable cardioverter defibrillator and resynchronization therapy in patients with overt chronic kidney disease: JACC state-of-the-art review. J Am Coll Cardiol. 2024;84(14):1342–62. https://doi.org/10.1016/j.jacc.2024.05.081.
120. Jukema JW, Timal RJ, Rotmans JI, Hensen LCR, Buiten MS, de Bie MK, et al. Prophylactic use of implantable cardioverter-defibrillators in the prevention of sudden cardiac death in dialysis patients. Circulation. 2019;139(23):2628–38. https://doi.org/10.1161/CIRCULATIONAHA.119.039818.

121. Pun PH, Hellkamp AS, Sanders GD, Middleton JP, Hammill SC, Al-Khalidi HR, et al. Primary prevention implantable cardioverter defibrillators in end-stage kidney disease patients on dialysis: a matchedcohort study. Nephrol Dial Transplant. 2015;30(5):829–35. https://doi.org/10.1093/ndt/gfu274.
122. Khan F, Adelstein E, Saba S. Implantable cardioverter defibrillators confer survival benefit in patients with renal insufficiency but not in dialysis-dependent patients. J Interv Card Electrophysiol. 2010;28(2):117–23. https://doi.org/10.1007/s10840-010-9484-6.
123. Hiremath S, Punnam SR, Brar SS, et al. Implantable defibrillators improve survival in end-stage renal disease: results from a multi-center registry. Am J Nephrol. 2010;32:305–10. https://doi.org/10.1159/000319461.
124. Herzog CA, Li S, Weinhandl ED, Strief JW, Collins AJ, Gilbertson DT. Survival of dialysis patients after cardiac arrest and the impact of implantable cardioverter defibrillators. Kidney Int. 2005;68(2):818–25. https://doi.org/10.1111/j.1523-1755.2005.00462.x.
125. Nakasuka K, Sakurai Y, Kawada Y, Mizoguchi T, Yokoi M, Mori K, et al. Secondary prevention implantable cardioverter-defibrillator for cardiac arrest survivors on hemodialysis in Japan—a nationwide claims-based analysis. Circulation Rep. 2026; https://doi.org/10.1253/circrep.CR-25-0209.
126. Charytan DM, Patrick AR, Liu J, Setoguchi S, Herzog CA, Brookhart MA, et al. Trends in the use and outcomes of implantable cardioverter-defibrillators in patients undergoing dialysis in the United States. Am J Kidney Dis. 2011;58(3):409–17. https://doi.org/10.1053/j.ajkd.2011.03.026.
127. Payne T, Waller J, Kheda M, Nahman NS Jr, Maalouf J, Gopal A, et al. Efficacy of implantable cardioverter-defibrillators for secondary prevention of sudden cardiac death in patients with end-stage renal disease. J Innov Card Rhythm Manag. 2020;11(8):4199–208. https://doi.org/10.19102/icrm.2020.110803.
128. Genovesi S, Porcu L, Luise MC, Riva H, Nava E, Stella A, Pozzi C, et al. Mortality, sudden death and indication for cardioverter defibrillator implantation in a dialysis population. Int J Cardiol. 2015;186:170–7. https://doi.org/10.1016/j.ijcard.2015.03.178.
129. Tangri N, Shastri S, Tighiouart H, Beck GJ, Cheung AK, Eknoyan G, et al. b-blockers for prevention of sudden cardiac death in patients on hemodialysis: a propensity score analysis of the HEMO study. Am J Kidney Dis. 2011;58(6):939–45. https://doi.org/10.1053/j.ajkd.2011.06.024.
130. Matsue Y, Suzuki M, Nagahori W, Ohno M, Matsumura A, Hashimoto Y. B-blocker prevents sudden cardiac death in patients with hemodialysis. Int J Cardiol. 2013;165(3):519–22. https://doi.org/10.1016/j.ijcard.2011.09.037.
131. Pun PH, Lehrich RW, Smith SR, Middleton JP. Predictors of survival after cardiac arrest in outpatient hemodialysis clinics. Clin J Am Soc Nephrol. 2007;2:491–500. https://doi.org/10.2215/CJN.02360706.

Chapter 9
Antithrombotic and Anticoagulant Therapy in Renal Dysfunction

Alexandru Burlacu and Crischentian Brinza

9.1 Introduction

Chronic kidney disease (CKD) affects more than 10% of the global adult population and is associated with a markedly elevated risk of cardiovascular morbidity and mortality [1]. In this context, patients with CKD often present with both prothrombotic and increased bleeding risk states, constituting a major challenge for antithrombotic and anticoagulant therapy [2, 3]. Renal impairment is frequently observed in cardiovascular disease patients, including those with coronary artery disease (CAD), atrial fibrillation (AF), or venous thromboembolism (VTE), and adapting antithrombotic strategies in the presence of renal dysfunction is of central importance [2, 3].

Alterations in hemostasis are frequent in CKD and involve both procoagulant and anticoagulant pathways. Endothelial dysfunction promotes increased expression of adhesion molecules and reduced nitric oxide availability, while circulating levels of fibrinogen, factor VIII, and von Willebrand factor are often elevated [4, 5]. Platelet activation is enhanced, yet platelet aggregation is paradoxically impaired by the retention of uremic toxins such as guanidinosuccinic acid and phenolic compounds, which interfere with receptor signaling [6–8]. The net result is a fragile equilibrium: CKD patients are at higher risk of arterial and venous thrombosis, but they also experience spontaneous bleeding, prolonged bleeding time, and an unpredictable response to antithrombotic drugs. This complex background explains

A. Burlacu (✉)
Institute of Cardiovascular Diseases "Prof. Dr. George I.M. Georgescu", Iasi, Romania

University of Medicine and Pharmacy "Grigore T Popa", Iasi, Romania
e-mail: alexandru.burlacu@umfiasi.ro

C. Brinza
Faculty of Medicine, University of Medicine and Pharmacy "Grigore T Popa", Iasi, Romania
e-mail: crischentian.brinza@d.umfiasi.ro

A. Covic, A. Burlacu (eds.), *Renal Dysfunction in Cardiovascular Pathologies*,
https://doi.org/10.1007/978-3-032-25434-4_9

why treatment protocols validated in populations with preserved renal function often cannot be directly applied in those with advanced kidney disease [5, 8].

Alterations in drug pharmacokinetics and pharmacodynamics are major determinants of both efficacy and safety in patients with CKD. Several antithrombotic agents, including low-molecular-weight heparins, direct oral anticoagulants, and certain $P2Y_{12}$ inhibitors, undergo renal excretion to varying degrees. When glomerular filtration rate declines, drug clearance is delayed, resulting in higher plasma exposure and prolonged biological effects that increase bleeding risk [3, 9]. On the other hand, the uremic milieu may attenuate the antiplatelet effect of clopidogrel in advanced CKD [10]. Because most pivotal cardiovascular trials have excluded patients with severe renal impairment or dialysis dependence, available evidence is derived mainly from pharmacokinetic analyses and limited observational cohorts [11]. Consequently, dose adjustment and close clinical monitoring remain essential when prescribing antithrombotic agents in the setting of renal dysfunction.

The close relationship between CKD and cardiovascular pathology makes the management of antithrombotic therapy particularly challenging. With the growing prevalence of CKD worldwide, clinical decisions must balance ischemic protection against bleeding risk in patients with impaired renal function. This chapter reviews the current evidence regarding the use of antiplatelet and anticoagulant agents across different stages of kidney dysfunction, emphasizing pathophysiological mechanisms, pharmacological considerations, and practical recommendations for clinical care. The objective is to provide a concise, evidence-based overview to guide individualized therapeutic decisions in this complex patient population.

9.2 Pathophysiological Background

Patients with CKD present a complex alteration of hemostasis in which thrombotic risk factors coexist with an increased bleeding risk [12]. On the one hand, markers of coagulation activation (e.g., elevated fibrinogen, factor VIII, von Willebrand factor) and delayed fibrinolysis support a prothrombotic milieu. On the other hand, primary hemostatic defects, notably platelet dysfunction and impaired platelet-vessel wall interaction, could contribute to bleeding risk despite normal or even elevated levels of clotting factors [13]. Recognition of this dual and opposing risk is essential to understanding how antithrombotic therapies must be customized in patients with renal dysfunction, especially in those with end-stage kidney disease (ESKD).

Endothelial injury constitutes a central feature of the hemostatic disturbance in CKD. In the large cross-sectional CRIB study, reduced estimated glomerular filtration rate (eGFR) was associated with impaired endothelial function and chronic low-grade inflammation [14]. Elevated circulating levels of von Willebrand factor and factor VIII have been documented in CKD patients, which could be linked to markers of vascular damage [5]. In one study, Huang and colleagues noted increased coagulation activity in CKD, particularly persistent elevation of factor VIII [5]. At the same time, nitric oxide-mediated antithrombotic mechanisms are impaired in CKD through both reduced bioavailability and increased endogenous inhibitors of endothelial nitric oxide synthase (eNOS) [15]. The net result is a vascular bed that is predisposed to thrombus formation but simultaneously prone to bleeding complications.

Platelet functional abnormalities in CKD are multifactorial. A meta-analysis of platelet function studies in CKD demonstrated that maximal aggregation (especially in response to collagen) is significantly reduced compared to controls [8]. In a flow-cytometry study of CKD patients, the authors found reduced P-selectin expression after CKD compared with healthy subjects [16]. These findings support the concept of impaired platelet reactivity despite preserved platelet count.

Diminished fibrinolytic capacity is another important element in CKD-associated hemostasis alteration. Elevated levels of plasminogen activator inhibitor-1 (PAI-1), together with decreased endogenous anticoagulant expression, have been documented in advanced renal disease [15]. Chronic inflammation, a state observed in CKD patients, could further promote procoagulant pathways by enhancing tissue factor expression on endothelial and monocyte surfaces, as well as by increasing oxidative stress [15]. These abnormalities not only promote thrombus formation but also reduce the capacity for timely clot resolution, thereby contributing to both macro- and microvascular complications [15].

The pathophysiological alterations translate into clinically relevant events. Patients with CKD are at higher risk of arterial thrombosis, including acute coronary syndromes (ACS), venous thromboembolism, and stent thrombosis. Simultaneously, they could have an elevated risk of spontaneous bleeding and procedural hemorrhage [15]. Because standard antithrombotic trials often exclude patients with advanced renal impairment, recommendations are frequently extrapolated from those with preserved kidney function (or less advanced CKD), which limits applicability. This underlines the need for an approach to antithrombotic therapy in renal dysfunction that is guided by the underlying hemostatic disturbances, renal clearance considerations and personalized risk-benefit assessment [15].

9.3 Antiplatelet Therapy in CKD

Patients with CKD experience a markedly increased incidence of atherothrombotic events compared with the general population. Both decreased renal function and albuminuria are independent predictors of myocardial infarction, stroke, and cardiovascular death [17]. The balance between ischemic benefit and bleeding risk may differ substantially across CKD stages, particularly in advanced kidney disease and dialysis patients. Observational data indicate that major bleeding rates increase progressively with declining eGFR, even at standard antiplatelet doses [18]. In addition, altered pharmacokinetics of some antiplatelet agents, variability in drug activation, and interactions with uremic toxins could influence both efficacy and safety profiles [19].

Despite these limitations, most guidelines endorse the use of antiplatelet therapy in secondary prevention of cardiovascular events among CKD patients, as the absolute ischemic risk remains high. However, evidence supporting its use for primary prevention is limited and inconsistent [20]. Clinical decision-making therefore requires careful individual risk stratification, considering eGFR, comorbidities, and concurrent anticoagulant therapy.

9.3.1 Aspirin Therapy

Aspirin remains the antiplatelet agent with the longest clinical experience in cardiovascular disease, and its role in secondary prevention is generally maintained across different stages of CKD. Several analyses highlighted that patients with reduced renal function continue to benefit from aspirin when used after the establishment of atherosclerotic cardiovascular disease (ASCVD) [21].

In a prospective observational analysis from the Chronic Renal Insufficiency Cohort (CRIC), investigators assessed the association between aspirin use and outcomes of all-cause mortality, major cardiovascular disease (CVD), kidney failure and major bleeding [22]. The primary prevention subgroup (participants without pre-existing CVD) comprised 2578 individuals, with a mean eGFR of 47.3 mL/min/1.73 m^2 [22]. Over a median follow-up of 11.5 years (interquartile range 7.4–13.0 years), aspirin use was not significantly associated with a lower risk of the composite cardiovascular endpoint in primary prevention (HR 0.97; 95% CI: 0.77–1.23; $P = 0.79$). Similarly, in the subgroup with known CVD, aspirin did not confer a statistically significant benefit (HR 0.88; 95% CI: 0.77–1.02; $P = 0.08$) for all-cause mortality [22].

The authors noted that aspirin use was likewise not associated with slowing progression to kidney failure or with a statistically significant elevation in major bleeding risk in this CKD cohort [1]. In the adjusted time-varying Cox model, aspirin did not provide a significant benefit in either primary or secondary prevention settings. Importantly, the authors emphasized the observational nature of the study as a key limitation, which precludes causal inference [22].

A recent meta-analysis synthesized evidence from five randomized controlled trials evaluating low-dose aspirin for primary prevention in individuals with CKD stages 3–5 [23]. Across these trials, aspirin use was associated with a statistically significant reduction in major adverse cardiovascular events, with a pooled relative risk (RR) of 0.76 (95% CI 0.62–0.94). Reductions in cardiovascular mortality (RR 0.60; 95% CI: 0.43–0.85) and all-cause mortality (RR 0.78; 95% CI: 0.63–0.96) were also observed, indicating a consistent direction of effect toward fewer fatal and non-fatal ischemic outcomes among aspirin-treated participants [23].

Subgroup analyses stratified by kidney function suggested that the magnitude of benefit differed by baseline eGFR. In the case of patients with eGFR <45 mL/

min/1.73 m², aspirin use was associated with a lower risk of non-fatal myocardial infarction (RR 0.47; 95% CI: 0.23–0.96) and cardiovascular mortality (RR 0.47; 95% CI: 0.24–0.92) [23]. These findings indicate that patients with more advanced renal impairment may experience a greater ischemic benefit from aspirin, although these data could be limited by the number of events and the heterogeneity of trial designs [23].

The favorable cardiovascular effect was counterbalanced by an increase in major bleeding risk. Across CKD stages 3–5, aspirin use was associated with a 50% relative increase in major bleeding events (RR 1.50; 95% CI: 1.12–2.02) [23]. The authors reported that bleeding risk tended to rise as eGFR declined, underscoring the need for individualized assessment, particularly in patients with additional risk factors for hemorrhage. Given the modest number of available trials and variability in outcome definitions, the precision of bleeding estimates remains limited, and the overall certainty of evidence is constrained by heterogeneity and risk-of-bias concerns [23].

In a propensity-score-matched cohort of 531 aspirin-users and 531 non-users drawn from a total of 2070 individuals with non-dialysis CKD (mean eGFR 53.1 ± 30.9 mL/min/1.73 m²), the investigators observed that low-dose aspirin (75–100 mg) was associated with an elevated risk of major cardiovascular events over a median follow-up of 51.8 months (HR 1.798; 95% CI: 1.146–2.819; $P = 0.011$) [24]. Within subgroups stratified by prior history of cardiovascular disease, the risk was particularly elevated among those with established CVD (in the matched sample the HR was 3.947; 95% CI: 1.343–11.598; $P = 0.013$). These findings challenge the assumption that low-dose aspirin uniformly reduces ischemic risk in patients with CKD and highlight the need to differentiate by clinical context [24].

The study further assessed bodyweight as a modifying factor and reported that among patients with bodyweight <60 kg (lowest quartile), aspirin use was associated with an adjusted HR of 4.014; 95% CI: 1.253–12.865; $P = 0.019$ for CVE in the matched cohort, whereas no significant risk difference was observed in higher weight strata. Secondary outcomes, including ≥50% eGFR decline, doubling of serum creatinine, initiation of kidney-replacement therapy, all-cause mortality, and major bleeding, did not differ significantly between aspirin users and non-users in matched analyses. However, the results are limited by the observational design, single-ethnicity (Korean) population, and potential residual confounding as limitations to causal interpretation [24].

Overall, aspirin use in CKD demonstrates a mixed risk-benefit profile shaped by clinical context, baseline cardiovascular risk, and renal function. Randomized evidence indicates that low-dose aspirin can reduce major adverse cardiovascular events, cardiovascular mortality, and all-cause mortality in CKD stages 3–5, with the possibility of greater benefit in patients with eGFR <45 mL/min/1.73 m². In contrast, observational data from large cohorts highlight the absence of benefit in primary prevention, the lack of clear survival advantage in secondary prevention, and a consistent signal toward increased bleeding or even higher cardiovascular event rates in specific subgroups such as low-body-weight patients. The aggregate evidence therefore supports a selective approach: aspirin remains reasonable for secondary prevention when ischemic risk is high, but should be used cautiously in primary prevention, in patients with advanced CKD and elevated bleeding susceptibility, and in individuals with low bodyweight. Individualized assessment remains essential, and routine prescribing in unselected CKD populations cannot be justified based on current data.

9.3.2 Clopidogrel and P2Y12 Inhibitor Therapy

Altered platelet biology in CKD reduces the antiplatelet effect of clopidogrel and contributes to high platelet reactivity. In the Assessment of Dual Antiplatelet Therapy With Drug-Eluting Stents registry, which included 8582 patients undergoing percutaneous coronary intervention (PCI), CKD was independently associated with high platelet reactivity on clopidogrel. Patients with CKD and HTPR had a higher incidence of stent thrombosis and ischemic events, underscoring the reduced pharmacodynamic responsiveness to clopidogrel in impaired renal function [25].

Randomized pharmacodynamic studies provide further insight into attenuated efficacy of clopidogrel in CKD patients. In the PIANO-2 CKD trial, patients with moderate-to-severe CKD receiving standard-dose clopidogrel after PCI showed persistently elevated platelet activity. Also adding cilostazol produced greater inhibition than increasing the clopidogrel dose alone, indicating impaired clopidogrel metabolism and persistent high platelet reactivity despite intensified dosing [26]. These findings support the concept that diminished responsiveness in CKD is driven by both uremia-related platelet alterations and reduced activation of clopidogrel's active metabolite [26].

More potent P2Y12 inhibition could overcome part of this resistance. In a randomized crossover study of 25 hemodialysis patients, ticagrelor achieved significantly greater platelet inhibition than clopidogrel after both loading and maintenance dosing [27]. Although the study was not powered for clinical outcomes, it provides mechanistic evidence that the antiplatelet effect of clopidogrel could be reduced in patients with advanced renal impairment, whereas ticagrelor maintains its inhibitory profile [27].

A detailed analysis from the PROMETHEUS study evaluated prasugrel versus clopidogrel in 19,832 patients undergoing PCI for ACS, of whom 28.3% had CKD [28]. CKD patients were older and had a higher prevalence of diabetes, multivessel disease, and other comorbid conditions that contributed to greater ischemic and bleeding risk. During the first year of follow-up, CKD was linked to a higher adjusted rate of major adverse cardiovascular events (MACE, HR 1.27; 95% CI: 1.18–1.37) and clinically significant bleeding (HR 1.46; 95% CI: 1.24–1.73). Although initial analysis favored prasugrel over clopidogrel in both CKD (18.3% vs. 26.5%; $P < 0.001$) and non-CKD patients (10.9% vs. 17.9%; $P < 0.001$) concerning adverse events, these differences were not significant after propensity score stratification [28]. Bleeding differences between prasugrel and clopidogrel were similarly attenuated after adjustment. Despite the higher baseline risk in CKD, prasugrel was used less frequently in the CKD group, reflecting clinicians' concern about bleeding risk. The overall findings suggest that although CKD amplifies both ischemic and hemorrhagic risk after ACS PCI, comparative effectiveness between prasugrel and clopidogrel remains uncertain once confounding factors are accounted for [28].

A meta-analysis of 15,664 patients with CKD and established CVD compared clinical outcomes between ticagrelor (n = 2456) and clopidogrel (n = 13,208). Across the included studies, ticagrelor did not demonstrate a statistically significant reduction in ischemic outcomes. The pooled estimates for MACE (RR 0.85; 95% CI: 0.71–1.03; P = 0.09), all-cause mortality (RR 0.82; 95% CI: 0.57–1.18; P = 0.29), and hemorrhagic stroke (RR 1.06; 95% CI: 0.38–2.99; P = 0.91) did not differ significantly between treatment groups [29]. Bleeding assessed using TIMI criteria was also comparable between groups. However, ticagrelor was associated with significantly higher bleeding when evaluated using BARC criteria. These results indicate that, within available observational and trial data, ticagrelor does not provide superior cardiovascular protection over clopidogrel in CKD, while potentially increasing clinically relevant bleeding as classified by BARC criteria [29].

A recent study evaluated ticagrelor versus clopidogrel as part of dual antiplatelet therapy (DAPT) in 18,579 adults with CKD undergoing PCI for ACS [30]. Over 1 year of follow-up, the risks of acute myocardial infarction (OR 0.912; 95% CI: 0.808–1.030), and all-cause mortality (OR 1.049; 95% CI: 0.892–1.235) did not differ significantly between treatment strategies. Notably, ticagrelor was associated with lower odds of cerebrovascular accident (OR 0.624; 95% CI: 0.493–0.788) and major bleeding (OR 0.804; 95% CI: 0.649–0.995). Although observational and dependent on electronic health record data, these findings suggest a potential cerebrovascular and bleeding advantage of ticagrelor over clopidogrel in CKD patients receiving DAPT after PCI for ACS [30].

A recent meta-analysis evaluated ticagrelor versus clopidogrel in patients with ESKD receiving chronic dialysis and presenting with acute or chronic coronary syndrome. Ticagrelor did not differ significantly from clopidogrel in the primary composite efficacy outcome, which included all-cause mortality, cardiovascular mortality, recurrent myocardial infarction, coronary revascularization, and ischemic or hemorrhagic stroke (P = 0.40). Safety outcomes were comparable across treatment groups. The pooled estimate for the composite bleeding endpoint did not indicate a significant difference between groups (P = 0.22), and major bleeding rates were comparable (P = 0.27). These findings suggest that, within the limits of observational evidence, ticagrelor does not offer superior efficacy or safety over clopidogrel in dialysis-dependent ESKD [31].

A recent secondary analysis of the TALOS-AMI randomized trial evaluated an unguided deescalation strategy from ticagrelor to clopidogrel in patients with CKD who had completed 1 month of ticagrelor-based DAPT after PCI for acute myocardial infarction [32]. A total of 2646 patients were analyzed and 305 had CKD. Among the CKD subgroup, deescalation (n = 160) was associated with fewer primary composite events, which included cardiovascular death, myocardial infarction, stroke, and BARC 2–5 bleeding, compared with continued ticagrelor (6.2% vs 13.1%; HR 0.45; 95% CI: 0.21–0.98; $P = 0.04$). The reduction was driven primarily by lower bleeding (2.5% vs 8.3%; HR 0.29; 95% CI: 0.09–0.89; $P = 0.03$), with no increase in ischemic events (4.4% vs 5.5%; HR 0.78; 95% CI: 0.28–2.16; $P = 0.64$). These findings suggest that a 1-month deescalation from ticagrelor to clopidogrel may reduce bleeding without compromising ischemic protection in stabilized patients with CKD after acute myocardial infarction, although larger studies are needed to confirm these results [32].

Overall, P2Y12 inhibitor therapy in CKD is characterized by reduced and heterogeneous responsiveness to clopidogrel, higher rates of high platelet reactivity, and uncertain clinical benefit compared with more potent agents. Pharmacodynamic trials consistently demonstrate impaired clopidogrel-induced platelet inhibition in moderate-to-severe CKD and in dialysis patients, whereas ticagrelor maintains more reliable platelet suppression. However, outcome data remain inconsistent. Meta-analyses assessing ticagrelor versus clopidogrel in CKD reported similar effects on MACE, mortality, myocardial infarction, and stroke, with variable bleeding results depending on the classification system used. In large matched datasets, ticagrelor has been associated with lower cerebrovascular event rates and reduced major bleeding, whereas in patients on dialysis the efficacy and safety profiles of ticagrelor and clopidogrel appeared similar. Taken together, these findings indicate that while more potent P2Y12 inhibition may offer pharmacologic advantages in CKD, robust evidence supporting superior clinical outcomes remains limited, and treatment decisions should be individualized to balance ischemic risk against bleeding susceptibility [31].

9.4 Oral Anticoagulant Therapy

Atrial fibrillation (AF) is frequent in CKD and significantly increases the risk of thromboembolic stroke and death, while renal impairment also amplifies bleeding risk. Observational cohorts and meta-analyses indicate that patients with CKD and AF have higher rates of stroke, major bleeding, and mortality than those without renal dysfunction, which complicates the risk-benefit assessment of oral anticoagulation in this population [33].

For vitamin K antagonists, data support a distinction between non-end-stage CKD and ESKD. In a meta-analysis of observational studies including more than 48,000 patients with AF and CKD, warfarin use in non-end-stage CKD was associated with lower risks of ischemic stroke or systemic embolism (HR 0.70; 95% CI: 0.54–0.89; $P = 0.004$) and all-cause mortality (HR 0.65; 95% CI: 0.59–0.72; $P < 0.00001$), without a significant increase in major bleeding (HR 1.15; 95% CI: 0.88–1.49; $P = 0.31$) [34].

In contrast, among patients with AF and ESKD, the same study reported no stroke or mortality benefit (stroke: HR 1.12; 95% CI: 0.69–1.82; $P = 0.65$; mortality: HR 0.96; 95% CI: 0.81–1.13; $P = 0.60$), but a higher risk of major bleeding with warfarin (HR 1.30; 95% CI: 1.08–1.56; $P = 0.005$) [34]. These findings are consistent with subsequent systematic reviews showing no reduction in ischemic stroke and an increased risk of hemorrhagic stroke with warfarin in AF patients receiving dialysis, without a clear effect on overall mortality [33, 35]. Other studies in hemodialysis cohorts similarly suggest that warfarin is associated with either neutral or higher stroke risk and more bleeding, particularly when INR monitoring is suboptimal [36, 37].

Direct oral anticoagulants (DOACs) have been evaluated in major randomized AF trials, with prespecified analyses across renal function strata. In ARISTOTLE, apixaban reduced stroke or systemic embolism and all-cause mortality compared with warfarin and was associated with less major bleeding. These benefits were preserved in patients with impaired renal function, with no efficacy loss at lower eGFR [38, 39]. In RE-LY, dabigatran (particularly the 150 mg twice-daily regimen) reduced stroke or systemic embolism versus warfarin, with similar bleeding risk at the 110 mg dose. Renal subgroup analyses confirmed that declining renal function increased the absolute risk of both thromboembolism and bleeding across all treatment arms [40]. In ROCKET AF, rivaroxaban was non-inferior to warfarin for prevention of stroke or systemic embolism in patients with nonvalvular AF, including those with moderate renal impairment, but bleeding rates were higher overall in the CKD subgroup irrespective of treatment allocation [41]. Collectively, these data suggest that in mild-to-moderate CKD, DOACs, especially apixaban, could provide at least comparable stroke prevention and often lower major bleeding risk than warfarin, although absolute event rates remain higher than in patients with preserved renal function.

Evidence in advanced CKD and dialysis is largely observational. In a US registry study of patients with AF and ESKD on dialysis, apixaban use was associated with a lower risk of major bleeding compared with warfarin (HR 0.72; 95% CI: 0.59–0.87; $P < 0.001$), with similar rates of stroke or systemic embolism and mortality [42]. Other data from systematic reviews and meta-analyses of apixaban versus warfarin in stage 4–5 CKD and dialysis populations report broadly comparable thromboembolic outcomes and a consistent trend toward less major bleeding with apixaban, though all underlying data are observational and susceptible to confounding by indication and dosing selection [43]. Data for dabigatran in ESKD are more limited, with some analyses suggesting similar stroke prevention but possible excess bleeding and concern about drug accumulation due to higher renal clearance, leading most guidelines to favor apixaban, if a DOAC is chosen, in severe CKD or dialysis [44].

A recent study compared apixaban with warfarin in patients with chronic AF occurring after the onset of stage 5 CKD or ESKD [45]. Following propensity matching, 1364 patients in each group were assessed. Across multiple cerebrovascular endpoints, apixaban demonstrated a consistent advantage over warfarin. Risks of cerebral infarction (SHR 0.72; 95% CI: 0.60–0.85), hemorrhagic stroke (SHR 0.42; 95% CI: 0.28–0.63), and the composite of cerebrovascular events (SHR 0.69; 95% CI: 0.59–0.81) were all significantly lower with apixaban. The investigators also noted that patients receiving warfarin had a time in therapeutic range of only

44.4%, which may have contributed to poorer outcomes. Overall, the study suggests that in advanced CKD and ESKD, apixaban may offer lower risks of cerebrovascular events and bleeding compared with warfarin, although optimal dosing remains uncertain [45].

Taken together, current evidence supports warfarin or DOAC therapy for stroke prevention in AF with mild-to-moderate CKD, with a shift in favor of apixaban in many settings because of a more favorable bleeding profile. In ESKD and dialysis, however, warfarin could offer neutral stroke benefit with higher hemorrhagic risk, and comparative data for DOACs are observational and heterogeneous. Anticoagulation decisions in advanced CKD should therefore be individualized, balancing high thromboembolic risk against substantial bleeding risk, and acknowledging the absence of robust randomized data in this subgroup [44].

Learning Objectives

- Understand the hemostatic disturbances associated with CKD, including endothelial dysfunction, altered platelet reactivity, impaired fibrinolysis, and increased procoagulant activity.
- Describe how reduced renal function modifies the pharmacokinetic and pharmacodynamic profiles of antiplatelet and anticoagulant agents, influencing both efficacy and bleeding risk.
- Differentiate the clinical effects of aspirin in CKD, recognizing where randomized evidence supports benefit and where observational data highlight inconsistent or harmful outcomes.
- Summarize the benefits and limitations of warfarin and DOAC therapy across CKD severity, with particular attention to differences between moderate CKD, stage 5 CKD, and dialysis-dependent patients.
- Recognize the challenges of anticoagulation in advanced CKD and ESKD, including elevated bleeding susceptibility, fluctuating drug clearance, and limited availability of randomized evidence.

Key Readings

- CKD increases both prothrombotic and bleeding risks through endothelial dysfunction, elevated coagulation factors, impaired nitric oxide signaling, and uremia-induced platelet abnormalities.
- Altered drug clearance in CKD enhances exposure to several antithrombotic agents, contributing to higher bleeding risk and requiring careful dose evaluation for both antiplatelet and anticoagulant therapies.
- Aspirin demonstrates heterogeneous effects across CKD stages: randomized evidence supports reduced cardiovascular and mortality risk in stage 3–5 CKD, whereas observational studies identify subgroups with no benefit or increased harm.
- Clopidogrel responsiveness could be reduced in CKD due to impaired metabolic activation and high on-treatment platelet reactivity, while ticagrelor preserves inhibitory activity even in advanced renal impairment.

- Deescalation from ticagrelor to clopidogrel after AMI reduces bleeding without increasing ischemic events in CKD patients, supporting individualized DAPT strategies.
- In mild-to-moderate CKD, DOACs, particularly apixaban, provide stroke prevention comparable or superior to warfarin, with lower rates of major bleeding.
- Optimal antithrombotic therapy in CKD requires balancing high cardiovascular risk against substantial bleeding susceptibility, emphasizing individualized clinical decision-making.

Declarations

Competing Interests The author(s) has no competing interests to declare that are relevant to the content of this manuscript.

Ethics Approval The author(s) declares that this manuscript does not include primary research with human participants.

The author(s) declares that this manuscript does not include primary studies involving animals.

References

1. Capodanno D, Angiolillo DJ. Antithrombotic therapy in patients with chronic kidney disease. Circulation. 2012;125(21):2649–61.
2. Lee KH, et al. Antithrombotic therapy for chronic kidney disease patients with concomitant atrial fibrillation and coronary artery disease. Front Cardiovasc Med. 2021;8:751359.
3. Montomoli M, et al. Anticoagulation in chronic kidney disease. Drugs. 2024;84(10):1199–218.
4. Dubin R, et al. Kidney function and multiple hemostatic markers: cross sectional associations in the multi-ethnic study of atherosclerosis. BMC Nephrol. 2011;12(1):3.
5. Huang MJ, et al. Blood coagulation system in patients with chronic kidney disease: a prospective observational study. BMJ Open. 2017;7(5):e014294.
6. Ocak G, et al. Chronic kidney disease and bleeding risk in patients at high cardiovascular risk: a cohort study. J Thromb Haemost. 2018;16(1):65–73.
7. Lutz J, et al. Haemostasis in chronic kidney disease. Nephrol Dial Transplant. 2013;29(1):29–40.
8. Baaten C, et al. Platelet function in CKD: a systematic review and meta-analysis. J Am Soc Nephrol. 2021;32(7):1583–98.
9. Lutz J, Jurk K, Schinzel H. Direct oral anticoagulants in patients with chronic kidney disease: patient selection and special considerations. Int J Nephrol Renovasc Dis. 2017;10:135–43.
10. Wu Y, et al. High on-clopidogrel platelet reactivity and chronic kidney disease: a meta-analysis of literature studies. Scand Cardiovasc J. 2019;53(2):55–61.
11. Chunduri S, Folstad JE, Vachharajani TJ. Antithrombotic therapy in end-stage renal disease. Hemodial Int. 2017;21(4):453–71.
12. Nunns GR, et al. The hypercoagulability paradox of chronic kidney disease: the role of fibrinogen. Am J Surg. 2017;214(6):1215–8.
13. Boccardo P, Remuzzi G, Galbusera M. Platelet dysfunction in renal failure. Semin Thromb Hemost. 2004;30(5):579–89.
14. Landray MJ, et al. Inflammation, endothelial dysfunction, and platelet activation in patients with chronic kidney disease: the chronic renal impairment in Birmingham (CRIB) study. Am J Kidney Dis. 2004;43(2):244–53.

15. Saeed Z, et al. Hallmarks for thrombotic and hemorrhagic risks in chronic kidney disease patients. Int J Mol Sci. 2024;25(16):8705.
16. van Bladel ER, et al. Platelets of patients with chronic kidney disease demonstrate deficient platelet reactivity in vitro. BMC Nephrol. 2012;13(1):127.
17. Go AS, et al. Chronic kidney disease and the risks of death, cardiovascular events, and hospitalization. N Engl J Med. 2004;351(13):1296–305.
18. Palmer SC, et al. Effects of antiplatelet therapy on mortality and cardiovascular and bleeding outcomes in persons with chronic kidney disease: a systematic review and meta-analysis. Ann Intern Med. 2012;156(6):445–59.
19. Lutz J, Jurk K. Antiplatelet agents and anticoagulants in patients with chronic kidney disease-from pathophysiology to clinical practice. Curr Pharm Des. 2017;23(9):1366–76.
20. Bilha SC, et al. Primary prevention of stroke in chronic kidney disease patients: a scientific update. Cerebrovasc Dis. 2018;45(1–2):33–41.
21. Collaborative meta-analysis of randomised trials of antiplatelet therapy for prevention of death, myocardial infarction, and stroke in high risk patients. BMJ. 2002;324(7329):71–86.
22. Taliercio JJ, et al. Aspirin for primary and secondary prevention of mortality, cardiovascular disease, and kidney failure in the chronic renal insufficiency cohort (CRIC) study. Kidney Med. 2022;4(11):100547.
23. Lin J, et al. Effect of low-dose aspirin on reducing cardiovascular events and mortality in individuals with CKD stages 3–5: a meta-analysis of randomized controlled trials. BMC Cardiovasc Disord. 2025;25(1):242.
24. Oh YJ, et al. Low-dose aspirin was associated with an increased risk of cardiovascular events in patients with chronic kidney disease and low bodyweight: results from KNOW-CKD study. Sci Rep. 2021;11(1):6691.
25. Baber U, et al. Prevalence and impact of high platelet reactivity in chronic kidney disease: results from the assessment of dual antiplatelet therapy with drug-eluting stents registry. Circ Cardiovasc Interv. 2015;8(6):e001683.
26. Woo JS, et al. Platelet reactivity in patients with chronic kidney disease receiving adjunctive cilostazol compared with a high-maintenance dose of clopidogrel: results of the effect of platelet inhibition according to clopidogrel dose in patients with chronic kidney disease (PIANO-2 CKD) randomized study. Am Heart J. 2011;162(6):1018–25.
27. Jeong KH, et al. Platelet reactivity after receiving clopidogrel compared with ticagrelor in patients with kidney failure treated with hemodialysis: a randomized crossover study. Am J Kidney Dis. 2015;65(6):916–24.
28. Baber U, et al. Associations between chronic kidney disease and outcomes with use of Prasugrel versus Clopidogrel in patients with acute coronary syndrome undergoing percutaneous coronary intervention: a report from the PROMETHEUS study. JACC Cardiovasc Interv. 2017;10(20):2017–25.
29. Guo Y, et al. Ticagrelor or Clopidogrel as antiplatelet agents in patients with chronic kidney disease and cardiovascular disease: a meta-analysis. Am J Cardiovasc Drugs. 2023;23(5):533–46.
30. Winson T, et al. D-47 | Ticagrelor versus Clopidogrel in dual antiplatelet therapy following percutaneous coronary intervention for acute coronary syndrome in chronic kidney disease. J Soc Cardiovasc Angiogr Intervent. 2025;4(5):103179.
31. Burlacu A, et al. Efficacy and safety of Ticagrelor versus Clopidogrel in dialysis patients with coronary syndromes: a systematic review and meta-analysis. J Clin Med. 2023;12(15):5011.
32. Kim SH, et al. Deescalation from Ticagrelor to Clopidogrel for myocardial infarction with chronic kidney disease: a secondary analysis of a randomized clinical trial. JAMA Netw Open. 2025;8(5):e2511297.
33. Tan J, et al. Warfarin use and stroke, bleeding and mortality risk in patients with end stage renal disease and atrial fibrillation: a systematic review and meta-analysis. BMC Nephrol. 2016;17(1):157.

34. Dahal K, et al. Stroke, major bleeding, and mortality outcomes in warfarin users with atrial fibrillation and chronic kidney disease: a meta-analysis of observational studies. Chest. 2016;149(4):951–9.
35. Randhawa MS, et al. Association between use of warfarin for atrial fibrillation and outcomes among patients with end-stage renal disease: a systematic review and meta-analysis. JAMA Netw Open. 2020;3(4):e202175.
36. Chan KE, et al. Warfarin use associates with increased risk for stroke in hemodialysis patients with atrial fibrillation. J Am Soc Nephrol. 2009;20(10):2223–33.
37. Shah M, et al. Warfarin use and the risk for stroke and bleeding in patients with atrial fibrillation undergoing dialysis. Circulation. 2014;129(11):1196–203.
38. Hohnloser SH, et al. Efficacy of apixaban when compared with warfarin in relation to renal function in patients with atrial fibrillation: insights from the ARISTOTLE trial. Eur Heart J. 2012;33(22):2821–30.
39. Hijazi Z, et al. Efficacy and safety of Apixaban compared with warfarin in patients with atrial fibrillation in relation to renal function over time: insights from the ARISTOTLE randomized clinical trial. JAMA Cardiol. 2016;1(4):451–60.
40. Hijazi Z, et al. Efficacy and safety of dabigatran compared with warfarin in relation to baseline renal function in patients with atrial fibrillation. Circulation. 2014;129(9):961–70.
41. Hori M, et al. Safety and efficacy of adjusted dose of rivaroxaban in Japanese patients with non-valvular atrial fibrillation: subanalysis of J-ROCKET AF for patients with moderate renal impairment. Circ J. 2013;77(3):632–8.
42. Siontis KC, et al. Outcomes associated with Apixaban use in patients with end-stage kidney disease and atrial fibrillation in the United States. Circulation. 2018;138(15):1519–29.
43. AlTurki A, et al. Meta-analysis evaluating apixaban in patients with atrial fibrillation and end-stage renal disease requiring dialysis. J Arrhythmia. 2024;40(3):440–7.
44. Parul F, et al. Anticoagulation in patients with end-stage renal disease: a critical review. Healthcare. 2025;13(12):1373.
45. Wu M-J, et al. Effectiveness and safety of apixaban and warfarin in patients with new- onset atrial fibrillation after advanced chronic kidney disease or end-stage kidney disease. Heart Rhythm. 2025;22(5):1197–209.

Chapter 10
Heart Failure and Renal Dysfunction

Ahmet Murt

10.1 Introduction

Chronic kidney disease (CKD) is a major global public health concern, affecting more than 10% of the adult population worldwide [1]. Owing to the close physiological communication between cardiovascular and renal systems, CKD is substantially more common among patients with heart failure (HF); over 40% of individuals with HF exhibit some degree of renal impairment [2]. In the other direction, patients with CKD also have a markedly elevated risk of developing HF—more than 20%, compared with only 5% among individuals without CKD [3].

The coexistence of heart failure and renal dysfunction represents one of the most challenging intersections in clinical medicine. These two conditions are profoundly interdependent, frequently coexist, and synergistically amplify each other's morbidity and mortality. CKD significantly increases the risk of hospitalization and death among patients with HF, while cardiovascular disease remains the leading cause of mortality in individuals with CKD and end-stage kidney disease (ESKD) [4].

Heart failure may present with reduced ejection fraction (HFrEF) or preserved ejection fraction (HFpEF). Traditionally, kidney injury in HF has been attributed to reduced cardiac output and subsequent renal hypoperfusion in HFrEF which is further complicated by induction of neurohormonal pathways—including the renin–angiotensin–aldosterone system (RAAS) and sympathetic nervous system. Although disease patterns may be slightly different, HFpEF is also an important entity, particularly among elderly, hypertensive, and diabetic individuals [5]. In HFpEF, renal dysfunction is driven primarily by venous congestion and elevated filling pressures.

A. Murt (✉)
Istanbul University-Cerrahpasa, Cerrahpasa Medical Faculty, Nephrology Department, Istanbul, Turkey
e-mail: ahmet.murt@iuc.edu.tr

A. Covic, A. Burlacu (eds.), *Renal Dysfunction in Cardiovascular Pathologies*,
https://doi.org/10.1007/978-3-032-25434-4_10

Importantly, both HF phenotypes are characterized by sodium and water retention, leading to progressive congestion.

Chronic kidney disease (CKD) symbolizes irreversible reduction in kidney function lasting more than 3 months, defined by a persistently reduced estimated glomerular filtration rate (eGFR <60 mL/min/1.73 m^2), evidence of kidney damage (e.g., albuminuria, structural abnormalities), or both. CKD reflects progressive loss of nephron mass driven by conditions such as diabetes, hypertension, glomerular diseases, and aging. CKD increases the risk of cardiovascular disease, hospitalization, and mortality, and may eventually lead to end-stage kidney disease requiring dialysis or transplantation.

Acute kidney injury (AKI), on the other hand, is a sudden decline in kidney function occurring over hours to days, characterized by a rapid rise in serum creatinine, a reduction in urine output, or both. It is common in hospitalized and critically ill patients and is associated with higher mortality, prolonged hospitalization, and an increased long-term risk of CKD.

Heart failure may be among the many other causes of both AKI and CKD. Such an interrelation may be attributed to reduced cardiac output, increased venous congestion and activation of neurohormonal pathways. It should be underlined here that recurrent episodes of AKI may be a reason for CKD progression, and HF patients often have hypertension, diabetes, older age, and vascular disease—each of which may accelerate the progression of CKD.

The bidirectional interaction between cardiac and renal dysfunction is captured by the concept of Cardiorenal Syndrome (CRS), encompassing disorders in which acute or chronic dysfunction of one organ precipitates acute or chronic dysfunction of the other. Recent understanding of CRS has evolved beyond simple hemodynamic explanations to cover a complex pathophysiological continuum involving neurohormonal dysregulation, inflammation, oxidative stress and endothelial dysfunction. In addition, as obesity and type 2 diabetes may be associated both with cardiovascular pathologies and CKD, there's an increasing research and data that accumulate around the terminology of cardiovascular-kidney-metabolic (CKM) syndrome.

Despite advances in HF and CKD management, outcomes still remain poor [6]. Patients with combined HF and renal impairment frequently face therapeutic limitations, including diuretic resistance, difficulty achieving adequate decongestion, and hesitancy to initiate guideline-directed therapies due to concerns about possible renal deterioration.

The aim of this chapter is to provide a brief overview of the pathophysiological interplay between the heart and kidneys, elucidate mechanisms underlying the maladaptive cross-talk, and offer practical, evidence-based strategies to optimize management in patients with concomitant HF and kidney diseases.

10.2 The Cardio-Renal Axis

10.2.1 The Cardiorenal Syndrome Concept

The cardiorenal syndrome involves a spectrum of disorders in which heart failure and chronic kidney disease interact through complex feedback mechanisms. The most widely used classification, proposed by Ronco and colleagues in 2008, categorizes CRS into five distinct subtypes based on the primary organ initiating the injury and the acuity of the process (Table 10.1) [7]. Patient history, physical examination, laboratory tests and imaging studies may help to reveal the initial pathology. However, as there are many additional pathways (neurohormonal and inflammatory) that are activated independent of any proposed CRS type, it's not always possible to define the triggering acute or chronic event and to exactly diagnose which type of CRS a patient has. The authors of this chapter do not recommend that physicians limit their clinical approach to a patient by trying to define the CRS type. An alternative, pathophysiology-based definition was proposed by Hatamizadeh et al., who categorized CRS as hemodynamic, uremic, vascular, neurohumoral, anemia-related, mineral metabolism-related or malnutrition/inflammation-related [8]. More than a trial to fit patients into some pre-defined concepts, these taxonomies emphasize that CRS is a pathophysiological spectrum, not a single-isolated disease, which necessitates tailored diagnostic and therapeutic approaches.

Among the 5 CRS classes, it's estimated that chronic forms, especially type 2, are generally more common. However, type 1 CRS is the one with the most available literature [9]. In type 1 CRS, acute decompensated heart failure is responsible for an acute kidney injury episode. This group of patients are frequently

Table 10.1 Five types of cardiorenal syndrome

Type	Primary organ affected	Sequence of injury	Clinical example
Type 1—acute	Heart (cardiorenal)	Acute HF or cardiogenic shock causing AKI	Acute decompensated HF with a rapid rise in serum creatinine
Type 2—chronic	Heart (cardiorenal)	Chronic HF leading to progressive CKD	Dilated cardiomyopathy with chronic, slow renal decline
Type 3—acute	Kidney (renocardiac)	AKI precipitating acute cardiac dysfunction	Contrast nephropathy leading to acute pulmonary edema or arrhythmia
Type 4—chronic	Kidney (renocardiac)	CKD promoting structural/functional cardiac disease	Left ventricular (LV) hypertrophy, myocardial fibrosis, and diastolic dysfunction in CKD
Type 5—secondary (systemic)	Both systems	Systemic disorder injuring both heart and kidney	Sepsis, amyloidosis, systemic lupus erythematosus, or advanced diabetes mellitus

Abbreviations: *AKI* acute kidney injury, *CKD* chronic kidney disease, *HF* heart failure hospitalized, resulting in the availability of large clinical datasets that make them common subjects of clinical research. Despite this, there are still major treatment uncertainties in the acute setting (mainly type 1 CRS), including optimal diuretic dosing and strategy, interpretation of worsening kidney functions during decongestive therapy, use of inotropes and use of ultrafiltration.

10.2.2 The Cardiovascular-Kidney-Metabolic Syndrome Concept

Cardiovascular–Kidney–Metabolic (CKM) syndrome is a recently formalized clinical concept that describes the interconnected and mutually reinforcing abnormalities of the cardiovascular system, kidneys, and metabolic pathways, particularly obesity, insulin resistance, and type 2 diabetes. Rather than viewing these conditions as separate entities, CKM syndrome recognizes their shared pathophysiology, which drives a markedly increased risk of cardiovascular events, chronic kidney disease (CKD) progression, heart failure, and all-cause mortality [10].

CKM syndrome is underpinned by chronic low-grade inflammation, oxidative stress, insulin resistance, endothelial dysfunction, activation of the RAAS, and adipose tissue dysregulation, all of which contribute to cardiovascular remodeling, renal microvascular injury, and metabolic deterioration [11]. These mechanisms create a multidirectional and self-perpetuating cycle in which metabolic dysfunction accelerates renal and cardiovascular disease, while both heart and kidney impairment further impair metabolic homeostasis.

Patients with CKM syndrome commonly have hypertension, albuminuria, atherosclerosis, HFpEF, arrhythmias, and progressive CKD—reflecting the systemic and multi-organ nature of the disorder [12]. The introduction of CKM staging by the American Heart Association provides a structured framework ranging from early metabolic risk (Stages 0–2) to advanced cardiovascular or kidney disease (Stage 4), underscoring that intervention opportunities exist across the disease continuum [11]. This model reshapes preventive cardiology and nephrology by highlighting the central role of metabolic disease as a driver of cardiorenal pathology, particularly in populations with obesity and diabetes.

Among the treatment strategies that are also shared in a separate section below, sodium–glucose cotransporter-2 inhibitors (SGLT2i), are the main drugs of CKM syndrome today, both with their antidiabetic characteristics and modulatory effects on hemodynamic and neurohormonal pathways. Glucagon-like peptide receptor agonists (GLP-1RA) also gained popularity, especially in patients with an obesity component. GLP-1RAs have the potential to exert protective effects for CKD as well [13].

10.3 Pathophysiology

The underlying mechanisms driving CRS are multifaceted and form a kind of vicious cycle of mutually destructive processes. Some main concepts should be reviewed to better delineate the treatment strategies.

10.3.1 Hemodynamic Mechanisms

While reduced cardiac output in HF leads to decreased renal perfusion pressure and a theoretical risk of ischemia, with many HF patients that have normal ejection pressure, current evidence shows that venous congestion plays a more prominent role [14]. Elevated central venous pressure (CVP) increases renal venous congestion. This congestion elevates renal interstitial pressure, compressing the tubules and reducing the transglomerular filtration gradient, which is now recognized as a stronger determinant of worsening renal function than low cardiac output alone. An increase in right atrial pressure is among the determinants of worsening kidney function, independent of cardiac output. That's why preservation of ejection fraction should not provide any reassurance in clinical evaluation to rule out CRS. One of the theoretically sound hemodynamic terms is kidney perfusion pressure, quantified as the difference between mean arterial pressure and CVP. Ideal kidney perfusion pressure is more than 60 mmHg.

Persistent congestion also impairs tubular oxygen delivery and triggers interstitial inflammation, leading to irreversible kidney damage over time. As there may also be a creatinine rise due to hemodynamic changes, distinguishing such pseudo-AKI from real AKI has gained popularity. Though none are perfect, many biomarkers, including Neutrophil Gelatinase-Associated Lipocalin (NGAL) or Kidney Injury Molecule-1 (KIM-1), might help to define true AKI (structural changes) [15]. On the other side, galectin-3 and BNP / NT-proBNP are markers of congestion. Their levels may fluctuate with impaired kidney function; however, a rising trend in subsequent measurements may point to sustained congestion.

Heart failure may cause abdominal ascites. An increase in intraabdominal pressure may cause compression of renal veins and other kidney structures, resulting in a decrease of GFR. Increasing levels of intraabdominal pressure can be related to a bad prognosis, and resultant kidney injury has been demonstrated with release of tubular injury markers [16]. When intraabdominal pressure exceeds 20 mmHg, the condition is called abdominal compartment syndrome, and this may eventually lead to a kind of "kidney tamponade" [17]. Especially for HF patients who start to have a gradual increase in their ascites volume, decongestion strategies (diuretics, paracentesis or ultrafiltration) should be commenced early to avoid intraabdominal hypertension, which is another risk factor for progressive kidney injury.

10.3.2 Neurohormonal and Inflammatory Pathways

The body's compensatory response to decreased cardiac output involves the robust activation of the RAAS and also the sympathetic nervous system. This leads to sodium and water retention and systemic vasoconstriction, initially aiming to maintain the systemic perfusion. These systems may help to compensate for initial changes to some extent. However, chronic activation of these systems promotes myocardial fibrosis, glomerulosclerosis, and endothelial dysfunction, perpetuating both cardiac and renal injuries.

In congested kidneys, interstitial edema leads to capillary compression, which causes the release of cytokines from endothelial injury. Inflammatory mediators such as IL-6 and IL-18 are elevated, promoting further endothelial injury, increased vascular permeability, and adverse myocardial remodeling [18]. Activation of RAAS, with resultant increase in angiotensin-2, is also a driver of inflammation. The chronic inflammatory milieu causes ongoing renal injury. Oxidative stress complicates the process by damaging renal tubular cells and reducing nitric oxide bioavailability, which further worsens vasoconstriction and tissue hypoxia.

10.4 Diagnostic Approach

The diagnostic evaluation in CRS aims to accurately quantify cardiac and renal function, assess volume status, and identify reversible causes of organ dysfunction.

10.4.1 Laboratory Assessment

Serum creatinine and eGFR still remain the standard laboratory tests but it should be underlined that creatinine is a relatively late marker of renal injury, and it only reflects changes once a substantial amount of kidney function is lost. Also, it may not differentiate between true AKI or reversible functional/hemodynamic changes. Cystatin C provides a potentially more accurate estimation of GFR, as it is less affected by muscle mass, age, or diet. Increased blood urea nitrogen (BUN) may also be related to poor prognosis in HF patients. A disproportionate increase in BUN relative to creatinine is a sign of reduced renal perfusion. In the outpatient management of heart failure, microalbuminuria should be carefully monitored and treated, as it is a marker of RAAS activation and is strongly associated with increased cardiovascular and renal events. Conventional definitions flag urine albümine-to-creatinine ratio (uACR) $\geq$ 30 mg/g as significant albuminuria [19]; however, in a cardiorenal context, any persistent or rising albuminuria should prompt closer monitoring and proactive management.

In the acute setting, for earlier detection of AKI in HF patients, markers like Neutrophil gelatinase–associated lipocalin (NGAL) and Kidney Injury Molecule-1 (KIM-1) are becoming increasingly important. NGAL rises in the first hours of tubular injury and may differentiate between true injury and hemodynamic creatinine fluctuations. NGAL may be measured in urine or serum. KIM-1 is highly specific for proximal tubular injury. Apart from biomarker-based approach, tracking changes in creatinine and urine output during aggressive decongestion may also help to differentiate true renal injury from the often-benign, hemodynamically mediated changes.

Pseudo-AKI (also called functional AKI or hemodynamic AKI) refers to an apparent rise in serum creatinine that does not represent true structural kidney injury.Instead, it reflects changes in renal hemodynamics and filtration pressure, often occurring during treatment of heart failure. Hemoconcentration with fluid removal also contributes to this phenomenon. Mild, transient rises in creatinine during decongestion (often defined as <30% increase or <0.3 mg/dL rise) are generally considered acceptable outcomes of effective volume removal and are also called permissive AKI. Hemoconcentration-associated pseudo-AKI is a sign of better decongestion and may be related to improved prognosis [20].

10.4.2 Imaging and Functional Assessment

Echocardiography is the essential imaging study in probable CRS patients for assessing left ventricular (LV) function, diastolic parameters, and the estimation of right-sided pressures and pulmonary hypertension. Right atrial pressure has been shown to be an important indicator of baseline renal function in CRS patients. In normal ultrasonographic evaluation, the inferior vena cava (IVC) is smaller than 2.1 cm in diameter and has more than 50% collapsibility. In systemic congestion, the IVC is found to be bigger in size with reduced collapsibility. When systemic venous pressure rises—evidenced by a dilated, non-collapsible (IVC)—this pressure is transmitted retrogradely through the renal veins into the renal capillaries and interstitium. In renal congestion, renal doppler ultrasound may detect renal venous pulsatility and increased resistivity indices that show congestion and kidney parenchymal injury, respectively. Lung ultrasound may help identify pulmonary congestion. B-lines, which are vertical hyperechoic lines arising from the pleural line, are the hallmarks of pulmonary congestion. The number of B-lines correlates with LV filling pressures, wedge pressure, and natriuretic peptide. With increasing congestion, pleural effusions additionally occur. Bioimpedance Analysis is a non-invasive method that quantifies total body water and may provide a dynamic assessment of volume status.

10.5 Clinical Management: Integrated Cardiorenal Care

Management of heart failure patients who also have CKD is complex, requiring a multidisciplinary approach involving cardiologists and nephrologists to achieve the treatment goals. There are three components of treatment for CRS from the acute period to the long-term follow-up (Fig. 10.1).

1. In the acute phase, the aim is to relieve congestion without inducing severe hypotension. The hemodynamic effect of decongestive therapy may cause elevations in the creatinine levels. Such elevations may mean that the decongestive therapy was clinically effective.
2. To improve long-term survival, evidence-based, guideline-directed medical therapies (GDMT) should be commenced for cardioprotection and nephroprotection.
3. Nephrotoxins should be avoided and comorbid conditions such as diabetes should be managed. Diabetes is a common etiology for cardiovascular and kidney diseases.

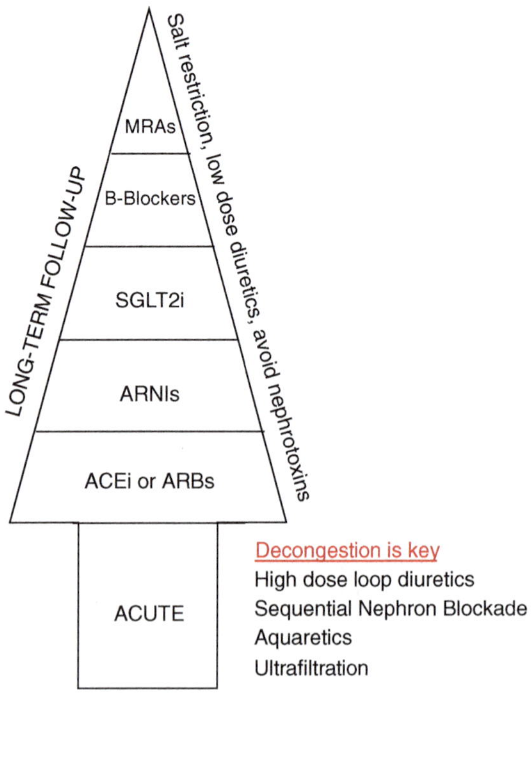

Fig. 10.1 The treatment approach in cardiorenal syndrome from acute setting to longer follow-up

10.5.1 Diuretic Therapy and Decongestion

Loop diuretics remain the cornerstone for achieving decongestion. Patients with CKD often require higher doses or more frequent dosing due to impaired tubular delivery and reduced nephron mass. The starting dose of loop diuretics in any acute decompensation of heart failure is at least 2.5 times their routinely prescribed dose. The starting dose should be between 40 and 80 mg if the patient was not taking furosemide before. The DOSE trial specifically evaluated this approach and found that such a dose resulted in better symptom relief and net fluid loss [21]. The intravenous (IV) route should be preferred for better pharmacodynamics, as gut edema may limit absorption. A common goal is to create 0.5 to 1 kg weight loss daily. However, 24 h may be a long period to wait for a diuretic response. Urine output less than 300 mL after 2 h of diuretic dosing may be a clue for reduced effect. Monitoring urine sodium concentrations is also helpful to check for diuretic efficiency and a concentration of less than 50 mmol/L 1–2 h after diuretic administration may be indicative of poor response. In the case of improper response, doubling the furosemide dose may be a good strategy and the total furosemide dose may be increased to 500 mg/day. Furosemide also has a ceiling dose (i.e., does not provide additional effect if that dose is exceeded). The ceiling dose of furosemide in patients with normal kidney function is 80 mg (dosed twice Daily—BID), while this increases to 240 mg BID in CKD stage 4. Although couldn't be proved by controlled trials, shifting from bolus to continuous infusion of loop diuretics can maintain steady natriuresis, potentially reducing the phenomenon of post-diuretic sodium retention. Torsemide may be an alternative with better bioavailability in the outpatient setting; however, a mortality benefit couldn't be shown in trials where torsemide was compared with furosemide [22].

When applied over their threshold dose, loop diuretics maintain natriuresis for some hours. After that, a period of very limited natriuresis is observed. That period is called post-diuretic sodium retention. To still maintain the negative sodium balance in this retention period, dietary salt restriction is quite important. Moderate sodium restriction—around 2 gr per day—is recommended in cardiorenal syndrome to reduce congestion, enhance the effectiveness of diuretics, and prevent neurohormonal activation.

Prolonged use of loop diuretics may cause distal tubular hypertrophy, which results in more sodium absorption via the thiazide-sensitive sodium chloride cotransporter in the distal convoluted tubule and epithelial sodium channel (ENaC) in the collecting duct. This is one of the reasons for diuretic resistance. Combining the loop diuretic with a thiazide may help alleviate this resistance, as shown in the CLOROTIC trial, which was on hospitalized patients with acute HF [23]. Limitations of such combinations are that creatinine levels may increase with increased diuresis and that thiazide diuretics may lose their effectiveness with decreasing GFR. Other strategies are combining loop diuretics with spironolactone, acetozolomide or SGLT2i. The strategy of combining diuretics of different classes for better decongestion is called sequential nephron blockade (SNB). All such combinations served for relief from congestion; only the addition of SGLT2i could provide a survival benefit.

The tubuloglomerular feedback (TGF) mechanism is one of the most important adaptive regulatory systems of the nephron. The macula densa in the distal tubule senses luminal NaCl concentration and adjusts afferent arteriolar tone accordingly. High NaCl delivery activates TGF and causes afferent vasoconstriction, reducing GFR, whereas low NaCl suppresses TGF, causing afferent vasodilation and an increase in GFR. Loop diuretics inhibit the Na^+–K^+–$2Cl^-$ cotransporter (NKCC2) in the thick ascending limb, which also serves as the sensing mechanism for NaCl at the macula densa. By blocking NKCC2, loop diuretics impair NaCl sensing, leading to suppression of TGF and afferent arteriolar vasodilation. This vasodilation increases GFR, enhances tubular flow, and initially augments the diuretic response. Thiazide diuretics, on the other hand, act distally and increase NaCl delivery to the macula densa, enhancing TGF activity, producing afferent vasoconstriction, and potentially lowering GFR, particularly in volume-depleted patients. In states of congestion, as in heart failure or cardiorenal syndrome, the normal TGF response becomes blunted due to neurohormonal activation, impaired renal perfusion, and elevated venous pressure. Acetazolamide, a proximal tubular carbonic anhydrase inhibitor, increases NaCl delivery to the macula densa but generates a bicarbonate-rich tubular fluid that modulates the macula densa signaling environment and prevents excessive TGF activation. This may explain the enhanced decongestion observed in the ADVOR trial [24], where acetazolamide improved natriuretic efficiency in acute decompensated heart failure. TGF triggered by different diuretics and their clinical effects are given in Table 10.2.

In HF patients, there's increased activity of antidiuretic hormone (vasopressin). Tolvaptan is a vasopressin 2 receptor antagonist that creates free water removal. Its mechanism of action makes it a preferred treatment for hyponatremia in HF. Tolvaptan was shown to induce an increase in urine output in the EVEREST trial, but this effect couldn't be extended to a positive effect on overall survival [25].

Dopamine does not provide any mortality benefit in acute CRS, even at low "renal" doses (i.e., 1–3 μg/kg/min) [26]. It may even have detrimental side effects

Table 10.2 Tubuloglomerular feedback (TGF) mechanisms by different diuretics

Drugs	Effect on macula densa	Effect on TGF	Resultant GFR	Clinical meaning
Loop diuretics	Block NKCC2	Disable TGF	Increase	Enhances diuretic efficiency
Thiazides	Increase NaCl delivery	Activate TGF	Decrease	Potent diuresis but creatinine may rise
Acetazolamide	Bicarbonate-rich NaCl delivery	Mild TGF effect	Generally neutral	Improves proximal natriuresis
SGLT2 inhibitors	Increase NaCl delivery	*Activate TGF*	Initial decline with decreased IGP.	Kidney-protective in the long term

Abbreviations: *IGP* intraglomerular pressure, *NKCC2* Na^+–K^+–$2Cl^-$ cotransporter, *SGLT2* sodium glucose cotransporter-2, *TGF* tubuloglomerular feedback, *GFR* glomerular filtration rate such as induction of arrhythmias and increasing myocardial oxygen demand. Another inotrope, dobutamine, which is a β-1 agonist, is also not recommended, but it can be considered only in cardiogenic shock.

10.5.2 Neurohormonal Modulation: Guideline-Directed Medical Therapy (GDMT)

As neurohormonal pathways are activated from the early stages of CRS, optimizing GDMT is also paramount for long-term survival.

ACE Inhibitors and angiotensin II receptor blockers (ARB) are essential for reducing afterload, inhibiting cardiac remodeling, and improving survival in HF, especially for HFrEF. A modest, asymptomatic rise in creatinine (up to 30% from baseline) is often acceptable and should not prompt discontinuation of these drugs, which have clear long-term survival benefits. The authors of this chapter recommend taking all precautions to sustain RAAS inhibition in CRS patients. Enalapril (BID) is the preferred ACE inhibitor in heart failure due to the strongest clinical trial evidence, while lisinopril and ramipril (both are dosed once daily—QD) are widely accepted alternatives. Among ARBs, valsartan (BID) and candesartan (QD) are the most effective choices in HF.

Angiotensin Receptor-Neprilysin Inhibitors (ARNIs), such as sacubitril/valsartan, offer additional survival benefit by providing dual neurohormonal modulation, especially in patients with HFrEF. This combination provided a lower eGFR decline when compared to RAAS inhibitors alone [27]. ARNIs are used twice daily to provide continuous neurohormonal modulation. ARNIs are found to be safe and effective also in later stages of CKD, but they're not recommended in the dialysis population yet. It should be noted that albuminuria may increase with the use of ARNIs. This may be related to a vasodilatory effect on the afferent arteriole.

β-Blockers are essential for the control of heart rate and inhibition of overactive sympathetic tone. Dosing often requires careful titration, but these are generally safe in moderate CKD. Carvedilol, bisoprolol, and metoprolol succinate are the three beta-blockers proven to reduce mortality in HFrEF. Among them, carvedilol is often considered the most potent due to additional α1-blocking effects and strong trial data, bisoprolol is the best tolerated and highly cardio-selective, and metoprolol succinate offers convenient once-daily dosing with proven survival benefit. Neither of these three needs dose reductions with decreasing eGFR in CRS patients. There's no evidence to recommend any other beta-blockers for HFrEF. Also, beta-blockers didn't provide a survival benefit for HFpEF. However, they should still be used in HFpEF patients when there's background ischemic heart disease.

Although many patients with CRS are already taking RAAS inhibitors, with a phenomenon called aldosterone breakthrough, some residual aldosterone activity persists. Spironolactone as a mineralocorticoid receptor antagonist (MRA) may provide additional mortality benefit, especially in HFrEF, by potentially blocking this aldosterone breakthrough effect [28]. Spironolactone may reduce congestion and further modulate RAAS activation. However, their use requires strict vigilance for hyperkalemia, particularly when the eGFR falls below 45 mL/min/1.73 m^2. A new class of MRAs, finerenone has a non-steroidal structure, is equally distributed between the heart and kidney, has higher MR selectivity, causes fewer side effects and causes relatively fewer hyperkalemia episodes than spironolactone. With these properties finerenone has provided benefits for renal and cardiac outcomes in many recent trials [29]. However, finerenone can't be used in CKD patients who have an eGFR of lower than 25 mL/min/1.73 m^2.

Patients with CRS experience higher rates of medication-related adverse events—such as worsening renal function, hyperkalemia, hypotension, and electrolyte imbalance—because of reduced kidney reserve, neurohormonal activation, and fluctuating hemodynamics. However, most adverse effects are predictable, preventable, and manageable. Every effort should be made to continue GDMT in HF patients as these treatments offer a clear survival benefit. Hyperkalemia is the main reason that limits the use of RAAS inhibitors and ARNIs. Starting with low doses, gradually increasing the dose, avoiding other K-raising agents (such as non-steroidal anti-inflammatory drugs- NSAIDs), correcting metabolic acidosis, a combination of diuretics (loop + thiazide) and relevant use of potassium binders may help to mitigate hyperkalemic effects. To limit the hemodynamic side effects, the volume status of the patients should be carefully followed up on, which will avoid unnecessary longer use of high-dose diuretics.

10.5.3 SGLT2 Inhibitors

SGLT2i, such as dapagliflozin and empagliflozin, demonstrated robust simultaneous cardiac and renal protection across all HF phenotypes (HFrEF and HFpEF). They induce osmotic diuresis, lower intraglomerular pressure (via afferent arteriolar vasoconstriction), improve myocardial energy balance, and possess anti-inflammatory and anti-fibrotic effects. Major trials consistently showed a lower risk of HF hospitalization and slowed progression of renal decline [30, 31]. SGLT2i can be safely initiated and continued in most patients until eGFR drops below 20 to 25 mL/min/1.73 m^2. An expected small fall in eGFR with the initiation of SGLT2i is typically transient and benign. An initial 30% increase in creatinine levels with 10% decline in eGFR is acceptable and should not prompt discontinuation of SGLT2i. Progressive increases in creatinine levels with hypotension, vomiting and dehydration should be warning signs to halt SGLT2i. The kidney-protective role of SGLT2i is obvious in the longer follow-ups. More importantly, with concomitant use of SGLT2i, hemodynamic stability is better preserved and adverse effects of GDMTs such as hyperkalemia and AKI had a decreasing trend. This is related to increased sodium delivery to distal nephron segments, which eventually promotes kaliuresis. Such effect is important for the continuous preservation of RAASi use

[32]. In a similar manner, use of SGLT2i also decreases the rate of MRA discontinuation [33].

10.5.4 Advanced Strategies

Ultrafiltration (UF): Mechanical fluid removal is reserved for patients with true diuretic resistance or persistent, refractory volume overload. Reasons for diuretic resistance include decreased absorption due to gut edema, reduced transport of furosemide in hypoalbuminemic conditions, free anions in the uremic milieu may compete for their release and drugs like NSAIDs may decrease their tubular secretion. CKD may be another factor for diuretic resistance with reduced nephron number. During decongestive therapy, diuretic resistance can be detected early by urine sodium level. If diuretic resistance can't be resolved by increasing doses of diuretics, SNB, or other strategies shared in Table 10.3, ultrafiltration may be preferred for decongestion. Earlier UNLOAD trial showed that UF could provide clinically significant fluid loss [34]. The CARRESS-HF trial, while showing no superiority to stepped pharmacologic therapy and a higher rate of adverse events, confirms that UF remains an option in carefully selected cases [35]. This should underline that UNLOAD and CARESS-HF trials used pre-defined UF rates; the need for UF may fluctuate on a daily basis. A later trial (AVOID) showed that adjustable UF according to patient needs could provide reduced hospitalizations [36].

Peritoneal dialysis (PD) may be another alternative. It may reduce chronic congestion, improve functional status, and lower rehospitalization rates. PD is especially useful in patients with diuretic resistance, recurrent admissions, or intolerance to intermittent hemodialysis. Although large randomized trials are lacking, observational data strongly support its role in managing advanced heart failure complicated by renal dysfunction [37]. Especially, the addition of icodextrin enhances

Table 10.3 Reasons for diuretic resistance in cardiorenal syndrome and possible solutions

Reasons of diuretic resistance	Solution
Low-dose administration (below threshold)	Doubling the dose
High-dietary sodium	Salt restriction
Diminished intestinal absorption	Preferring the IV route
Impaired drug secretion in the tubules	Abstaining from competing drugs (e.g., NSAIDs)
More distal sodium delivery	Sequential nephron blockade
Hypoalbuminemia	Albumin replacement
Neurohormonal activation	Using baseline RAASi
Severe uremia	Consider hemodialysis, peritoneal dialysis or ultrafiltration

Abbreviations: *IV* intravenous, *NSAID* non-steroidal anti-inflammatory drugs, *RAAS* renin-angiotensin-aldosterone system long-dwell ultrafiltration, improves volume control in fast peritoneal transporters, reduces glucose load, and allows for better long-term management of fluid overload.

10.6 Prognosis and Conclusion

Key clinical outcomes in patients with heart failure and CKD include; mortality (mortality risk rises progressively with declining eGFR and increasing albuminuria), higher rates of hospitalization and rehospitalization, progression of kidney disease, diuretic resistance (leads to refractory congestion, more frequent hospitalizations, and need for advanced therapies), higher risk of hyperkalemia and metabolic complications, increased risk of arrhythmias and reduced quality of life.

Renal dysfunction remains one of the strongest independent predictors of adverse outcomes and mortality in HF. Even a mild decline in eGFR confers substantial risk. Key prognostic indicators in CRS include: persistent congestion after discharge, high levels of NT-proBNP, a progressive eGFR decline (>5 mL/min/year), and the presence of albuminuria.

The modern management of CRS requires early recognition, integrated multidisciplinary care, and the judicious use of therapies that simultaneously protect both the heart and the kidney. The emergence of SGLT2 inhibitors, new non-steroidal MRA finerenone and refined decongestive strategies has substantially improved outcomes, marking a new era in cardiorenal care. However, CRS remains a major cause of morbidity and mortality, making collaborative heart–kidney programs and ongoing research essential for improving patient survival.

Conflicts of Interest None declared.

Declarations

Competing Interests The author(s) has no competing interests to declare that are relevant to the content of this manuscript.

Ethics Approval The author(s) declares that this manuscript does not include primary research with human participants.

The author(s) declares that this manuscript does not include primary studies involving animals.

References

1. Francis A, Harhay MN, Ong ACM, et al. Chronic kidney disease and the global public health agenda: an international consensus. Nat Rev Nephrol. 2024;20(7):473–85.
2. Parmar SS, Muthuppalaniappan V, Banerjee D. Gaps in modern heart failure and chronic kidney disease research. Eur Cardiol. 2023;18:e51. https://doi.org/10.15420/ecr.2022.64.

3. House AA, Wanner C, Sarnak MJ, et al. Heart failure in chronic kidney disease: conclusions from a kidney disease: improving global outcomes (KDIGO) controversies conference. Kidney Int. 2019;95(6):1304–17.
4. Bhandari SK, Zhou H, Shaw SF, et al. Causes of death in end-stage kidney disease: comparison between the United States renal data system and a large integrated health care system. Am J Nephrol. 2022;53(1):32–40.
5. Sobue Y, Watanabe E, Yanase M, Izawa H. Distinct mortality patterns and sudden cardiac death mechanisms in heart failure with a preserved ejection fraction. Sci Rep. 2025;15(1):37048.
6. Woodruff RC, Tong X, Khan SS, et al. Trends in cardiovascular disease mortality rates and excess deaths, 2010-2022. Am J Prev Med. 2024;66(4):582–9.
7. Ronco C, Haapio M, House AA, Anavekar N, Bellomo R. Cardiorenal syndrome. J Am Coll Cardiol. 2008;52(19):1527–39.
8. Hatamizadeh P, Fonarow GC, Budoff MJ, Darabian S, Kovesdy CP, Kalantar-Zadeh K. Cardiorenal syndrome: pathophysiology and potential targets for clinical management. Nat Rev Nephrol. 2013;9(2):99–111.
9. Uduman J. Epidemiology of cardiorenal syndrome. Adv Chronic Kidney Dis. 2018;25(5):391–9.
10. Ndumele CE, Neeland IJ, Tuttle KR, et al. A synopsis of the evidence for the science and clinical management of Cardiovascular-Kidney-Metabolic (CKM) syndrome: a scientific statement from the American Heart Association. Circulation. 2023;148(20):1636–64.
11. Zhang H, Huang S, Fang Y, Zhang H, Yang W, Yu M. Insulin resistance assessed by estimated glucose disposal rate predicts cardiovascular disease in stages 0-3 of cardiovascular-kidney-metabolic syndrome: a UK biobank cohort study. Cardiovasc Diabetol. 2025;24(1):360. https://doi.org/10.1186/s12933-025-02860-z.
12. Bansal N, Weiner D, Sarnak M. Cardiovascular-kidney-metabolic health syndrome: what does the American Heart Association framework mean for nephrology? J Am Soc Nephrol. 2024;35(5):649–52.
13. Taal MW, Selby NM. Glucagon-like peptide-1 receptor agonists: new evidence of kidney and cardiovascular protection from the FLOW and SELECT trials. Am J Kidney Dis. 2025;85(1):115–8.
14. Anju N, Vic H, Amanda S, et al. Cardiorenal interactions. J Am Coll Cardiol. 2008;51:1268–74.
15. Bhavsar NA, Köttgen A, Coresh J, Astor BC. Neutrophil gelatinase-associated lipocalin (NGAL) and kidney injury molecule 1 (KIM-1) as predictors of incident CKD stage 3: the Atherosclerosis Risk in Communities (ARIC) study. Am J Kidney Dis. 2012 Aug;60(2):233–40.
16. Muğlu H, İnan Kahraman E, Sünger E, Murt A, Bilici A, Görgülü N. Acute kidney injury secondary to abdominal compartment syndrome: biomarkers, pressure variability, and clinical outcomes. Medicina (Kaunas). 2025;61(3):383.
17. Boorsma EM, Ter Maaten JM, Voors AA, van Veldhuisen DJ. Renal compression in heart failure: the renal tamponade hypothesis. JACC Heart Fail. 2022;10(3):175–83.
18. Virzì GM, Breglia A, Brocca A, et al. Levels of proinflammatory cytokines, oxidative stress, and tissue damage markers in patients with acute heart failure with and without cardiorenal syndrome type 1. Cardiorenal Med. 2018;8(4):321–31.
19. Kidney Disease: Improving Global Outcomes (KDIGO) CKD Work Group. KDIGO 2024 Clinical Practice Guideline for the Evaluation and Management of Chronic Kidney Disease. Kidney Int. 2024;105(4S):S117–314.
20. Martins JL, Santos L, Faustino A, Viana J, Santos J. Worsening or 'pseudo-worsening' renal function? The prognostic value of hemoconcentration in patients admitted with acute heart failure. Rev Port Cardiol (Engl Ed). 2018;37(7):595–602.
21. Felker GM, Lee KL, Bull DA, et al. Diuretic strategies in patients with acute decompensated heart failure. N Engl J Med. 2011;364(9):797–805.
22. Effect of torsemide vs furosemide after discharge on all-cause mortality in patients hospitalized with heart failure: the TRANSFORM-HF randomized clinical trial. JAMA. 2023;329(3):214–23.

23. Trullàs JC, Morales-Rull JL, Casado J, et al. Combining loop with thiazide diuretics for decompensated heart failure: the CLOROTIC trial. Eur Heart J. 2023;44(5):411–21.
24. Mullens W, Dauw J, Martens P, et al. Acetazolamide in acute decompensated heart failure with volume overload. N Engl J Med. 2022;387(13):1185–95.
25. Konstam MA, Gheorghiade M, Burnett JC Jr, et al. Efficacy of Vasopressin Antagonism in Heart Failure Outcome Study With Tolvaptan (EVEREST) Investigators. Effects of oral tolvaptan in patients hospitalized for worsening heart failure: the EVEREST outcome trial. JAMA. 2007;297(12):1319–31.
26. Chen HH, Anstrom KJ, Givertz MM, et al. Low-dose dopamine or low-dose nesiritide in acute heart failure with renal dysfunction: the ROSE acute heart failure randomized trial. JAMA. 2013;310(23):2533–43.
27. Covic A, Voroneanu L, Stefan AE, et al. Comparative renal effects of angiotensin receptor neprilysin inhibitors and ACEi/ARB: a systematic review and meta-analysis. Clin Kidney J. 2025;18(8):sfaf224.
28. Pitt B, Zannad F, Remme WJ, et al. The effect of spironolactone on morbidity and mortality in patients with severe heart failure. Randomized Aldactone Evaluation Study Investigators. N Engl J Med. 1999;341(10):709–17.
29. Vaduganathan M, Filippatos G, Claggett BL, et al. Finerenone in heart failure and chronic kidney disease with type 2 diabetes: FINE-HEART pooled analysis of cardiovascular, kidney and mortality outcomes. Nat Med. 2024;30(12):3758–64.
30. Solomon SD, McMurray JJV, Claggett B, et al. Dapagliflozin in heart failure with mildly reduced or preserved ejection fraction. N Engl J Med. 2022;387(12):1089–98.
31. Packer M, Anker SD, Butler J, et al. Cardiovascular and renal outcomes with Empagliflozin in heart failure. N Engl J Med. 2020;383(15):1413–24.
32. Fletcher RA, Jongs N, Chertow GM, et al. Effect of SGLT2 inhibitors on discontinuation of renin-angiotensin system blockade: a joint analysis of the CREDENCE and DAPA-CKD trials. J Am Soc Nephrol. 2023;34(12):1965–75.
33. Ferreira JP, Butler J, Zannad F, et al. Mineralocorticoid receptor antagonists and Empagliflozin in patients with heart failure and preserved ejection fraction. J Am Coll Cardiol. 2022;79(12):1129–37.
34. Costanzo MR, Guglin ME, Saltzberg MT, et al. Ultrafiltration versus intravenous diuretics for patients hospitalized for acute decompensated heart failure. J Am Coll Cardiol. 2007;49(6):675–83.
35. Bart BA, Goldsmith SR, Lee KL, et al. Ultrafiltration in decompensated heart failure with cardiorenal syndrome. N Engl J Med. 2012;367(24):2296–304.
36. Costanzo MR, Negoianu D, Jaski BE, et al. Aquapheresis versus intravenous diuretics and hospitalizations for heart failure. JACC Heart Fail. 2016;4(2):95–105.
37. Timóteo AT, Mano TB. Efficacy of peritoneal dialysis in patients with refractory congestive heart failure: a systematic review and meta-analysis. Heart Fail Rev. 2023;28(5):1053–63.

Chapter 11
Acute and Chronic Coronary Syndromes in Chronic Kidney Disease: Challenges and Strategies

Cristian Mornoş and Sebastian Zus

11.1 Introduction

Chronic kidney disease (CKD) represents a major and growing global health burden, affecting an estimated 10–15% of adults worldwide and imposing a heavy toll of morbidity and mortality [1, 2]. Cardiovascular disease and coronary artery disease (CAD), in particular, are the principal causes of death in patients with CKD [3]. The risk of cardiovascular events escalates in parallel with declining glomerular filtration rate (GFR), yet importantly the excess risk is already apparent early in the course of renal impairment [4]. This heightened vulnerability cannot be explained solely by traditional risk factors such as hypertension, diabetes, dyslipidemia or smoking. Rather, CKD introduces a set of interacting pathophysiological processes that together produce an aggressive and distinctive form of cardiovascular disease: systemic inflammation, endothelial dysfunction, mineral metabolism derangements, accumulation of uremic toxins, and accelerated vascular calcification [5, 6]. Even at eGFR 45–59, albuminuria independently amplifies cardiovascular risk and should be co-indexed with eGFR in risk discussions [7].

Acute coronary syndromes (ACS) and chronic coronary syndromes (CCS) in patients with CKD display important differences in clinical presentation, diagnostic behavior, and therapeutic outcomes when compared with persons with preserved renal function. Contemporary international guidelines and recent high-quality evidence emphasize the need for tailored, kidney-aware approaches to both diagnosis and management [8, 9].

C. Mornoş (✉) · S. Zus
"Victor Babeş" University of Medicine and Pharmacy, Timisoara, Romania

A. Covic, A. Burlacu (eds.), *Renal Dysfunction in Cardiovascular Pathologies*,
https://doi.org/10.1007/978-3-032-25434-4_11

11.2 Epidemiology and Risk Factors

The prevalence of coronary atherosclerosis in patients with CKD is strikingly high and rises with disease severity and dialysis dependence [5, 10]. Estimates vary by population and method of ascertainment, but many cohorts report that a large minority of patients with advanced CKD have angiographic or clinically manifest CAD. Mortality from cardiovascular causes in end-stage kidney disease is dramatically higher than in the general population, and even moderate CKD (for example, stage 3, eGFR 30–59 ml/min/1.73 m^2) is associated with a two- to threefold increased risk of myocardial infarction [4, 11].

The excess cardiovascular risk in CKD stems from both conventional and kidney-specific factors. Traditional drivers including hypertension, diabetes mellitus, dyslipidemia and advancing age, remain highly prevalent and important contributors. Yet they operate on a background of CKD-specific mechanisms that amplify vascular injury and myocardial vulnerability. Uremic toxins such as indoxyl sulfate and p-cresyl sulfate impair endothelial repair and promote vascular smooth muscle proliferation; abnormalities of mineral metabolism including hyperphosphatemia and elevations of fibroblast growth factor-23 promote medial arterial calcification and arterial stiffening [7, 12]; anemia and chronic volume overload increase myocardial workload and foster left ventricular hypertrophy; and a persistent pro-inflammatory milieu and oxidative stress drive plaque progression, microvascular dysfunction and thrombogenicity [8, 13]. In addition, more subtle contributors such as protein–energy wasting, autonomic dysfunction, impaired vascular repair mechanisms, and heightened sympathetic tone help shape a distinctive cardio-renal phenotype that is at once atherosclerotic, calcific and fibrotic [5, 13, 14].

11.3 Pathophysiology

The pathophysiology that links CKD with CAD is multifactorial and operates at systemic, vascular and myocardial levels. Endothelial dysfunction is a pervasive early abnormality: reduced nitric oxide bioavailability, increased oxidative stress, and impaired endothelial repair mechanisms render the vasculature pro-atherogenic and less able to adapt to hemodynamic stress [15]. Beyond intimal atherosclerosis, medial (Mönckeberg-type) calcification stiffens arteries, widens pulse pressure, and impairs diastolic coronary perfusion [10, 14]. This medial calcification increases arterial stiffness, widens pulse pressure, and reduces coronary perfusion reserve, particularly during diastole, thereby increasing ischemic vulnerability even in the absence of focal obstructive lesions [11, 12].

At the myocardial level, pressure and volume overload, anemia, and uremic cardiomyopathy collectively promote concentric hypertrophy, interstitial fibrosis and impaired myocardial energetics. These structural changes reduce coronary flow reserve, increase oxygen demand, and predispose to both ischemia and heart failure.

The myocardial substrate in CKD is therefore characterized by overlapping ischemic, fibrotic and hypertrophic processes [5, 7, 11].

Hemostatic abnormalities in CKD create a well-recognized prothrombotic–bleeding paradox [15]. Uremia alters platelet function and coagulation factor activity: patients may display enhanced platelet activation and impaired fibrinolysis, contributing to thrombotic risk, while at the same time qualitative platelet dysfunction and abnormal interactions with the vessel wall increase bleeding susceptibility. This duality complicates decisions around antithrombotic and antiplatelet regimens [7]. Additionally, Klotho deficiency and phosphate-driven osteogenic switching of vascular smooth muscle cells accelerate medial calcification in CKD [12, 13].

11.4 Clinical Presentation

The clinical expression of coronary syndromes in CKD is often atypical. In the setting of ACS, classic ischemic chest pain may be absent; patients frequently present with dyspnea, profound fatigue, gastrointestinal symptoms such as nausea, or syncope. In many instances, heart failure exacerbation or arrhythmia is the first clinical manifestation of an underlying ischemic event, particularly among those with advanced renal dysfunction [6, 16].

Troponin elevations are common in CKD even in the absence of an acute coronary occlusion, reflecting chronic myocardial injury, reduced renal clearance and comorbid structural heart disease; hence, the interpretation of troponin levels must rely on serial measurements and assessment of dynamic changes rather than single absolute values [17–19].

CCS in CKD are likewise frequently concealed. Many patients do not report typical angina, whether due to autonomic neuropathy, the presence of concomitant diabetic neuropathy, or because exertional symptoms are ascribed to anemia or fluid overload [16, 20]. Exertional intolerance, limited functional capacity, or nonspecific fatigue commonly mask myocardial ischemia. Silent ischemia is therefore common, and clinical vigilance combined with appropriate non-invasive testing is often required to unmask clinically significant CAD [21–23].

11.5 Diagnostic Considerations

Diagnosing coronary disease in patients with CKD is intrinsically challenging because many conventional tests have reduced specificity or sensitivity in this population, and because the stakes of invasive evaluation include potential renal injury.

Biomarkers retain a central role but must be interpreted with caution. High-sensitivity cardiac troponins are frequently chronically elevated in CKD; therefore, clinicians should prioritize dynamic change over single measurements when diagnosing ACS [17, 19]. Natriuretic peptides (BNP, NT-proBNP) remain useful indicators of myocardial stress and heart failure, but their concentrations are influenced by both volume status and reduced renal clearance; some groups have explored indices adjusted for creatinine to improve discrimination, although these require further validation [18, 20, 23].

Electrocardiography remains the ubiquitous first-line test but is limited by a high rate of false positives and negatives in CKD. Conduction abnormalities, left ventricular hypertrophy and nonspecific ST–T changes complicate interpretation, and small subendocardial ischemic signals may be missed. Recent work exploring artificial-intelligence algorithms applied to ECGs shows potential for detecting more subtle ischemic patterns in high-risk populations, including CKD, but these tools are not yet widely validated for routine clinical use [20].

Non-invasive imaging must be selected with careful attention to the diagnostic question, renal function, and local resources. Stress echocardiography remains a practical and radiation-free first choice in many patients, but its sensitivity declines in the setting of chronic ventricular dysfunction and concentric left ventricular hypertrophy, both of which are common in CKD [24]. Myocardial perfusion imaging by scintigraphy can be limited by artifacts from vascular and thoracic calcification; positron emission tomography myocardial perfusion imaging, where available, offers superior spatial resolution, quantitation of myocardial blood flow, and reduced susceptibility to these artifacts [21, 24]. Cardiac magnetic resonance imaging offers powerful tissue characterization; non-contrast T1/T2 mapping often suffices. When gadolinium is essential, modern macrocyclic (group II) agents confer very low nephrogenic systemic fibrosis risk even in eGFR<30, so benefits may outweigh risks with appropriate selection [21]. Non-invasive coronary angiography is a highly accurate anatomic tool in patients with low to intermediate pretest probability, and recent technical advances (low-contrast protocols, deep-learning denoising algorithms) allow meaningful reductions in iodinated contrast volume while preserving diagnostic quality; nevertheless, the heavy burden of vascular calcification in CKD often limits coronary CT angiography's utility [21, 24]. Future directions could be in the sphere of artificial intelligence reconstruction/denoising to cut both contrast and radiation [24, 25].

When non-invasive testing points to a high probability of obstructive coronary disease and revascularization is being considered, clinicians must undertake a careful, CKD-specific appraisal of the risks and benefits of *invasive angiography*. Coronary calcification is a dominant and defining feature in many patients with renal impairment, often extensive, concentric, and it substantially complicates every step of the invasive pathway [21, 24]. Heavy calcification (Fig. 11.1) degrades angiographic image quality, obscures vessel contours, and limits the diagnostic value of contrast injections. Intravascular ultrasound (IVUS) and optical coherence tomography (OCT) provide indispensable information about calcium distribution, thickness and arc, guiding decisions on plaque modification and optimal stent sizing (Fig. 11.2).

Risk stratification tools commonly used in ACS and stable CAD (for example, TIMI or GRACE scores) do not incorporate the full spectrum of CKD-specific variables such as albuminuria, inflammatory burden or uremic markers. Several investigators have therefore proposed CKD-adapted risk models that include measures of renal function, albuminuria and biomarkers of inflammation.

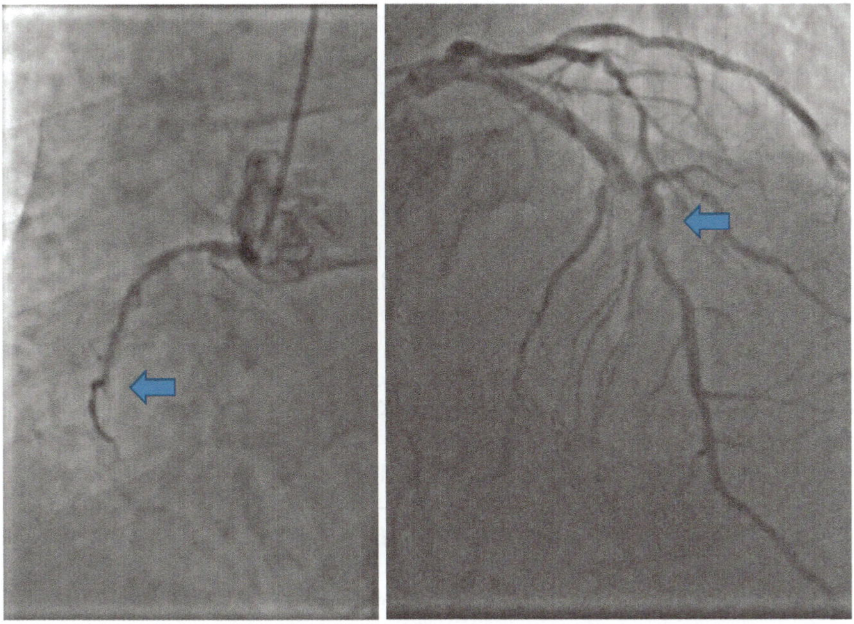

Fig. 11.1 Invasive coronary angiography in a CKD patient demonstrating complex CAD: chronic total occlusion of the right coronary artery (left) and severe mid-LAD stenosis (right)

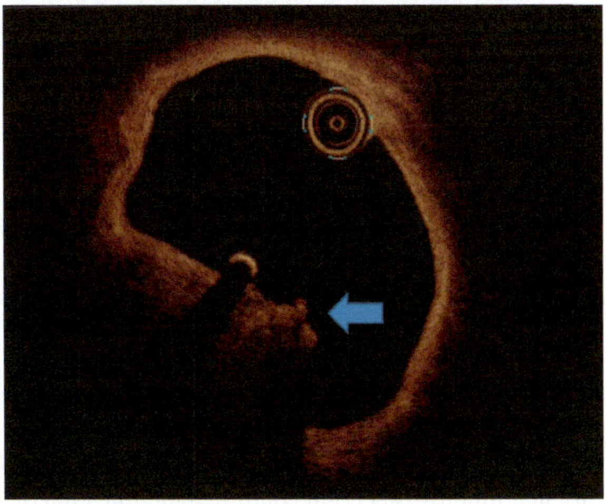

Fig. 11.2 Optical coherence tomography (OCT) of a right coronary artery showing a protruding calcific nodule (blue arrow)

11.6 Management of Acute Coronary Syndromes in CKD Patients

Treatment of ACS in patients with CKD requires a nuanced balance between providing effective ischemic protection and minimizing iatrogenic harm.

Antiplatelet therapy is central to secondary prevention following ACS, but CKD complicates drug selection and duration. Contemporary randomized trials and meta-analyses have explored abbreviated dual antiplatelet therapy (DAPT) regimes and de-escalation strategies to reduce bleeding without compromising ischemic protection [26, 27]. Notably, unguided de-escalation from ticagrelor to clopidogrel after a short initial period has been shown in recent randomized work to reduce bleeding events while maintaining ischemic efficacy in stabilized patients, a strategy that may be particularly relevant for CKD patients at elevated bleeding risk. Similarly, trials of very short DAPT (1 to 3 months) followed by P2Y12 monotherapy or early de-escalation have reported reductions in bleeding with neutral effects on ischemic endpoints in selected high-bleeding-risk populations; these findings support a flexible, risk-adapted approach to DAPT duration in renal patients, rather than a one-size-fits-all prescription.

Anticoagulation in ACS also requires caution. Unfractionated heparin is often preferred in advanced CKD because of hepatic clearance and full reversibility, whereas low-molecular-weight heparins require careful dose adjustment and are often avoided in severe renal impairment [27]. Direct oral anticoagulants retain utility in many patients with moderate CKD, but their use in eGFR <15 ml/min or in dialysis remains limited or off-label, so multidisciplinary discussion and individualized risk assessment are essential.

Revascularization strategy, whether to pursue percutaneous coronary intervention (PCI) or coronary artery bypass grafting (CABG), should be individualized and based on coronary anatomy, comorbidities, and patient-centered goals. Contemporary meta-analyses suggest that in selected patients with multivessel disease and moderate CKD, CABG may confer superior long-term survival compared with PCI, but the perioperative risk of acute kidney injury and requirement for postoperative dialysis are meaningful and must be weighed [28–30]. For many patients, especially those with focal disease or prohibitive surgical risk, PCI remains the preferred option; in such settings, adoption of minimal-contrast or zero-contrast PCI guided by IVUS/OCT and physiologic indices has expanded the feasibility of percutaneous revascularization with a reduced risk of contrast-associated renal decline [28, 29]. Adjunctive technologies (rotational or orbital atherectomy, excimer laser, and intravascular lithotripsy) permit controlled modification of rigid calcific plaques to facilitate stent delivery and achieve adequate radial expansion [30].

Recent registries and small randomized studies suggest that in selected lesions, especially in small vessels or in-stent restenosis, drug-coated balloons-only PCI may achieve comparable short- and mid-term outcomes to drug-eluting stents, even in ACS presentations. However, robust data specific to advanced CKD or dialysis populations are scarce, and the high burden of calcified, thrombus-rich lesions in these patients limits widespread applicability. Current guidelines, therefore, do not recommend routine use of drug-coated balloons in ACS with CKD, but acknowledge their potential role in niche situations, particularly when stent implantation is technically unfeasible or when minimizing DAPT duration is a clinical priority [26, 27, 30].

Adjunctive pharmacotherapies with dual renal and cardiovascular benefits have become central to comprehensive care. Statins remain a cornerstone for secondary prevention in non-dialysis CKD [6, 31–33]. The emergence of therapies such as sodium–glucose cotransporter-2 (SGLT2) inhibitors and glucagon-like peptide-1 (GLP-1) receptor agonists has transformed cardio-renal management. The recent data support incorporation of such agents into the secondary prevention armamentarium for appropriate patients with CKD, albeit with attention to tolerability and individual contraindications [30, 31].

Anti-inflammatory strategies targeting the interleukin-6 pathway and other inflammatory mediators represent a promising avenue in CKD-associated atherosclerosis. Early randomized data have shown that selective interleukin-6 inhibition markedly reduces circulating inflammatory biomarkers and favorably modulates surrogate measures of vascular disease; however, large outcome trials in CKD populations specifically powered for hard cardiovascular endpoints are still needed before routine clinical adoption [30].

11.7 Management of Chronic Coronary Syndromes (CCS) in CKD Patients

Unlike the acute setting, where decisions are often urgent and centered on stabilizing ischemia, management of CCS in CKD emphasizes sustained reduction of atherosclerotic progression, optimization of myocardial oxygen supply–demand balance, and mitigation of adverse remodeling. Patients on dialysis and those with advanced CKD warrant particular attention. Interventions should, whenever possible, be planned for non-dialysis days; peri-procedural hemodynamics and volume status must be tightly controlled, and contrast use minimized.

Pharmacological therapy remains the foundation of CCS management. Beta-blockers, nitrates, and calcium-channel blockers retain a central role in angina relief and ischemia control [31, 34]. However, their use in CKD must be carefully tailored: beta-blockers may accumulate in advanced renal failure depending on lipophilicity and route of clearance, while long-acting nitrates require vigilance for hypotension in volume-depleted or dialyzed patients. Ivabradine, where available, may serve as an adjunct in patients with preserved sinus rhythm and high resting heart rates, although robust data in advanced CKD are limited.

Antiplatelet therapy in CCS is usually limited to aspirin monotherapy, though in selected patients with high ischemic burden and low bleeding risk, extended dual therapy or aspirin plus low-dose rivaroxaban has shown benefit in the general population [31, 35, 36]. Extrapolation to CKD populations, however, must be cautious. Observational analyses suggest that advanced CKD substantially increases bleeding risk without a proportionate ischemic benefit, favoring conservative antiplatelet strategies in this setting.

Lipid-lowering therapy is a cornerstone of CCS care in CKD, though evidence varies by disease stage. Large randomized trials such as SHARP have demonstrated significant reductions in atherosclerotic events with statins in non-dialysis CKD, whereas the benefits appear attenuated in dialysis-dependent populations [37, 38]. Nonetheless, guidelines continue to endorse statin therapy in earlier CKD stages and in transplant candidates [6, 31, 32]. Recent trials exploring PCSK9 inhibitors in high-risk populations have included subsets of CKD patients, showing effective LDL-C lowering and potential event reduction, though long-term renal-specific outcomes remain under investigation [37].

Antianginal strategies beyond conventional pharmacotherapy are also relevant in CKD [31, 34]. Ranolazine, which acts by inhibiting the late sodium current, has theoretical appeal given its lack of significant hemodynamic effects; however, concerns about QT prolongation and limited data in advanced CKD necessitate cautious use. Trimetazidine, a metabolic modulator, may improve exercise tolerance and angina frequency in some patients, though its role in CKD-specific practice remains exploratory. Rounding up cardiometabolic therapy, SGLT2 inhibitors (EMPA KIDNEY; DAPA CKD) and semaglutide (FLOW 2024) reduce kidney disease progression and CV events—consider as foundational therapy when tolerated [34, 37, 38].

Risk factor control and renal–cardiovascular interaction represent a crucial dimension of CCS management [7, 20]. Rigorous blood pressure control using renin–angiotensin–aldosterone system blockade when feasible, slows both cardiovascular and renal disease progression, though clinicians must monitor for hyperkalemia and worsening renal function. Glycemic optimization is equally vital, and the advent of SGLT2 inhibitors and GLP-1 receptor agonists has shifted the paradigm toward agents that provide both renal preservation and cardiovascular protection. Evidence from large cardiovascular outcome trials, including EMPA-KIDNEY and FLOW, suggests that these therapies reduce cardiovascular events and slow CKD progression, making them central to contemporary CCS management in patients with diabetes and renal impairment.

Revascularization in chronic coronary syndromes (CCS) among patients with CKD remains less well defined than in acute coronary syndromes (ACS); however, symptomatic patients with refractory angina or a substantial ischemic burden may derive meaningful benefit. Contemporary practice increasingly relies not merely on limiting contrast volume but on meticulous pre-procedural planning, intravascular imaging, and lesion-modification strategies [24, 25, 29]. Coronary calcification, a hallmark of CKD-associated vasculopathy, represents a major challenge by reducing the accuracy of angiographic lesion assessment, impairing stent deliverability and expansion, and substantially increasing the risk of stent underexpansion, restenosis, and acute procedural complications, including dissection, perforation, and slow-flow phenomena [21, 28, 31].

To address these challenges, calcium modification techniques have become central. Rotational and orbital atherectomy allow controlled debulking of rigid plaques, while intravascular lithotripsy (IVL) fractures both intimal and medial calcium through acoustic pressure waves, facilitating optimal stent expansion with minimal vessel trauma. Scoring and cutting balloons serve as adjuncts in fibrotic or moderately calcified lesions. Widespread adoption of IVUS and OCT guidance enables precise characterization of calcium distribution, plaque morphology, and stent apposition, thereby mitigating the risk of suboptimal results. Furthermore, stent optimization strategies, including high-pressure post-dilatation and stent boost imaging, are increasingly used to ensure adequate expansion in heavily calcified vessels [21, 31, 38].

Zero- or ultra-low-contrast PCI protocols [28], guided by intravascular imaging and physiologic indices, are now applied not only in ACS but also in CCS, offering a feasible revascularization option for patients with advanced CKD and eGFR <20 ml/min/1.73 m^2. Observational registry data indicate that both PCI and CABG can improve symptoms in this population; however, procedural risks (including peri-procedural acute kidney injury, contrast-induced nephropathy, and higher perioperative mortality with surgery) must be carefully considered. In multivessel disease, CABG may provide superior long-term outcomes, particularly in younger or less frail patients, but its higher perioperative risk necessitates individualized assessment, especially in dialysis-dependent or highly comorbid patients [31, 34, 38].

While structured programs and new technologies have expanded revascularization options for patients with severe CKD, the burden of coronary calcification remains a primary determinant of procedural complexity and prognosis [38]. Its presence should be explicitly incorporated into individualized treatment planning, patient counseling, and informed consent, with close collaboration between interventional cardiology and nephrology teams to optimize both cardiac and renal outcomes.

Although indications for coronary interventions in CKD patients are less clear, symptomatic patients with refractory angina or large ischemic burdens may benefit. Contemporary revascularization in advanced CKD increasingly relies on meticulous pre-procedural planning, intravascular imaging, and lesion-modification strategies rather than on contrast volume alone. Data from observational registries suggest that PCI and CABG can both improve symptoms in CKD, though procedural risks (including peri-procedural acute kidney injury, contrast-induced nephropathy, and higher perioperative mortality) must be carefully weighed. Zero-contrast PCI techniques, guided by intravascular imaging, are increasingly applied in chronic settings as well, offering an option for patients with advanced renal dysfunction. Heavy calcification reduces the accuracy of lesion severity assessment, impairs stent deliverability and expansion (Fig. 11.3), and markedly increases the risk of stent underexpansion, restenosis and procedural complications (including dissection, perforation and slow-flow). In multivessel disease, CABG may offer superior long-term outcomes, but its higher perioperative risk profile demands individualized assessment, particularly in frail or dialysis-dependent patients [34, 37]. Although such programs expand revascularization options for patients with severe CKD, the

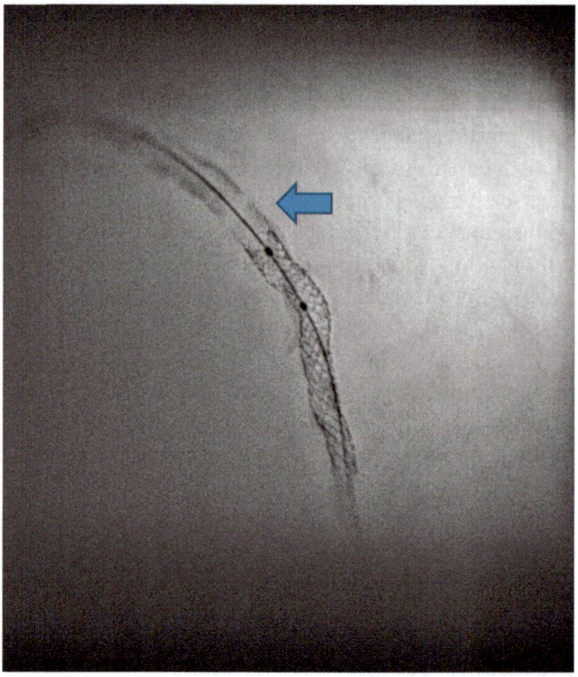

Fig. 11.3 Coronary angioplasty with stent boost imaging: severe proximal coronary calcifications (blue arrow) adjacent to deployed stents and stent underexpansion

presence of heavy calcification remains a major determinant of procedural complexity and prognosis and should be explicitly factored into individualized decision-making and informed consent.

CKD patients present a therapeutic challenge because heavy coronary calcification, small vessel disease, and high bleeding risk often complicate percutaneous coronary intervention with stent implantation. Drug-coated balloons offer the theoretical advantage of delivering potent antiproliferative drugs without leaving a permanent metallic scaffold, thereby reducing the long-term risks of in-stent restenosis, late stent thrombosis, and prolonged DAPT [31, 34, 38].

Novel and emerging therapies may reshape CCS care in CKD. Anti-inflammatory agents such as colchicine and interleukin-6 inhibitors, currently tested in post-ACS populations, hold promise for chronic atherosclerotic disease [31]. Similarly, research into antifibrotic and anti-calcification agents may eventually provide disease-modifying options specifically tailored to CKD patients, though robust outcome data are awaited [39].

11.8 Challenges, Gaps and Research Directions

Despite important advances, several major gaps persist [40]. One of the most critical is the underrepresentation of patients with advanced CKD and dialysis dependence in cardiovascular clinical trials, which forces clinicians to extrapolate from non-CKD populations and leaves many questions unanswered about safety and efficacy in true renal practice. Registries provide useful real-world data but are limited by heterogeneity and residual confounding.

Diagnostic dilemmas endure: biomarkers such as troponin and natriuretic peptides lack the same specificity they have in non-renal populations, and imaging strategies are constrained by calcification and concerns about contrast and gadolinium exposure. Translationally, key mechanistic pathways (including effects of uremic toxins, klotho deficiency, and fibroblast growth factor-23-mediated vascular remodeling) are incompletely targeted by current therapies [39]. Therapeutically, optimal antiplatelet regimens (type and duration), the relative merits of CABG versus PCI across CKD stages, and the use of emerging agents such as SGLT2 inhibitors or GLP-1 receptor agonists in the immediate post-ACS setting remain areas of active investigation [41].

11.9 Future Directions

The coming years should see a progressive integration of molecular biomarkers, advanced non-contrast imaging modalities, AI-assisted risk modelling and precision pharmacotherapy into routine care for CKD patients with coronary disease [40, 41]. Trials that explicitly include CKD and dialysis populations are essential. Device innovations that facilitate safe revascularization with minimal nephrotoxic exposure, and pharmacologic strategies that target inflammation and fibrosis in addition to atherothrombosis, hold promise for closing the outcome gap between CKD and non-CKD populations [41, 42].

11.10 Conclusion

Coronary syndromes in CKD patients constitute a uniquely high-risk clinical constellation in which atypical presentations, altered biomarker kinetics, and competing risks complicate diagnosis and management. Although advances in imaging, antithrombotic strategy, contrast-sparing interventions, and cardio-renal therapies provide important new tools, patients with advanced renal disease remain vulnerable and are underrepresented in the evidence base. Progress will require a dual approach: broaden inclusion of CKD patients in rigorous cardiovascular research, and translate mechanistic and translational insights into tailored diagnostic and therapeutic algorithms that acknowledge the distinct biology of the cardio-renal patient. Multidisciplinary, patient-centered care remains the cornerstone for improving outcomes in this challenging population.

Declarations

Competing Interests The author(s) has no competing interests to declare that are relevant to the content of this manuscript.

Ethics Approval The author(s) declares that this manuscript does not include primary research with human participants.

The author(s) declares that this manuscript does not include primary studies involving animals.

References

1. Go AS, et al. Chronic kidney disease and the risks of death, cardiovascular events, and hospitalization. N Engl J Med. 2004;351(13):1296–305.
2. Fox CS, et al. Associations of kidney disease measures with mortality and cardiovascular events: a meta-analysis. Lancet. 2012;380(9854):1662–73.
3. Matsushita K, et al. Association of estimated glomerular filtration rate and albuminuria with all-cause and cardiovascular mortality. JAMA Cardiol. 2020;5(5):507–17.
4. Sarnak MJ, et al. Kidney disease as a risk factor for development of cardiovascular disease: a statement from the American Heart Association. Circulation. 2003;108(17):2154–69.
5. Shroff GR, et al. Chronic kidney disease and coronary artery disease: shifting paradigms. Am J Kidney Dis. 2017;70(1):111–21.
6. Wanner C, et al. KDIGO clinical practice guideline for lipid management in CKD: summary of recommendations and rationale. Kidney Int Suppl. 2014;4(1):1–15.
7. Jankowski J, et al. Cardiovascular disease in chronic kidney disease: pathophysiological insights and therapeutic options. Nat Rev Nephrol. 2021;17(8):519–34.
8. Vaziri ND. Oxidative stress in uremia: nature, mechanisms, and potential consequences. Kidney Int. 2004;66(5):1719–33.
9. Stenvinkel P, et al. Inflammation in end-stage renal disease: the hidden enemy. Lancet. 2005;365(9456):945–55.
10. London GM, et al. Arterial stiffness and function in end-stage renal disease. Hypertension. 2004;43(3):320–6.
11. Herzog CA, et al. Cardiovascular disease in chronic kidney disease: a clinical update from Kidney Disease: Improving Global Outcomes (KDIGO). Kidney Int. 2011;80(6):572–86.
12. Lerman LO, et al. Mechanisms of disease progression in CKD and cardiovascular risk. Kidney Int. 2022;101(4):662–75.
13. Lanzer P, et al. Medial vascular calcification revisited: review and perspectives. Eur Heart J. 2014;35(30):1990–2001.
14. Di Lullo L, et al. Pathophysiology of cardiovascular disease in chronic kidney disease. Cardiorenal Med. 2015;5(2):76–80.
15. Drechsler C, et al. Impact of abnormal coagulation and inflammation on cardiovascular outcomes in CKD. Kidney Int. 2009;75(1):22–30.
16. Chen SC, et al. Autonomic dysfunction in CKD: implications for clinical outcomes. Nephrology (Carlton). 2021;26(6):535–42.

17. Apple FS, et al. Cardiac troponin assays: guide to understanding analytical characteristics and clinical use. Clin Chem. 2012;58(1):157–64.
18. DeFilippi CR, et al. Cardiac biomarkers in renal disease: state of the art. J Am Coll Cardiol. 2021;77(5):560–70.
19. Hickman PE, et al. Biochemical markers of myocardial damage. Clin Biochem Rev. 2010;31(1):15–25.
20. Szummer K, et al. Relation between renal function, presentation, use of therapies and in-hospital complications in acute coronary syndrome: data from the SWEDEHEART register. J Intern Med. 2010;268:40–9. https://doi.org/10.1111/j.1365-2796.2009.02204.x.
21. Charytan DM, et al. Advances in coronary imaging in patients with CKD. Circ Cardiovasc Interv. 2017;10(8):e004494.
22. Chapman AR, et al. High-sensitivity cardiac troponin and the early rule-out pathway. Eur Heart J. 2020;41(14):1404–13.
23. McCullough PA, et al. B-type natriuretic peptides in cardiovascular disease in patients with CKD. Clin J Am Soc Nephrol. 2007;2(2):207–15.
24. Cowan BR, et al. Imaging advances in heart disease with renal dysfunction. J Cardiovasc Magn Reson. 2019;21(1):1–17.
25. Mehran R, et al. Contrast-induced nephropathy: definition, epidemiology, and implications. J Am Coll Cardiol. 2004;44(7):1393–9.
26. Mega JL, et al. Comparative effectiveness of antiplatelet therapy in CKD. N Engl J Med. 2009;360(4):354–62.
27. Lim W, et al. Prevention and management of bleeding complications in CKD. Chest. 2012;141(2 Suppl):e591S–606S.
28. Ali ZA, et al. Zero-contrast PCI: feasibility and safety. JACC Cardiovasc Interv. 2020;13(24):3053–63.
29. Solomon RJ, et al. Contrast nephropathy: latest evidence. N Engl J Med. 2018;378(7):603–14.
30. Byrne RA, et al. 2023 ESC Scientific Document Group. 2023 ESC guidelines for the management of acute coronary syndromes. Eur Heart J. 2023;44(38):3720–826.
31. Vrints C, et al. 2024 ESC guidelines for the management of chronic coronary syndromes. Eur Heart J. 2024;45(36):3415–537.
32. Baigent C, et al. The effects of lowering LDL cholesterol in CKD. Lancet. 2011;377(9784):2181–92.
33. Wanner C, et al. Atorvastatin in patients with type 2 diabetes and end-stage renal disease. N Engl J Med. 2005;353(3):238–48.
34. Bangalore S, et al. Management of coronary disease in advanced CKD. N Engl J Med. 2020;382(17):1608–18.
35. Bonaca, et al. Long-term use of ticagrelor in patients with prior myocardial infarction. N Engl J Med. 2015;372:1791–800. https://doi.org/10.1056/NEJMoa1500857.
36. Eikelboom JW, et al. Rivaroxaban with or without aspirin in stable cardiovascular disease. N Engl J Med. 2017;377:1319–30. https://doi.org/10.1056/NEJMoa1709118.
37. Pecoits-Filho R, et al. Cardiovascular clinical trials and CKD: inclusion needed. Nephrol Dial Transplant. 2023;38(4):739–47.
38. Hickson LJ, et al. Long-term outcomes after coronary intervention in ESKD. Kidney Int. 2019;96(5):1029–38.
39. Sangaralingham SJ, et al. Novel biomarkers in cardiorenal disease. Circ Res. 2021;128(10):1404–25.
40. Khera R, et al. Artificial intelligence in cardiovascular care. JAMA Cardiol. 2021;6(1):9–10.
41. Stevens PE, et al. Evaluation and management of CKD: integrative perspectives. Lancet. 2013;382(9889):339–52.
42. Ridker PM, et al. IL-6 inhibition with ziltivekimab in patients at high atherosclerotic risk (RESCUE): a double-blind, randomised, placebo-controlled, phase 2 trial. Lancet. 2021;397:2060–9. https://doi.org/10.1016/S0140-6736(21)00520-1.

Chapter 12
Myocardial Infarction with Non-obstructive Coronary Arteries in End-Stage Kidney Disease: Pathophysiology, Diagnosis and Management

Vasile Bogdan Halațiu and Theodora Benedek

12.1 Epidemiology

Myocardial infarction with non-obstructive coronary arteries (MINOCA) is currently recognized as a well-defined subset of acute myocardial infarction (AMI), characterized by clinical, electrocardiographic, and biochemical criteria of infarction in the absence of ≥50% epicardial coronary stenoses on coronary angiography [1]. Although initially regarded as a rare and relatively benign phenomenon, contemporary data indicate that MINOCA accounts for approximately 3–15% of all AMI cases, with a prevalence of approximately 8%, and is associated with a non-neglectable burden of morbidity and mortality [2].

Observational studies and recent meta-analyses have shown that patients with MINOCA are, on average, younger than those with myocardial infarction with obstructive coronary artery disease (MIOCA), and that they include a higher proportion of women, individuals without a prior history of coronary disease, and patients with a lower prevalence of diabetes mellitus or traditional dyslipidemia [3]. Nevertheless, the risk profile is heterogeneous, including both patients with microvascular coronary disease or vasospasm and those with non-coronary causes (e.g., spontaneous coronary artery dissection, myocarditis, Takotsubo syndrome, etc.) [4]. From a prognostic standpoint, contemporary data contradict the perception of MINOCA as a "mild infarction." One- to five-year rates of major adverse cardiovascular events (MACE)—including cardiovascular death, reinfarction, and heart

V. B. Halațiu · T. Benedek (✉)
George Emil Palade University of Medicine, Pharmacy, Science, and Technology of Targu Mures, Targu Mures, Romania

Cardiology Department, County Emergency Clinical Hospital of Targu Mures, Targu Mures, Romania

A. Covic, A. Burlacu (eds.), *Renal Dysfunction in Cardiovascular Pathologies*,
https://doi.org/10.1007/978-3-032-25434-4_12

failure, are comparable to, or only slightly lower than, those seen in patients with MIOCA, particularly in subgroups with markedly elevated troponin levels or significant comorbidities [3]. Thus, MINOCA should be regarded as a high-risk syndrome requiring the same diagnostic rigor and therapeutic attention as classic AMI.

Chronic kidney disease (CKD) is one of the most important independent risk factors for AMI, and progression to end-stage renal disease (ESRD) requiring renal replacement therapy (dialysis or transplantation) dramatically amplifies the risk of coronary events. In large AMI registries, renal impairment, most often defined as an eGFR <60 mL/min/1.73 m^2, is reported in 30–40% of patients [5]. In MINOCA, the prevalence of renal dysfunction appears to be even higher. One observational study showed that approximately one-third of MINOCA patients have chronic renal dysfunction, which is associated with significantly worse short and long-term outcomes [6]. Recent data from the KAMIR-NIH registry suggest that the presence of CKD in the context of MINOCA is linked to a marked increase in all-cause mortality and non-fatal cardiovascular events at 3 years, reaching levels comparable to those observed in patients with MIOCA and CKD [7].

Patients with ESRD exhibit some of the highest incidences of AMI reported in cardiovascular populations. A classic study among individuals initiating hemodialysis showed that the incidence of AMI is approximately three times higher in those with a documented history of coronary artery disease compared with those without, and both in-hospital and long-term mortality are exceptionally high [8]. Analyses from dialysis registries have demonstrated that dialysis patients hospitalized for AMI differ substantially from non-dialysis patients: they tend to be younger, have a heavier comorbidity burden, and experience markedly higher mortality at 30 days and 1 year [9]. Moreover, the clinical presentation of acute coronary syndromes (ACS) in dialysis patients is frequently atypical, with absent or non-specific chest pain, subtle ECG changes, and chronically elevated troponin levels, all of which complicate diagnosis and often delay referral for coronary angiography [10]. For this reason, the true proportion of MINOCA among patients with ESRD is likely underestimated, as a subset of episodes labeled as "myocardial injury" or "angiographically unconfirmed AMI" are, in reality, undiagnosed cases of MINOCA.

Several recent analyses have evaluated the impact of renal function on outcomes in patients with MINOCA. *Kim YH* et al. demonstrated that in both MINOCA and MIOCA, the presence of CKD is associated with a significant increase in all-cause mortality and non-fatal cardiovascular events at 3 years, and that the adverse effect of CKD is of comparable magnitude in both entities [7]. Other data suggest that among patients with MINOCA and renal dysfunction, 3-year mortality is similar to that observed in patients with CKD and MIOCA, contradicting any perception of "protection" conferred by the absence of significant coronary stenoses [6]. In the subgroup of patients with ESRD, the risk appears to be even higher due to the overlap of traditional and non-traditional risk factors (inflammation, oxidative stress, vascular calcification, coagulation abnormalities, arrhythmias, intradialytic hypotension, etc.). Although data specifically addressing MINOCA in ESRD remain limited, it is plausible and partly supported by registry analyses that these patients experience some of the poorest outcomes, with high rates of cardiovascular death and reinfarction [9].

From an epidemiological standpoint, MINOCA in the context of ESRD represents an important “blind spot.” On one hand, patients with ESRD carry an extremely high burden of coronary events, present with atypical symptoms, and have elevated mortality [8]. On the other hand, they are less frequently referred for angiography and the systematic use of intracoronary techniques is limited, which leads to underdiagnosis of MINOCA and incomplete reporting of its underlying causes [11, 12]. Moreover, most MINOCA studies include patients with varying degrees of CKD but do not provide dedicated analyses of the ESRD subgroup, and dialysis patients are often excluded from randomized trials or prospective registries [3]. Available data come predominantly from retrospective observational analyses, characterized by substantial heterogeneity in definitions and diagnostic approaches. These methodological limitations make it difficult to accurately determine the incidence and prevalence of MINOCA in ESRD.

12.2 Clinical Presentation

In registries comparing ACS in patients with and without CKD, it has been observed that patients with CKD (including those with end-stage disease) more frequently present with non-ST-segment elevation myocardial infarction (NSTEMI) and show a relatively higher incidence of MINOCA than patients without CKD [13]. This means that a dialysis patient presenting with suspected ACS has a higher likelihood, compared with the general population, of having either a NSTEMI or MINOCA, rather than a classic STEMI caused by epicardial coronary artery occlusion. The main clinical presentation forms of MINOCA in ESRD patients are presented in Table 12.1.

Retrosternal, constrictive chest pain remains a frequent, though not dominant, symptom of ACS in patients with ESRD. Several studies have shown that patients with ESRD experience “typical” chest pain (retrosternal, radiating to the arm or jaw, described as “pressure” or “tightness”) less often than patients without kidney disease [14]. Autonomic neuropathy (particularly in diabetics), altered pain thresholds, and the concomitant presence of other causes of chest discomfort (uremic pericarditis, left ventricular hypertrophy, volume overload) contribute to this blunting of the clinical picture. In the case of MINOCA, the presentation is even more heterogeneous. Large MINOCA series show that chest pain is often less intense, of variable duration, and sometimes associated with emotional or physiological triggers (acute emotional stress, sepsis, tachyarrhythmias, hypertensive crises) [15, 16]. In dialysis patients, such triggering factors overlap with episodes of intradialytic hypotension, rapid shifts in circulating volume, hypoxia, and electrolyte disturbances, which may lead to silent or pauci-symptomatic ischemic episodes.

Dyspnea, marked fatigue, asthenia, and exertional intolerance are extremely common symptoms in ESRD, caused by volume overload, anemia, and diastolic

Table 12.1 Key clinical presentation forms of MINOCA in ESRD patients

	Characteristics in ESRD-MINOCA patients
Chest pain (angina)	*Less typical or absent:* Retrosternal, constrictive chest pain is less frequent or dominant. *Variable intensity and duration:* Often less intense, of variable duration, sometimes associated with emotional or physiological triggers (acute emotional stress, sepsis, tachyarrhythmias, hypertensive crises). *Blunted by comorbidities:* Autonomic neuropathy, altered pain thresholds, and coexisting causes of chest discomfort (uremic pericarditis, left ventricular hypertrophy, volume overload) complicate the clinical picture.
Atypical/non-specific symptoms	*Dyspnea:* May be the predominant or initial manifestation through worsening dyspnea, orthopnea, peripheral edema, or interdialytic weight gain, often mistaken for heart failure decompensation. *Generalized symptoms:* Marked fatigue, asthenia, exertional intolerance, weakness, nausea, or hypotension. *Diagnostic challenge:* This non-specific presentation complicates differentiation between true myocardial infarction (type 1 or 2) and other causes of myocardial injury (e.g., sepsis, pulmonary embolism, rapid tachyarrhythmias).
Silent or pauci-symptomatic ischemia	*"Silent" events:* A substantial proportion of ischemic events remain clinically "silent" or manifest as arrhythmias and sudden death, without clear preceding chest pain. *Underdiagnosis:* Many MINOCA episodes likely remain undiagnosed, inferred retrospectively from necropsy findings or echocardiographic changes. *Dialysis-triggered:* Episodes often occur during or immediately after hemodialysis sessions, in the setting of intradialytic hypotension, rapid circulating volume reduction, hypovolemia, electrolyte shifts, and blood pressure fluctuations.

ESRD end-stage renal disease, *MINOCA* myocardial infarction with non-obstructive coronary arteries

dysfunction. Consequently, an episode of MINOCA may begin or manifest predominantly through worsening dyspnea, orthopnea, peripheral edema, or interdialytic weight gain, and may be easily mistaken for a "simple" episode of heart failure decompensation [13]. In studies examining ACS presentation in dialysis patients, a substantial proportion present without chest pain, instead exhibiting isolated dyspnea or generalized symptoms (weakness, nausea, hypotension) [17]. In the context of MINOCA, this non-specific presentation complicates the distinction between a true myocardial infarction (type 1 or type 2) and other causes of myocardial injury (e.g., sepsis, pulmonary embolism, rapid tachyarrhythmias) [17].

A substantial proportion of ischemic events in patients with ESRD remain clinically "silent" or manifest through arrhythmias and sudden death, without a clearly documented preceding episode of chest pain. A significant percentage of deaths among dialysis patients are classified as sudden cardiac death [18]. In this context, it is likely that some episodes of MINOCA remain completely undiagnosed, being inferred only retrospectively from necropsy findings or from echocardiographic evolution (the emergence of new hypokinetic segments).

At presentation, the ECG may show both STEMI and NSTEMI patterns; however, patients with MINOCA and CKD tend to exhibit ST-segment elevations or diffuse T-wave inversions more frequently, accompanied by higher troponin levels, findings that suggest more extensive ischemia despite the absence of significant angiographic stenosis. Nevertheless, in patients with ESRD, ECG interpretation is complicated by left ventricular hypertrophy, conduction abnormalities, and non-specific changes related to electrolyte disturbances (hyperkalemia, hypocalcemia) [19, 20]. In patients with advanced CKD and ESRD, troponin levels are frequently elevated even in the absence of acute AMI, due to reduced clearance and chronic myocardial injury (fibrosis, micro-ischemia, pressure and volume overload) [21]. Cohort studies in dialysis populations have shown that a significant proportion have persistently elevated hs-cTnT or hs-cTnI levels, and that these values are associated with adverse cardiovascular prognosis even without evident ACS [22].

In patients with ESRD, a substantial proportion of ischemic episodes occur during hemodialysis sessions, in the setting of intradialytic hypotension and rapid reduction of circulating volume, or immediately after dialysis, when relative hypovolemia, electrolyte shifts, and blood pressure fluctuations may coexist [23]. These episodes can lead to type 2 myocardial ischemia, sometimes fulfilling AMI criteria, yet without significant epicardial stenosis, which, after exclusion of other causes, places them within the MINOCA spectrum. In addition, patients with ESRD frequently undergo major surgical procedures (e.g., nephrectomies, vascular interventions), where perioperative hypotension, anemia, and adrenergic stress may precipitate MINOCA. Typical precipitating factors in MINOCA (intense emotional stress, coronary spasm, microembolization, rapid tachyarrhythmias, hypertensive crises) often occur in amplified form in dialysis patients, explaining the high prevalence of myocardial injury and, likely, the underdiagnosis of MINOCA in this population [4, 24].

12.3 Pathophysiology: Coronary Microvascular Dysfunction and Inflammation

The pathogenesis of MINOCA in patients with ESRD revolves around a complex interaction between coronary microvascular dysfunction and an altered systemic inflammatory status associated with advanced uremia. Coronary microvascular dysfunction is highly prevalent in ESRD and mediates a significant part of the relationship between renal impairment, ventricular remodeling, and cardiovascular events. This creates a conducive substrate for myocardial infarction in the absence of significant epicardial stenosis [25, 26].

Coronary microvascular dysfunction is defined by structural and/or functional abnormalities of the coronary microcirculation, leading to reduced coronary flow reserve and an inadequate vasomotor response to stimuli, in the absence of significant epicardial stenosis. In MINOCA, coronary microvascular dysfunction may represent both a primary mechanism (pure microvascular ischemia) or a precipitating factor in contexts of epicardial spasm or different coagulopathies, resulting in focal or subendocardial myocardial necrosis [2, 25, 27, 28]. Recent studies addressing MINOCA from a pathophysiological perspective have identified coronary microvascular dysfunction as a common mechanism, alongside plaque disruption, epicardial vasospasm, and coronary embolism. Notably, coronary microvascular dysfunction includes functional components (such as vasoconstrictor hyperreactivity, endothelial dysfunction, and altered endothelial-dependent and independent vasodilation) and structural components (including diffuse luminal narrowing, arteriolar remodeling, microthrombi, and extravascular compression). These changes lead to increased microvascular resistance and perfusion heterogeneity, explaining why ischemia and infarction may occur in the absence of angiographically significant lesions [29–31].

Chronic kidney disease, particularly in its end-stage, is associated with a gradual reduction in coronary microvascular function, correlated with the severity of decreased eGFR. Studies assessing coronary flow reserve through positron emission tomography or echocardiographic techniques have demonstrated that coronary microvascular dysfunction is a major mediator of the relationship between impaired renal function, ventricular dysfunction, and major cardiovascular events, accounting for up to a quarter of the effect of renal failure on diastolic and systolic dysfunction [26, 32]. The mechanisms by which ESRD induces coronary microvascular dysfunction (Fig. 12.1) are multifaceted: chronic hypertension with arteriolar remodeling, heightened oxidative stress, the accumulation of uremic toxins, uremia-specific dyslipidemia, hyperphosphatemia, and vascular calcification, all contributing to thickening of the resistance vessel walls and rigidity of the microcirculation. Anemia and volume overload, highly prevalent in ESRD, lead to sympathetic

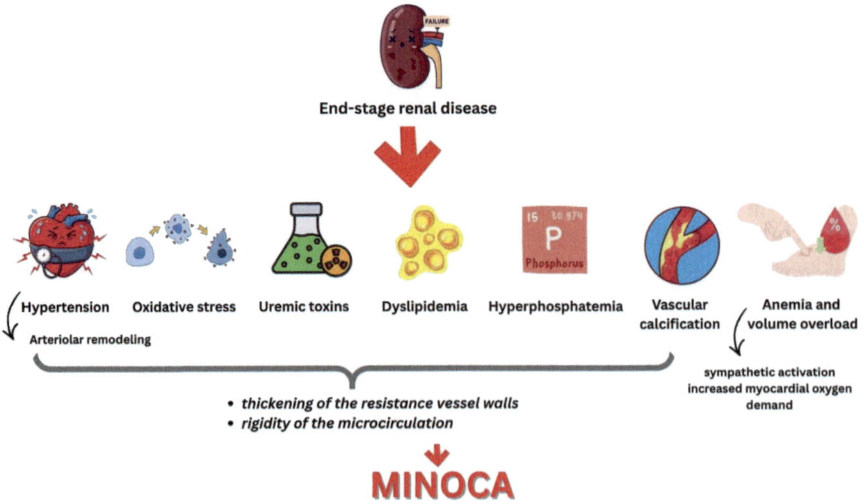

Fig. 12.1 Mechanisms of ESRD-induced coronary microvascular dysfunction

activation and increased myocardial oxygen demand on a pre-existing compromised microvascular substrate, promoting repeated episodes of silent microvascular ischemia and, ultimately, MINOCA [32–35].

The coronary endothelium is profoundly affected in ESRD, both at the epicardial and microvascular levels, characterized by reduced bioavailability of nitric oxide (NO), increased production of reactive oxygen species (ROS), and elevated expression of adhesion molecules (VCAM-1, ICAM-1) and pro-inflammatory receptors. In MINOCA, this endothelial dysfunction translates into an inability to adequately regulate microvascular tone, facilitating episodes of diffuse vasoconstriction, perfusion heterogeneity, and microvascular "no-reflow," even in the absence of epicardial obstruction [25, 29, 31, 33]. A recent study involving patients with MINOCA found that the progression of subclinical coronary atherosclerosis is closely correlated with elevated levels of pro-inflammatory endothelial biomarkers such as soluble VCAM-1 (sVCAM-1) and chemokine CCL-21, suggesting that endothelial and microcirculatory alterations play a distinct central role compared to MIOCA [36]. In patients with CKD, these same mediators are chronically elevated, which enhances the vulnerability of the microvasculature to acute ischemic stimuli and may explain the increased susceptibility to MINOCA events.

End-stage renal disease represents a prototypical state of chronic low-grade inflammation, characterized by persistently elevated levels of ultra-sensitive C-reactive protein (CRP), interleukin-6 (IL-6), tumor necrosis factor-alpha (TNF-α), and other pro-inflammatory mediators, further compounded by acute episodes of inflammatory activation associated with infections, dialysis, or ischemic events [32, 33, 36]. Inflammation induces coronary microvascular dysfunction through several interrelated mechanisms: activation of adhesion molecules and recruitment of leukocytes to the vessel wall, release of cytokines and ROS that impair endothelial and smooth muscle cell function, and structural remodeling characterized by perivascular fibrosis and intimal thickening. The model proposed by experimental and clinical studies suggests that the infiltration of monocytes and neutrophils into the coronary microcirculation is accompanied by increased expression of ICAM-1 and VCAM-1, exacerbating endothelial injury and impairing the physiological vasodilatory response [29].

In advanced CKD, uremic toxins (such as indoxyl sulfate and p-cresyl sulfate), advanced glycation end-products, and systemic oxidative stress act synergistically with inflammation to impair microcirculation. These substances induce mitochondrial dysfunction in endothelial and smooth muscle cells, increase vascular permeability, and predispose to micro-thrombosis, thereby reducing coronary flow reserve even in the absence of unstable epicardial plaques [33, 34]. Moreover, dialysis itself can amplify inflammatory and microvascular stress: the contact of blood with dialysis membranes, fluctuations in volume and osmotic pressure, and repeated episodes of intradialytic hypotension led to repeated ischemia-reperfusion injury of the myocardium and microcirculation. This creates a vicious cycle in which coronary microvascular dysfunction and inflammation perpetuate themselves, gradually increasing the vulnerability of the myocardium to acute ischemic episodes that may manifest as MINOCA [26, 32, 33, 35].

In addition to altered vasomotor mechanisms, coronary microvascular dysfunction in ESRD is characterized by a prothrombotic state, with increased platelet aggregation, activation of the coagulation cascade, and relative inhibition of endogenous anticoagulant pathways. Calcium and phosphorus imbalances, uremic hyperlipidemia, and inflammation promote the formation of microthrombi and fibrin-thrombotic deposits at the arteriolar level, which can lead to segmental occlusion of coronary arterioles and micro-focal infarcts, consistent with the presentation of MINOCA [32–34]. In MINOCA, advanced imaging techniques (such as cardiac magnetic resonance and intracoronary optical coherence tomography) have demonstrated the presence of microvascular lesions and distal embolization even when conventional coronary angiography does not reveal significant stenosis. Patients with ESRD are particularly susceptible to such phenomenon, due to the combination of hyperreactive platelets, periodic use of heparin during dialysis, and the presence of calcific or thrombotic micro-emboli originating from peripheral circulation or from dialysis access sites [2, 22, 33, 35].

Chronic coronary microvascular dysfunction in ESRD leads to "uremic cardiomyopathy," characterized by concentric left ventricular hypertrophy, diffuse interstitial fibrosis, and increased stiffness, compromising subendocardial coronary reserve. In this context, transient decreases in microvascular coronary flow, triggered by microvascular spasms, episodes of hypotension, or acute increases in oxygen demand, can exceed the critical perfusion threshold, resulting in limited myocardial necrosis detectable as MINOCA [25, 26, 32]. Imaging studies have shown that patients with coronary microvascular dysfunction and CKD frequently exhibit patterns of diffuse or subendocardial late gadolinium enhancement on cardiac magnetic resonance, corresponding to diffuse fibrosis and repeated silent infarcts. This explains why a proportion of MINOCA cases in ESRD exhibit a substrate of "cumulative ischemia" rather than a single major thrombotic event. This structural substrate amplifies the impact of any acute microvascular or inflammatory insult, transforming otherwise "minor" episodes of supply-demand mismatch into clinical infarcts [25, 26, 32, 34].

Based on current data, an integrated model can be proposed in which ESRD induces coronary microvascular dysfunction through structural remodeling, endothelial dysfunction, and micro-thrombosis, all amplified by chronic systemic inflammation and uremic toxins. In light of these factors, acute stimuli such as hemodynamic fluctuations during dialysis, intercurrent infections, hypertensive crises, or even modest subcritical coronary plaques become sufficient to cause a focal or diffuse ischemic episode, clinically manifesting as MINOCA [25, 26, 32, 33].

12.4 Diagnostic Challenges and Imaging Considerations

It is estimated that 5–15% of patients with myocardial infarction meet the criteria for MINOCA, but the proportion of those in whom a clear ischemic cause is subsequently identified through advanced imaging or functional testing is significant.

Recent guidelines and reviews emphasize that the term MINOCA should not be considered a final diagnosis, but rather a starting point for a detailed etiological evaluation. The diagnosis of MINOCA in patients with ESRD presents one of the most complex challenges in contemporary cardiology. On one hand, MINOCA is a "framework diagnosis" that requires a stepwise algorithmic approach, systematically excluding other causes of myocardial injury and extensively utilizing advanced imaging techniques. On the other hand, ESRD and hemodialysis profoundly alter clinical presentation, biomarker interpretation, risk assessment, and the feasibility of invasive investigations, as well as the safety of imaging modalities, often leading to under-investigation and incomplete diagnoses [37–40].

In patients with advanced CKD, the significance of ECG changes is often ambiguous. Left ventricular hypertrophy, conduction disturbances, anemia, hypertension, and electrolyte imbalances (especially hyperkalemia) produce ST-T and QRS changes that can mimic acute ischemia. Consequently, the sensitivity and specificity of the ECG for detecting AMI are reduced, and non-specific patterns are common, leading to both underdiagnosis and unnecessary initiation of invasive investigations [13, 41]. Cardiac biomarkers also undergo significant alterations in ESRD. High-sensitivity troponin levels are often chronically elevated even in the absence of acute ischemia, while N-terminal pro-BNP reflects both volume overload and ventricular dysfunction, rather than solely ischemia. Guidelines for myocardial ischemia in CKD emphasize that the diagnosis of infarction should be based on the dynamics of troponin values (significant increase/decrease) in correlation with clinical presentation and imaging results, not on a single value above the reference threshold. In the context of MINOCA, where necrosis is often limited, these background disturbances make it challenging to differentiate between "uremic troponin elevation" and true AMI, necessitating additional imaging investigations [13, 38, 41].

Main imaging modalities for diagnosing MINOCA in ESRD patients are presented in Fig. 12.2. Confirmation of the "non-obstructive" criterion typically requires invasive coronary angiography, a standard procedure for patients with ACS, including those with ESRD. In advanced CKD and dialysis patients, angiography faces two major challenges: the risk of further deteriorating residual kidney function due to exposure to iodinated contrast and the underestimation of diffuse atherosclerotic burden, which can be hemodynamically significant even when appearing "non-obstructive" angiographically [13, 40–42]. Computed coronary tomography angiography (CCTA) offers a non-invasive alternative for assessing coronary anatomy, but its use is severely limited in ESRD due to the need for iodinated contrast and extensive coronary calcifications that reduce image quality and may overestimate the severity of stenosis. Additionally, CCTA is less useful for the etiological characterization of MINOCA (for example, distinguishing between myocarditis, Takotsubo syndrome, or microvascular infarction), serving primarily to rule out obstructive coronary disease in lower-risk patients with moderately impaired renal function [38, 40, 41, 43].

Intravascular ultrasound (IVUS) and optical coherence tomography (OCT) are effective modalities for identifying plaque disruption, erosion, intracoronary thrombus, or spontaneous dissection in patients with MINOCA. These imaging

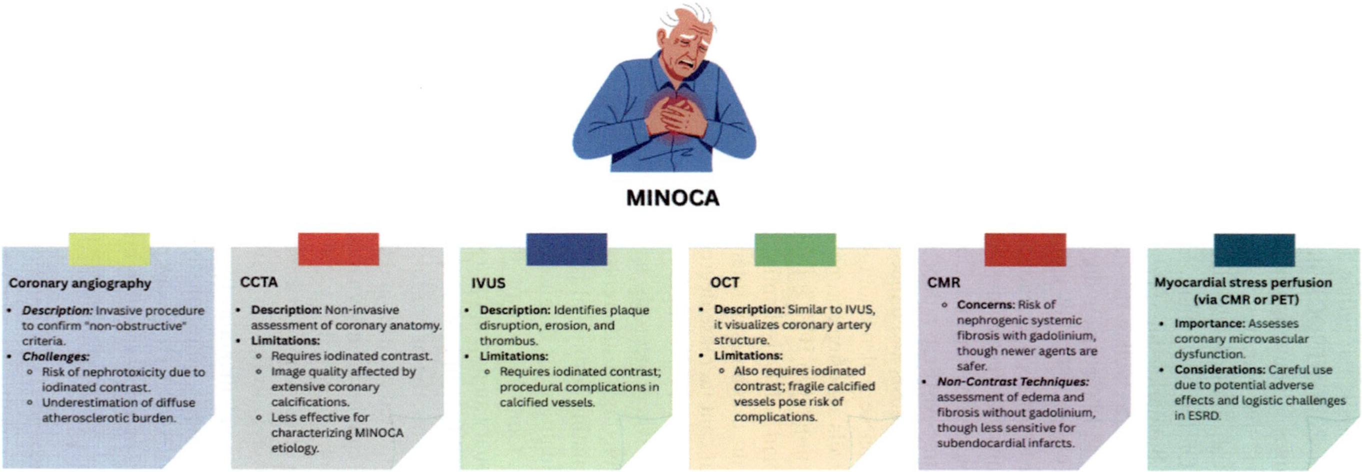

Fig. 12.2 Imaging modalities for diagnosing MINOCA in ESRD patients

techniques can reclassify a significant percentage of cases as "atherothrombotic" infarctions exhibiting angiographically subcritical lesions. Recent reviews concerning MINOCA emphasize the critical role of intracoronary imaging as a fundamental component of the diagnostic algorithm, particularly in younger patients or in instances where cardiac magnetic resonance imaging fails to clarify the underlying etiology [37, 38, 44].

However, in patients with CKD, the use of IVUS and OCT is constrained by the additional requirement for iodinated contrast, especially for OCT, and the fragility of calcified vessels, which may be more susceptible to procedural complications. Recent studies focusing on imaging-guided percutaneous coronary intervention (PCI) in patients presenting with complex coronary lesions and CKD suggest that the prognostic benefits of IVUS and OCT may be less pronounced when eGFR falls below 30 mL/min/1.73 m^2 or in those requiring dialysis. This likelihood may be attributed to an extremely elevated baseline cardiovascular risk and limitations concerning contrast volume. Nonetheless, in selected patients with ESRD, intracoronary imaging can elucidate whether MINOCA has an atherothrombotic or non-atherosclerotic substrate, which has direct implications for the intensity of antiplatelet and lipid-lowering therapy [40, 44–46].

Cardiac magnetic resonance imaging is recognized as the "cornerstone" of the diagnostic algorithm for MINOCA. It enables the differentiation of various conditions, including infarction, myocarditis, Takotsubo cardiomyopathy, infiltrative cardiomyopathies, and other potential causes. Recent data advocate for the performance of cardiac magnetic resonance imaging within the first 7–14 days following an acute event to maximize diagnostic yield. This is achieved through a combination of T2 imaging (edema), late gadolinium enhancement (LGE), and ideally, T1/T2 mapping as well as stress perfusion imaging [38, 39, 47]. In patients with ESRD, a significant concern arises regarding the use of gadolinium-based contrast agents, given the risk of nephrogenic systemic fibrosis and gadolinium tissue deposition. Current consensus guidelines from the American College of Radiology (ACR) and the National Kidney Foundation (NKF), along with contemporary reviews of gadolinium use, emphasize that the risk of NSF is exceedingly low when utilizing new-generation macrocyclic agents (referred to as "Group II GBCM"), even in patients with an eGFR below 30 mL/min/1.73 m^2 or those on dialysis. Research on gadopiclenol and gadobutrol indicates that there is no further deterioration in renal function and that elimination occurs efficiently via hemodialysis, without documented cases of nephrogenic systemic fibrosis in a cohort of patients with ESRD [48–50]. Consequently, cardiac magnetic resonance with contrast, utilizing macrocyclic agents, is increasingly accepted in the ESRD population when the diagnostic benefit is considerable, as seen in cases of suspected MINOCA, with recommendations for one or more dialysis sessions shortly after administration. Additionally, non-contrast techniques, such as native T1 mapping, T2 imaging, and cine-sequences, can provide valuable information regarding edema, diffuse fibrosis, and ventricular function, occasionally allowing for an adequate assessment even without gadolinium, although sensitivity for detecting small subendocardial infarcts may be diminished [39, 47–49].

Myocardial stress perfusion assessment via cardiac magnetic resonance or positron emission tomography is crucial for documenting coronary microvascular dysfunction, a key component in the pathogenesis of MINOCA, including in patients with ESRD. A recent study demonstrated that patients with MINOCA exhibit reduced global stress perfusion compared to age and sex-matched volunteers, suggesting the persistence of coronary microvascular dysfunction even after the acute event has resolved. In ESRD, coronary flow reserve is often diminished independent of the presence of epicardial stenoses, reflecting microvascular remodeling and chronic hemodynamic burden [26, 32, 51]. In clinical practice, when evaluating stress perfusion in patients with ESRD and MINOCA, careful consideration is necessary due to examination time, the potential need for contrast agents, for cardiac magnetic resonance, and comorbidities such as hypotension and arrhythmias, which may limit the use of pharmacological vasodilators. Positron emission tomography using perfusion radiotracers remains the gold standard for measuring flow reserves; however, its routine application in ESRD is constrained by limited accessibility, radiation exposure, and complex logistical requirements [26, 32, 50].

Transthoracic echocardiography is often the initial imaging investigation for patients presenting with ACS, including MINOCA. It provides valuable information regarding ventricular function, segmental kinetic abnormalities, valvular regurgitation, and pulmonary systolic pressure. In patients with advanced CKD, concentric hypertrophy, atrial dilation, and pulmonary hypertension are common and may diminish or alter typical ischemic signs, particularly when the infarction is limited or microvascular [13, 41].

Speckle-tracking techniques and global longitudinal strain analysis can identify subclinical dysfunction and regional patterns suggestive of infarction or Takotsubo syndrome, even when ejection fraction remains preserved. In ESRD, serial monitoring of strain can assist in differentiating between progressive deterioration associated with uremic cardiomyopathy and acute injuries correlated with a MINOCA event. However, standardization of thresholds and correction for hemodynamic changes (pre- and post-dialysis) continue to pose significant challenges [13, 28, 32, 35].

12.5 Management Approaches and Prognosis

The management of MINOCA in patients with ESRD lies at the intersection of two "gray zones": the lack of standardized guidelines for MINOCA and the underrepresentation of ESRD patients in ACS trials. This results in significant variability in clinical practices, underutilization of invasive strategies, and inadequate secondary prevention therapy, all of which have a clear impact on prognosis.

Current recommendations (AHA/ESC) consider MINOCA as an "umbrella term" that necessitates identifying the underlying mechanism (plaque disruption, epicardial spasm, embolism/thrombosis, dissection, microvascular dysfunction, non-ischemic causes) before initiating targeted treatment [1, 52, 53]. The 2025

ACC/AHA/ACEP/NAEMSP/SCAI guideline for the management of patients with ACS [53] recommends that patients with MINOCA initially receive standard AMI management (antiplatelets, statins, beta-blockers, angiotensin-converting enzyme inhibitors/angiotensin receptor blockers when not contraindicated) until imaging and invasive evaluations clarify the etiology and allow for therapy adjustment. Recent data emphasize that the approach should be individualized, but secondary prevention treatment is associated with better prognosis, even when the exact mechanism is not fully understood. Registries suggest that patients with MINOCA are less likely to receive complete "cardioprotective" therapies compared to those with MIOCA, a phenomenon that is more pronounced in patients with CKD, which may contribute to their increased mortality rates [54–56].

Patients with ESRD present an increased risk of bleeding, altered volume distribution, reduced drug clearance, and multiple comorbidities, which necessitate careful dosage adjustments and therapeutic combinations. Recent reviews on ACS in hemodialysis patients indicate that they are treated less aggressively than patients with normal kidney function (fewer angiographies, PCIs, statins, and antiplatelets at optimal doses), even though the relative benefit of evidence-based therapies is often similar [17, 55, 57]. In ESRD, the cardiologist must balance the extremely high ischemic risk with the risk of bleeding (including gastrointestinal bleeding, bleeding at the fistula site, and intracranial hemorrhages), considering the patient's age, frailty, and life expectancy. Guidelines for coronary artery disease in patients with chronic kidney disease support the use of all major classes of cardioprotective medications, with dosage adjustments and careful monitoring, rather than systematic avoidance of these therapies [17, 57, 58].

There are currently no specific randomized studies on the duration and intensity of antiplatelet therapy in MINOCA, particularly in the subgroup with CKD/ESRD, so recommendations are drawn from registries and extrapolated from guidelines for MIOCA. AHA position papers suggest that patients with an identified atherothrombotic mechanism (plaque disruption/erosion confirmed by IVUS/OCT) should receive dual antiplatelet therapy for at least 12 months, similar to MIOCA, while those with non-atherosclerotic mechanisms (pure spasm, microvascular dysfunction, Takotsubo, myocarditis) may receive single antiplatelet therapy or none, depending on the context [37, 44, 52]. In ESRD, dual antiplatelet therapy is associated with a significantly increased risk of major bleeding; however, observational studies show that dialysis patients with acute coronary syndromes who receive aspirin have lower mortality, and the addition of a P2Y12 inhibitor may be beneficial in the initial months, especially after PCI. Guidelines for ACS in ESRD often suggest a shorter duration of dual antiplatelet therapy (e.g., 3–6 months) for patients with very high bleeding risk and without complex stents, followed by monotherapy with either aspirin or P2Y12 inhibitors, but specific data on MINOCA is lacking, and the decision should be individualized [1, 17, 55, 57, 59–62]. Long-term anticoagulation in MINOCA patients is reserved for those with documented coronary embolism, atrial fibrillation, or intracavitary thrombosis; for patients with ESRD, the use of oral anticoagulants (especially vitamin K antagonists) must be considered very carefully, and direct oral anticoagulants may be partially or completely contraindicated in dialysis depending on the specific agent [17, 52].

Registry studies in MINOCA have shown that the use of statins, angiotensin-converting enzyme inhibitors/angiotensin receptor blockers, and beta-blockers is associated with a reduction in MACE and mortality, suggesting that these therapies are beneficial even in the absence of significant epicardial stenosis. A large cohort study reported that patients with MINOCA treated with statins had a lower risk of mortality and recurrent myocardial infarction, and the benefit of angiotensin-converting enzyme inhibitors/angiotensin receptor blockers was similar to that observed in MIOCA [17, 18, 52]. In CKD/ESRD, the role of statins is well established for cardiovascular prevention up to the dialysis stage, but data from large studies suggest a more modest benefit after the initiation of dialysis; nonetheless, guidelines recommend maintaining treatment in patients with manifest coronary artery disease. Renin-Angiotensin-Aldosterone system inhibitors remain essential for blood pressure control, regression of left ventricular hypertrophy, and cardiovascular protection, but in ESRD, potassium levels and blood pressure must be closely monitored, with dose adjustments made accordingly [17, 57, 58, 63]. Beta-blockers reduce mortality after AMI and are particularly useful in patients with ventricular dysfunction or microvascular ischemia. However, in dialysis patients, the risk of bradycardia and intradialytic hypotension is higher; therefore, molecules with non-renal elimination are preferred [17, 55].

In patients where investigations indicate plaque disruption or intracoronary thrombosis, management should follow treatment guidelines for obstructive ACS: PCI when feasible, complete dual antiplatelet therapy, and intensification of lipid-lowering therapy (including consideration of PCSK9 inhibitors in patients with persistently elevated LDL-cholesterol). In ESRD, the selection of patients for PCI must take into account fragile vascular anatomy, the risk of complications at the dialysis access site, and the potential prognostic benefit. However, recent data show that dialysis patients with ACS remain under-revascularized compared to the general population [17, 18, 64]. For MINOCA due to epicardial spasm or microvascular dysfunction, therapy includes calcium channel blockers, nitrates, selected beta-blockers, and possibly ranolazine, along with the avoidance of triggering factors (such as cocaine use, vasoconstrictors, and severe intradialytic hypotension). In ESRD patients, fine control of volume and blood pressure during dialysis is essential to reduce episodes of microvascular ischemia and hypotension that can precipitate ischemic recurrences [17, 37, 52, 58]. In cases of Takotsubo or myocarditis identified via CMR, treatment is primarily supportive (beta-blockers, renin-angiotensin-aldosterone system inhibitors, volume control, immunosuppression when indicated), but in patients with ESRD, the regimen must be integrated with the dialysis schedule and involve careful monitoring of ventricular function and arrhythmias [39, 47].

Recent data on ACS in hemodialysis patients emphasize the importance of establishing an interdisciplinary protocol to coordinate the timing of dialysis with cardiology interventions (angiography, PCI, CMR) to minimize hemodynamic fluctuations and cumulative contrast exposure [65]. It is generally recommended to schedule a dialysis session shortly after the administration of iodinated or gadolinium contrast to facilitate elimination and reduce the risks of volume overload and complications [66]. In the acute post-MINOCA phase, dialysis parameters (duration, ultrafiltration, dialysate composition, temperature) should be adjusted to avoid hypotension and reflex tachycardia, which can exacerbate microvascular ischemia [67, 68]. Close monitoring of dry weight is recommended, along with the use of slower ultrafiltration rates [69]. For patients with reduced ejection fraction or recent ischemia, more frequent dialysis with shorter sessions may be considered to alleviate hemodynamic stress.

Cohort studies indicate that patients with MINOCA and renal impairment have a significantly worse prognosis compared to those with MINOCA and normal kidney function. An analysis from 2021 revealed that approximately 1/3 of patients with MINOCA have renal dysfunction, and these individuals experience markedly higher short and long-term mortality, comparable to or even exceeding that of patients with obstructive infarction and similar renal impairment [6]. A study comparing outcomes at 3 years between MINOCA and MIOCA, stratified by renal function, found that overall and cardiovascular mortality rates were similar between MINOCA and MIOCA regardless of renal status. However, patients with CKD in both groups had significantly higher mortality than those without CKD. Within the CKD subgroup, a higher rate of non-cardiovascular deaths (particularly from sepsis) was observed in MINOCA patients compared to those with MIOCA, reflecting the fragility and burden of comorbidities in this population [7].

The data on ACS in patients with ESRD demonstrates that in-hospital and 30-day mortality rates are 2–4 times higher compared to patients with normal kidney function, with high rates of heart failure, cardiogenic shock, and malignant arrhythmias. Although these data primarily include MIOCA, it is reasonable to assume that patients with MINOCA and ESRD share a similar risk profile, in the absence of dedicated studies [17, 55, 58, 64]. In the long term, patients with ESRD and documented ischemia have a very high cumulative risk of cardiovascular mortality, and even those with "normal" myocardial scintigraphy have a higher risk than the general population, while perfusion abnormalities are associated with particularly unfavorable prognoses. Prognostic studies on dialysis patients with ACS have reported significantly lower 5-year survival rates, especially in the presence of STEMI or extensive coronary artery disease [58, 64, 70].

Recent data on the management of MINOCA highlight the need for specific randomized studies for this condition, including dedicated sub-analyses for patients with CKD and end-stage renal disease ESRD, to define the optimal duration of dual antiplatelet drug therapy, the intensive role of statins, and the effect of anti-inflammatory or vascular-protective therapies (such as colchicine, IL-1 inhibitors, targeted therapies on microcirculation) [6, 71, 72]. Additionally, risk scores dedicated to MINOCA are being developed, integrating clinical, imaging, and biological variables, and including renal impairment as a major determinant of prognosis is widely recognized [73]. In the field of nephrology, the impact of optimizing dialysis regimens (such as nocturnal dialysis, short daily dialysis, and online hemodiafiltration) on silent myocardial ischemia and acute events is being explored, along with the role of nutritional interventions and reduction of systemic inflammation in lowering coronary risk [74–76]. The integration of these research directions with a better understanding of MINOCA mechanisms is likely to enable the development of personalized therapeutic strategies for patients with ESRD, with the potential to significantly improve the prognosis of this highly vulnerable population.

12.6 Conclusions

The management of MINOCA in patients with ESRD remains a significant and complex challenge. This population exists within a "gray area" of clinical practice due to the lack of standardized guidelines specific to MINOCA, particularly compounded by the underrepresentation of ESRD patients in acute coronary syndrome trials.

Key issues include the atypical clinical presentation of MINOCA in ESRD, which often leads to delayed diagnosis and under-revascularization. Diagnostic precision is hampered by the altered physiological milieu of ESRD, affecting biomarker interpretation and limiting the safe application of advanced imaging techniques. The underlying pathophysiology is an intricate interplay of coronary microvascular dysfunction, chronic inflammation, uremic toxins, and a prothrombotic state, all exacerbated by the hemodynamic stresses of dialysis. This creates a highly vulnerable myocardium prone to ischemic events.

From a therapeutic perspective, clinicians must delicately balance the extremely high ischemic risk against a significantly increased bleeding risk, necessitating individualized approaches, careful dose adjustments, and meticulous monitoring of cardioprotective medications. Despite these challenges, evidence suggests that standard cardiac therapies, when adapted, can still offer benefit. Moreover, an interdisciplinary approach coordinating dialysis with cardiac interventions is paramount to minimize complications.

The prognosis for MINOCA patients with ESRD is considerably poorer than for those with normal renal function, with mortality rates often comparable to or exceeding those of obstructive myocardial infarction in similar renal impairment. This highlights the urgent need for dedicated research, including randomized controlled trials, to establish evidence-based guidelines for optimal antiplatelet, lipid-lowering, and anti-inflammatory strategies. Furthermore, the development of specific risk stratification tools and the exploration of optimized dialysis regimens hold promise for developing personalized therapeutic strategies. Addressing these gaps will be crucial to improve the outcomes and quality of life for this highly vulnerable patient group.

Declarations

Competing Interests The author(s) has no competing interests to declare that are relevant to the content of this manuscript.

Ethics Approval The author(s) declares that this manuscript does not include primary research with human participants.

The author(s) declares that this manuscript does not include primary studies involving animals.

References

1. Byrne RA, Rossello X, Coughlan JJ, ESC Scientific Document Group, et al. 2023 ESC Guidelines for the management of acute coronary syndromes. Eur Heart J. 2023;44(38):3720–826. https://doi.org/10.1093/eurheartj/ehad191. Erratum in: Eur Heart J. 2024 Apr 1;45(13):1145. https://doi.org/10.1093/eurheartj/ehad870.
2. Yildiz M, Ashokprabhu N, Shewale A, et al. Myocardial infarction with non-obstructive coronary arteries (MINOCA). Front Cardiovasc Med. 2022;9:1032436. https://doi.org/10.3389/fcvm.2022.1032436.
3. Reynolds HR, Smilowitz NR. Myocardial infarction with nonobstructive coronary arteries. Annu Rev Med. 2023;74:171–88. https://doi.org/10.1146/annurev-med-042921-111727.
4. Tognola C, Maloberti A, Varrenti M, et al. Myocardial infarction with nonobstructive coronary arteries (MINOCA): current insights into pathophysiology, diagnosis, and management. Diagnostics (Basel). 2025;15(7):942. https://doi.org/10.3390/diagnostics15070942.
5. Walendy V, Stang A, Girndt M. Management of acute myocardial infarction in chronic kidney disease in Germany: an observational study. BMC Nephrol. 2025;26(1):15. https://doi.org/10.1186/s12882-025-03943-5.
6. Zalewska-Adamiec M, Malyszko J, Grodzka E, et al. The outcome of patients with myocardial infarction with non-obstructive coronary arteries (MINOCA) and impaired kidney function: a 3-year observational study. Int Urol Nephrol. 2021;53(12):2557–66. https://doi.org/10.1007/s11255-021-02794-x.
7. Kim YH, Her AY, Rha SW, et al. The impact of renal function on the three-year outcomes in patients with myocardial infarction with nonobstructive coronary arteries. Hell J Cardiol. 2024;77:13–26. https://doi.org/10.1016/j.hjc.2023.08.001.
8. Sánchez-Perales C, Vázquez-Ruiz de Castroviejo E, Segura-Torres P, et al. Incidence of acute myocardial infarction in the evolution of dialysis patients. Nefrologia. 2012;32(5):597–604. English, Spanish. https://doi.org/10.3265/Nefrologia.pre2012.Jun.11464.
9. Herzog CA, Littrell K, Arko C, et al. Clinical characteristics of dialysis patients with acute myocardial infarction in the United States: a collaborative project of the United States Renal Data System and the National Registry of Myocardial Infarction. Circulation. 2007;116(13):1465–72. https://doi.org/10.1161/CIRCULATIONAHA.107.696765.
10. Scott J. Acute coronary events in kidney patients: the dialysis dilemma. Br J Cardiol. 2025;32:3–5. https://doi.org/10.5837/bjc.2025.012.
11. Karamasis G, Xenogiannis I, Varlamos C, et al. Use of optical coherence tomography in MI with non-obstructive coronary arteries. Interv Cardiol. 2022;17:e06. https://doi.org/10.15420/icr.2021.31.
12. Illum E, Kofod DH, Ballegaard EF, et al. Coronary angiography in patients with kidney dysfunction and myocardial injury: a retrospective cohort study on management of myocardial injury in hospitalized patients with kidney disease. Cardiovasc Revasc Med. 2024;63:59–65. https://doi.org/10.1016/j.carrev.2024.01.001.
13. Moisi MI, Rus M, Bungau S, et al. Acute coronary syndromes in chronic kidney disease: clinical and therapeutic characteristics. Medicina (Kaunas). 2020;56(3):118. https://doi.org/10.3390/medicina56030118.
14. Sarnak MJ, Amann K, Bangalore S, et al. Chronic kidney disease and coronary artery disease: JACC state-of-the-art review. J Am Coll Cardiol. 2019;74(14):1823–38. https://doi.org/10.1016/j.jacc.2019.08.1017.

15. Montone RA, Cosentino N, Gorla, PROMISE Trial Investigators, et al. Stratified treatment of myocardial infarction with non-obstructive coronary arteries: the PROMISE trial. Eur Heart J. 2025:ehaf917. https://doi.org/10.1093/eurheartj/ehaf917.
16. Pasupathy S, Tavella R, Beltrame JF. Myocardial infarction with nonobstructive coronary arteries (MINOCA): the past, present, and future management. Circulation. 2017;135(16):1490–3. https://doi.org/10.1161/CIRCULATIONAHA.117.027666.
17. Haider MA, Shah MU, Kassianides X. Diagnosis and management of ACS in patients with ESRD on haemodialysis: a comprehensive review. Br J Cardiol. 2025;32:7–11. https://doi.org/10.5837/bjc.2025.011.
18. Jankowski J, Floege J, Fliser D, Böhm M, Marx N. Cardiovascular disease in chronic kidney disease: pathophysiological insights and therapeutic options. Circulation. 2021;143(11):1157–72. https://doi.org/10.1161/CIRCULATIONAHA.120.050686.
19. Mancebo NG, Caballero RM, Sanz AF, et al. Impact of chronic kidney disease on patients with myocardial infarction with non obstructive coronary arteries (MINOCA). Eur Heart J. 2024;45(Supplement_1):ehae666.3267.
20. Hao K, Takahashi J, Sato K, et al. Clinical characteristics and outcome of patients with myocardial infarction with nonobstructive coronary arteries in Japan: insights from the Miyagi acute myocardial infarction registry study. J Am Heart Assoc. 2025;14(5):e036802. https://doi.org/10.1161/JAHA.124.036802.
21. Long B, Belcher CN, Koyfman A, Bronner JM. Interpreting troponin in renal disease: a narrative review for emergency clinicians. Am J Emerg Med. 2020;38(5):990–7. https://doi.org/10.1016/j.ajem.2019.11.041.
22. Huang HL, Zhu S, Wang WQ, et al. Diagnosis of acute myocardial infarction in hemodialysis patients with high-sensitivity cardiac troponin T assay. Arch Pathol Lab Med. 2016;140(1):75–80. https://doi.org/10.5858/arpa.2014-0580-OA.
23. Howard CE, McCullough PA. Decoding acute myocardial infarction among patients on dialysis. J Am Soc Nephrol. 2017;28(5):1337–9. https://doi.org/10.1681/ASN.2017030226.
24. Fang X, Mei W. Myocardial infarction with non-obstructive coronary arteries in a patient undergoing nephrectomy under general anesthesia. J Anesthesia Transl Med. 2025;4:50–4.
25. Khattab E, Karelas D, Pallas T, et al. MINOCA: a pathophysiological approach of diagnosis and treatment-a narrative review. Biomedicine. 2024;12(11):2457. https://doi.org/10.3390/biomedicines12112457.
26. Bajaj NS, Singh A, Zhou W, et al. Coronary microvascular dysfunction, left ventricular remodeling, and clinical outcomes in patients with chronic kidney impairment. Circulation. 2020;141(1):21–33. https://doi.org/10.1161/CIRCULATIONAHA.119.043916.
27. Galante D, La Vecchia G, Leone AM, Crea F. Coronary microvascular dysfunction in angina and non-obstructive coronary arteries: pathophysiology, diagnosis, novel markers and therapy. Kardiol Pol. 2025;83(3):269–76. https://doi.org/10.33963/v.phj.105217.
28. Rocco M, Flavia N, Margherita L, et al. Coronary microvascular dysfunction: searching the strongest imaging modality in different scenarios. Echocardiography. 2024;41(11):e70022. https://doi.org/10.1111/echo.70022.
29. Guo Z, Yang Z, Song Z, et al. Inflammation and coronary microvascular disease: relationship, mechanism and treatment. Front Cardiovasc Med. 2024;11:1280734. https://doi.org/10.3389/fcvm.2024.1280734.
30. Borkowski P, Maliha M, Borkowski M, et al. Myocardial infarction with non-obstructive coronary arteries (MINOCA): a case report and comprehensive discussion of pathophysiology and risk factors. Cureus. 2024;16(8):e67144. https://doi.org/10.7759/cureus.67144.
31. Scarica V, Rinaldi R, Animati FM, et al. Coronary microvascular dysfunction: pathophysiology, diagnosis, and therapeutic strategies across cardiovascular diseases. EXCLI J. 2025;24:454–78. https://doi.org/10.17179/excli2025-8285.
32. Parnham SF, Gleadle JM, De Pasquale CG, Selvanayagam JB. Myocardial ischemia assessment in chronic kidney disease: challenges and pitfalls. Front Cardiovasc Med. 2014;1:13. https://doi.org/10.3389/fcvm.2014.00013.

33. Krishnan S, Suarez-Martinez AD, Bagher P, et al. Microvascular dysfunction and kidney disease: challenges and opportunities? Microcirculation. 2021;28(3):e12661. https://doi.org/10.1111/micc.12661.
34. Feuer DS, Handberg EM, Mehrad B, et al. Microvascular dysfunction as a systemic disease: a review of the evidence. Am J Med. 2022;135(9):1059–68. https://doi.org/10.1016/j.amjmed.2022.04.006.
35. Radhakrishnan A, Pickup LC, Price AM, et al. Coronary microvascular dysfunction is associated with degree of anaemia in end-stage renal disease. BMC Cardiovasc Disord. 2021;21(1):211. https://doi.org/10.1186/s12872-021-02025-2.
36. Ryabov VV, Vorobeva DA, Kologrivova IV, Suslova TE. Pro-inflammatory biomarkers and progression of atherosclerosis in patients with myocardial infarction with non-obstructive coronary artery disease: 1-year follow-up. J Pers Med. 2023;13(12):1669. https://doi.org/10.3390/jpm13121669.
37. Ezhumalai B, Modi R, Chidambaram S. A comprehensive review on myocardial infarction with non-obstructive coronary arteries (MINOCA): one size does not fit all. Indian Heart J. 2025;77(4):318–25. https://doi.org/10.1016/j.ihj.2025.05.013.
38. Thurmann KE, Bellamkonda P, Kalinkin OM. A stepwise diagnostic approach to transmural myocardial infarction with non-obstructive coronary arteries with microvascular obstruction highlighting the role of cardiac MRI in suspected thrombolysis. Cureus. 2025;17(6):e85489. https://doi.org/10.7759/cureus.85489.
39. Riahi F, Tooyserkani SH, Mojahedi A, et al. Cardiac magnetic resonance imaging in myocardial infarction with non-obstructed coronary arteries: diagnostic and prognostic value. Am J Cardiovasc Dis. 2025;15(2):56–68. https://doi.org/10.62347/FCDC4114.
40. Ananthakrishna R, Liang Z, Raman B, et al. Long-term clinical outcomes in patients with a working diagnosis of myocardial infarction with non-obstructed coronary arteries (MINOCA) assessed by cardiovascular magnetic resonance imaging. Int J Cardiol. 2022;349:12–7. https://doi.org/10.1016/j.ijcard.2021.11.088.
41. Zoccali C, Chinnappa S, Fernández-Fernández B, et al. Myocardial Ischaemic syndromes in chronic kidney disease: risky pathways from non-acute to acute events. Nephrol Dial Transplant. 2025:gfaf142. https://doi.org/10.1093/ndt/gfaf142.
42. Zghyer F, Ziada KM. The diagnostic dilemma of myocardial infarction without obstructive coronary artery disease: advanced imaging to the rescue! Cleve Clin J Med. 2024;91(12):755–61. https://doi.org/10.3949/ccjm.91a.24106.
43. Kato K, Yonetsu T, Jia H, et al. Nonculprit coronary plaque characteristics of chronic kidney disease. Circ Cardiovasc Imaging. 2013;6(3):448–56. https://doi.org/10.1161/CIRCIMAGING.112.000165.
44. Squires I, Khalil S, Patel A, Katukari N. MINOCA: predictors and future management. Indian J Cardiovasc Dis Women. 2025;10:45–50. https://doi.org/10.25259/IJCDW_50_2024.
45. Kwon W, Choi KH, Song YB, et al. Intravascular imaging in patients with complex coronary lesions and chronic kidney disease. JAMA Netw Open. 2023;6(11):e2345554. https://doi.org/10.1001/jamanetworkopen.2023.45554.
46. Lin CP, Hsiao FC, Tung YC, et al. Intravascular imaging-guided percutaneous coronary intervention in patients with end-stage renal disease on maintenance dialysis. JACC Asia. 2024;5(1):28–41. https://doi.org/10.1016/j.jacasi.2024.10.006.
47. Párraga R, Real C, Fernández-Jiménez R. Cardiovascular magnetic resonance in the working diagnosis of MINOCA: the sooner, the better? Rev Esp Cardiol (Engl Ed). 2024;77(7):524–6. English, Spanish. https://doi.org/10.1016/j.rec.2023.12.013.
48. Alsogati E, Ghandourah H, Bakhsh A. Review of the efficacy and safety of Gadopiclenol: a newly emerging gadolinium-based contrast agent. Cureus. 2023;15(8):e43055. https://doi.org/10.7759/cureus.43055.
49. Weinreb JC, Rodby RA, Yee J, et al. Use of intravenous gadolinium-based contrast media in patients with kidney disease: consensus statements from the American College of Radiology

and the National Kidney Foundation. Radiology. 2021;298(1):28–35. https://doi.org/10.1148/radiol.2020202903.
50. Iyad N, S Ahmad M, Alkhatib SG, Hjouj M. Gadolinium contrast agents- challenges and opportunities of a multidisciplinary approach: literature review. Eur J Radiol Open. 2023;11:100503. https://doi.org/10.1016/j.ejro.2023.100503.
51. Steffen Johansson R, Tornvall P, Sörensson P, Nickander J. Reduced stress perfusion in myocardial infarction with nonobstructive coronary arteries. Sci Rep. 2023;13(1):22094. https://doi.org/10.1038/s41598-023-49223-w.
52. Tamis-Holland JE, Jneid H, Reynolds HR, American Heart Association Interventional Cardiovascular Care Committee of the Council on Clinical Cardiology; Council on Cardiovascular and Stroke Nursing; Council on Epidemiology and Prevention; and Council on Quality of Care and Outcomes Research, et al. Contemporary diagnosis and management of patients with myocardial infarction in the absence of obstructive coronary artery disease: a scientific statement from the American Heart Association. Circulation. 2019;139(18):e891–908. https://doi.org/10.1161/CIR.0000000000000670.
53. Rao SV, O'Donoghue ML, Ruel M, et al. 2025 ACC/AHA/ACEP/NAEMSP/SCAI guideline for the management of patients with acute coronary syndromes: a report of the American College of Cardiology/American Heart Association joint committee on clinical practice guidelines. Circulation. 2025;151(13):e771–862. https://doi.org/10.1161/CIR.0000000000001309.
54. Haertel F, Montag C, Kraeplin T, et al. Management of myocardial infarction with non-obstructive coronary arteries (MINOCA) in Germany: a single-center study on hospital resources and healthcare economics. Front Public Health. 2024;12:1407568. https://doi.org/10.3389/fpubh.2024.1407568.
55. Santolucito PA, Tighe DA, McManus DD, et al. Management and outcomes of renal disease and acute myocardial infarction. Am J Med. 2010;123(9):847–55. https://doi.org/10.1016/j.amjmed.2010.04.025.
56. Pacheco C, Coutinho T, Bastiany A, et al. Canadian cardiovascular society/Canadian women's heart health Alliance clinical practice update on myocardial infarction with no obstructive coronary artery disease (MINOCA). Can J Cardiol. 2024;40(6):953–68. https://doi.org/10.1016/j.cjca.2024.02.032.
57. Kim JA, Kim SE, El Hachem K, et al. Medical management of coronary artery disease in patients with chronic kidney disease. Am J Med. 2023;136(12):1147–59. https://doi.org/10.1016/j.amjmed.2023.06.013.
58. Kwon W, Choi KH, Jeong DS, et al. Comparison of long-term cardiovascular and renal outcomes between percutaneous coronary intervention and coronary artery bypass grafting in multi-vessel disease with chronic kidney disease. Front Cardiovasc Med. 2022;9:951113. https://doi.org/10.3389/fcvm.2022.951113.
59. Li S, Wang D, Han X, et al. Antiplatelet strategy for patients with acute coronary syndrome and chronic kidney disease: a systematic review and meta-analysis. Front Cardiovasc Med. 2025;12:1527667. https://doi.org/10.3389/fcvm.2025.1527667.
60. Burlacu A, Covic A. Longer or shorter dual antiplatelet therapy in dialysis patients receiving a coronary drug-eluting stent? A rope game still ongoing. Clin Kidney J. 2020;13(5):749–52. https://doi.org/10.1093/ckj/sfaa040.
61. Ortega-Paz L, Galli M, Capodanno D, et al. The role of antiplatelet therapy in patients with MINOCA. Front Cardiovasc Med. 2022;8:821297. https://doi.org/10.3389/fcvm.2021.821297.
62. Mantzouranis E, Leontsinis I, Vlachakis PK, et al. Antiplatelet treatment strategy in MINOCA patients: predictors of decision making in clinical practice and prognostic implications. J Clin Med. 2025;14(11):3984. https://doi.org/10.3390/jcm14113984.
63. Zhao L, Li S, Gao Y. Efficacy of statins on renal function in patients with chronic kidney disease: a systematic review and meta-analysis. Ren Fail. 2021;43(1):718–28. https://doi.org/10.1080/0886022X.2021.1915799.

64. Nakao S, Ishihara T, Okada K, et al. Long-term prognosis after acute coronary syndrome due to de novo coronary artery lesions and stent thrombosis in patients on hemodialysis. Sci Rep. 2025;15:26063. https://doi.org/10.1038/s41598-025-11968-x.
65. Şener YZ, Erdogdu T. Acute coronary syndrome in hemodialysis patients: a look from a broad perspective. Acta Cardiol Sin. 2024;40(4):467. https://doi.org/10.6515/ACS.202407_40(4).20240521C.
66. Deray G. Dialysis and iodinated contrast media. Kidney Int Suppl. 2006;100:S25–9. https://doi.org/10.1038/sj.ki.5000371.
67. Tsujimoto Y, Tsujimoto H, Nakata Y, et al. Dialysate temperature reduction for intradialytic hypotension for people with chronic kidney disease requiring haemodialysis. Cochrane Database Syst Rev. 2019;7(7):CD012598. https://doi.org/10.1002/14651858.CD012598.pub2. PMID: 31273758; PMCID: PMC6609546.
68. Stuard S, Ridel C, Cioffi M, et al. Hemodialysis procedures for stable incident and prevalent patients optimize hemodynamic stability, dialysis dose, electrolytes, and fluid balance. J Clin Med. 2024;13(11):3211. https://doi.org/10.3390/jcm13113211.
69. Sinha AD, Agarwal R. Setting the dry weight and its cardiovascular implications. Semin Dial. 2017;30(6):481–8. https://doi.org/10.1111/sdi.12624.
70. Park GH, Song JW, Lee CM, et al. Long-term prognosis of end-stage renal disease patients with normal myocardial perfusion as determined by single photon emission computed tomography. Korean J Intern Med. 2018;33(1):148–56. https://doi.org/10.3904/kjim.2016.116.
71. Montenegro Sá F, Carvalho R, Santos L, Portuguese Registry of Acute Coronary Syndromes, et al. Dual antiplatelet therapy in myocardial infarction with non-obstructive coronary artery disease - insights from a nationwide registry. Rev Port Cardiol (Engl Ed). 2020;39(12):679–84. English, Portuguese. https://doi.org/10.1016/j.repc.2020.05.008.
72. Oro P, Vignarajah A, El Dahdah J, et al. Colchicine and cardiovascular outcomes in MINOCA: a retrospective cohort study. Am Heart J Plus. 2025;60:100643. https://doi.org/10.1016/j.ahjo.2025.100643.
73. Xia J, Deng C, Yang C, et al. Clinical characteristics and prognosis of myocardial infarction with nonobstructive coronary arteries evaluated by optical coherence tomography. Sci Rep. 2025;15:9962. https://doi.org/10.1038/s41598-025-91865-5.
74. Narula AS, Bali HS, Sakhuja V, et al. Silent myocardial ischemia in hemodialysis patients – factor fiction? Med J Armed Forces India. 1996;52(2):110–2. https://doi.org/10.1016/S0377-1237(17)30855-9.
75. Dasselaar JJ, Slart RH, Knip M, et al. Haemodialysis is associated with a pronounced fall in myocardial perfusion. Nephrol Dial Transplant. 2009;24(2):604–10. https://doi.org/10.1093/ndt/gfn501.
76. McIntyre CW. Update on hemodialysis-induced multiorgan ischemia: brains and beyond. J Am Soc Nephrol. 2024;35(5):653–64. https://doi.org/10.1681/ASN.0000000000000299.

Chapter 13
Cardiac Stunning During Haemodialysis: Pathophysiology, Risk Stratification, and Management

Beata Franczyk, Anna Gluba-Sagr, Abdusalam Sagr, and Jacek Rysz

13.1 Introduction

Cardiovascular disease (CVD) remains the leading cause of death in patients receiving maintenance haemodialysis, accounting for roughly 40% of all-cause mortality in contemporary cohorts [1, 2]. Sudden cardiac death (SCD), often presumed arrhythmic, represents a substantial proportion of these events (commonly estimated at ~20–30% of all deaths in haemodialysis populations), although the exact contribution varies across studies and method of assessment [2–4]. Observational data further suggest that cardiovascular (CV) risk peaks around the initiation of dialysis, with early mortality several-fold higher than in the general population and CV and SCD deaths are over-represented [5–7]. Intradialytic myocardial stunning has emerged as a plausible mechanistic link between the haemodialysis procedure and downstream heart failure (HF), arrhythmias, and SCD.

The concept of myocardial stunning originated in general cardiology and refers to a reversible form of post-ischemic left ventricular (LV) dysfunction. Experimental work from the 1970s and 1980s, consolidated by Braunwald and Kloner, showed that brief periods of coronary occlusion followed by timely reperfusion could leave myocardium viable but mechanically depressed for hours to days, despite restoration of normal blood flow. This "stunned myocardium" was defined as prolonged, reversible contractile dysfunction after ischemia without irreversible necrosis [8, 9]. Subsequent clinical observations in patients with coronary artery disease (CAD) confirmed analogous transient regional wall motion abnormalities that recover over time in the absence of infarction [10]. The phenomenon remains closely associated

B. Franczyk · A. Gluba-Sagr (✉) · A. Sagr · J. Rysz
Department of Nephrology, Hypertension and Family Medicine, Medical University of Lodz, Lodz, Poland
e-mail: anna.gluba-brzozka@umed.lodz.pl

A. Covic, A. Burlacu (eds.), *Renal Dysfunction in Cardiovascular Pathologies*,
https://doi.org/10.1007/978-3-032-25434-4_13

with reperfusion injury mechanisms, including oxidative stress and disturbed calcium handling [9].

Over the last two decades, a similar pattern of transient LV dysfunction has been recognized in patients undergoing haemodialysis. Using intradialytic echocardiography, Selby and colleagues demonstrated that standard haemodialysis frequently provokes new regional LV wall motion abnormalities, consistent with myocardial stunning, and that these abnormalities can be attenuated by interventions such as biofeedback-guided ultrafiltration or dialysate cooling [1, 11]. McIntyre, Burton, and co-workers further demonstrated that haemodialysis-induced LV dysfunction is accompanied by acute reductions in global and regional myocardial blood flow, supporting the concept that repetitive intradialytic ischemia is common in routine practice [12, 13]. In clinical cohorts, Burton et al. found that approximately two-thirds of patients exhibited significant intradialytic myocardial stunning and that its presence was independently associated with lower LV ejection fraction (LVEF) at follow-up and higher 12-month mortality [1]. In a 12-month follow-up of prevalent haemodialysis patients, those who developed intradialytic regional wall motion abnormalities also experienced a greater decline in LVEF and significantly higher mortality and time to first CV event compared with patients without stunning [1]. Another study has shown that stunning is common, that its severity correlates with intradialytic hypotension, ultrafiltration volume and rate, and biomarkers such as cardiac troponin T, and that its presence is associated with worse survival and progressive LV dysfunction [1, 14]. Collectively, these mechanistic and clinical studies underpin recognition of "haemodialysis-induced myocardial (cardiac) stunning" as a dialysis-related manifestation of ischemic myocardial injury [15, 16].

More recent prospective and interventional data strengthen the link between dialysis-induced stunning and clinically relevant endpoints by demonstrating modifiability of the phenomenon. Frequent haemodialysis schedules and strategies that improve hemodynamic stability, such as cooler dialysate or ultrafiltration profiling, reduce the burden of intradialytic stunning and are associated with lower levels of dialysis-induced cardiac injury [17, 18]. Intradialytic exercise programs have been shown to attenuate stunning and improve measures of cardiac structure and function, and are now being evaluated specifically for their ability to reduce CV events [19–22]. Experimental data further support a mechanistic role for mitochondrial dysfunction and ion flux disturbances in haemodialysis-induced myocardial stunning, providing biologic plausibility for its progression to chronic myocardial injury and arrhythmogenic remodelling [16].

Taken together, contemporary evidence supports viewing cardiac stunning during dialysis not merely as an imaging curiosity but as a central pathophysiologic process at the interface of the failing heart and kidney. It provides a mechanistic framework linking intradialytic hemodynamic stress and ischemia to the high incidence of HF, malignant arrhythmias, and sudden death in the haemodialysis population, and it represents an attractive target for treatment strategies aimed at improving cardiovascular outcomes in CKD and ESKD.

Definitions

In this chapter, "cardiac" or "myocardial stunning during dialysis" refers to transient regional or global LV systolic dysfunction that arises during a haemodialysis session as a consequence of intradialytic ischemia, in the absence of irreversible myocardial necrosis, and that shows partial or complete recovery between treatments. In most clinical series, stunning is operationalized as the development of new or worsening regional wall motion abnormalities or a $\geq$15–20% reduction in segmental or global systolic strain during dialysis, with subsequent improvement on post-dialysis or interdialytic imaging [1, 23, 24]. Repetition of this acute insult over months to years is hypothesized to contribute to a progressive decline in resting LV function and the development of a characteristic haemodialysis-associated cardiomyopathy [15, 18, 25]. This intradialytic entity needs to be distinguished from other forms of myocardial dysfunction frequently observed in chronic kidney disease (CKD) and end-stage kidney disease (ESKD):

1. Chronic uremic cardiomyopathy/CKD-related cardiomyopathy is characterized by concentric or eccentric LV hypertrophy, chamber dilation, fibrosis, and diastolic and/or systolic dysfunction that develop over time in response to long-standing pressure and volume overload, anaemia, neurohumoral activation, and uremic toxins [1, 6, 18]. This remodelling is present at baseline, persists between dialysis sessions, and does not by itself imply an acute ischemic trigger linked to an individual treatment.
2. Hibernating myocardium represents chronically hypoperfused but viable tissue, in which resting flow and contractile function are both reduced due to severe, typically fixed coronary stenosis. Contractile function can recover after successful revascularization [26]. In contrast, stunned myocardium, whether in coronary disease or during dialysis, has relatively preserved resting perfusion at the time of assessment, but exhibits disproportionate, reversible contractile depression following transient ischemia [8, 9].
3. Fixed infarction denotes non-viable scar tissue formed after prolonged ischemia with myocyte necrosis. Infarcted segments lack contractile reserve and typically show reduced tracer uptake on perfusion or metabolic imaging, even long after revascularization [8]. Haemodialysis-induced myocardial stunning, by definition, occurs in viable tissue and is distinguished from silent or overt infarction by its reversibility and by the absence of new irreversible scar on appropriate imaging [1, 15, 27].

Recognizing these distinctions is crucial: intradialytic stunning is an acute, treatment-linked process superimposed on a background of CKD-related structural heart disease and, in many patients, coexisting coronary atherosclerosis or prior infarction.

13.2 Concept of Myocardial Stunning

13.2.1 General Principles

Myocardial stunning denotes a state in which regional or global systolic function remains depressed after an ischemic episode even though coronary flow has been re-established (or is close to normal). In this setting, the affected myocardium is still viable, but mechanical performance lags behind the recovery of perfusion, hence the concept of a perfusion-contraction mismatch following ischemia-reperfusion. This phenomenon is most often discussed as a reperfusion-related functional deficit rather than permanent loss of contractile tissue [28–30]. The hallmark of stunning is delayed functional recovery: contractility may improve over hours, but full normalization commonly requires days, particularly when ischemia is longer or more severe (while still short of causing extensive irreversible necrosis). Experimental and clinical descriptions emphasize a graded relationship, more intense/prolonged ischemia generally produces deeper dysfunction and slower recovery, and recovery may be heterogeneous across myocardial layers/regions. Recurrent episodes ("repetitive" stunning) can prolong dysfunction and are being studied with modern metabolic and mechanistic profiling [28, 31, 32].

13.2.2 Mechanistic Underpinnings

Restoration of coronary blood flow after a prolonged ischemic episode is indispensable for myocardial salvage, yet the sudden reintroduction of oxygen and substrates initiates a complex cascade of biochemical events collectively termed myocardial ischemia–reperfusion injury (MIRI). Clinically, reperfusion injury contributes to final infarct size, early post-ischemic dysfunction, and downstream remodelling in patients with acute myocardial infarction (AMI) treated with reperfusion therapies [33–35]. During ischemia, reduced oxygen delivery rapidly constrains oxidative phosphorylation, forcing a shift toward anaerobic glycolysis with accumulation of lactate and protons, depletion of high-energy phosphates, and progressive failure of ATP-dependent ion transport. ATP depletion impairs sarcolemmal and sarcoplasmic reticulum (SR) transporters and destabilizes cytoskeletal and membrane integrity. Intracellular Na^+ rises in part through activation of the Na^+/H^+ exchanger (NHE1) during acidosis, which, together with impaired Na^+/K^+-ATPase activity, predisposes to Ca^{2+} overload via reverse-mode Na^+/Ca^{2+} exchange (NCX) when extracellular conditions normalize at reperfusion [33, 36].

A large part of the harmful biology occurs when oxygen delivery is restored. Reperfusion reactivates mitochondrial respiration in a metabolically primed cardiomyocyte, producing an early burst of reactive oxygen species (ROS) that can convert potentially reversible injury into irreversible cardiomyocyte death and dysfunction. Contemporary models place mitochondria among the key early ROS sources, particularly through ischemia-driven accumulation of succinate and its rapid oxidation at reperfusion. Succinate oxidation can drive reverse electron transport (RET) at respiratory complex I, promoting superoxide generation during the first minutes of reperfusion [37–40]. This mitochondrial ROS pulse is complemented by extramitochondrial sources, including NADPH oxidases (NOX family), xanthine oxidase (activated in the context of ischemic purine catabolism), uncoupled endothelial nitric oxide synthase, and activated leukocytes recruited to the reperfused territory. Superoxide and downstream radicals can react with nitric oxide to form peroxynitrite and other reactive nitrogen species (RNS), amplifying nitrosative stress. When ROS/RNS exceeds endogenous antioxidant and redox-buffering capacity, oxidative stress promotes MIRI via direct molecular injury (lipid peroxidation; oxidative/nitrative modification of proteins and nucleic acids) and indirect activation of regulated injury pathways [33, 41, 42]. Importantly, oxidative stress in MIRI is time-structured and compartmentalized rather than uniform: redox-proteomics in murine reperfusion models demonstrates prominent reversible thiol oxidation early after reperfusion, with later reversal, whereas protein carbonylation and glutathione depletion increase progressively, consistent with an early mitochondrial-centred oxidant burst followed by broader oxidative/inflammatory contributions [43]. At the mitochondrion, ROS and Ca^{2+} dysregulation converge on the mitochondrial permeability transition (mPT). Sustained opening of the mitochondrial permeability transition pore (mPTP) collapses membrane potential, uncouples oxidative phosphorylation, induces matrix swelling, and precipitates rapid energetic failure. Although mitochondrial permeabilization can contribute to apoptotic signalling under some conditions, early reperfusion infarct expansion is most consistently linked to necrotic/regulated necrotic mechanisms driven by mitochondrial dysfunction and bioenergetic collapse [33, 44, 45]. These concepts also help explain why broad, non-selective antioxidant strategies have often shown limited clinical benefit despite strong preclinical effects. The biology is highly source-, compartment-, and timing-dependent, and ROS also participate in signalling required for repair/adaptation. Consequently, current translational approaches increasingly focus on targeting specific ROS sources (including mitochondria/RET), modulating redox-sensitive signalling, and combining redox interventions with anti-inflammatory, metabolic, or microvascular strategies [35, 41].

Calcium overload is a canonical trigger and amplifier of reperfusion injury and is tightly linked with redox signalling. During ischemia, acidosis and ATP depletion impair SR Ca^{2+} reuptake (SERCA2a) and promote Na^+ accumulation. At reperfusion, rapid pH normalization and renewed Na^+ entry via NHE can drive NCX into reverse mode, worsening cytosolic Ca^{2+} loading. In parallel, ROS can modify key Ca^{2+}-handling proteins (including RyR2 and SR/mitochondrial targets), promoting SR Ca^{2+} leak, impaired Ca^{2+} sequestration, and diastolic Ca^{2+} accumulation, thereby linking the oxidant burst to Ca^{2+} overload and hypercontracture [33, 36, 41]. A pivotal downstream event is mitochondrial Ca^{2+} overload. Ca^{2+} entry into mitochondria (via MCU-dependent and context-dependent alternative routes) sensitizes permeability transition, especially in the presence of oxidative stress and rapid pH recovery. Thus, Ca^{2+}, ROS, and pH behave as an interdependent triad: Ca^{2+}-loaded mitochondria generate more ROS, ROS further destabilize Ca^{2+} handling and lower the threshold for mPTP opening, and rapid pH normalization removes an inhibitory constraint on pore opening and contractile activation [44, 46, 47]. Beyond cell death, Ca^{2+} overload contributes to post-ischemic mechanical dysfunction ("stunning"), in which viable myocardium remains mechanically depressed for hours to days despite restored perfusion and absence of extensive necrosis. Stunning reflects impaired excitation-contraction coupling (abnormal Ca^{2+} transients and SR dysfunction) and reduced responsiveness of the contractile apparatus to Ca^{2+} (altered myofilament Ca^{2+} sensitivity) [29, 48]. Myofilament sensitivity is governed by thin-filament regulation (troponin–tropomyosin), thick-filament state, titin-based mechanics, and post-translational modifications that shift cross-bridge kinetics and Ca^{2+} binding/activation. Ischemia-reperfusion disturbs these determinants through combined effects of acidosis, inorganic phosphate accumulation, kinase signalling (PKA/PKC/CaMKII), and oxidative/nitrosative modifications. Acidosis during ischemia depresses myofilament Ca^{2+} sensitivity and may transiently limit force development and energetic demand. At reperfusion, rapid pH recovery can unmask Ca^{2+} overload and precipitate forceful contraction in structurally vulnerable sarcomeres [33, 48]. Evidence supports both biochemical modification and proteolysis of sarcomeric proteins in post-ischemic dysfunction including Ca^{2+}-activated calpain–mediated troponin I proteolysis, which correlates with reduced myofilament Ca^{2+} responsiveness in stunned myocardium [48, 49]. Finally, impaired myofilament sensitivity should be regarded as a dynamic context-dependent phenotype: β-adrenergic phosphorylation can reduce Ca^{2+} sensitivity to accelerate relaxation, whereas specific oxidative modifications may either sensitize or desensitize myofilaments depending on the target and residue. Regional heterogeneity is expected, and persistence of Ca^{2+} handling abnormalities with sarcomeric remodelling contributes to adverse remodelling and heart failure risk [29, 33].

13.3 Haemodialysis as a Trigger

13.3.1 Hemodynamic Changes During Standard HD

Standard intermittent haemodialysis (HD) imposes a repetitive, time-compressed circulatory challenge in which rapid fluid and solute shifts must be buffered by cardiac reserve, autonomic reflexes, and microvascular vasomotor control. The most immediate hemodynamic perturbation is the reduction in effective circulating volume driven by ultrafiltration (UF). UF removes plasma water faster than many patients can achieve compensatory plasma refilling from the interstitium, particularly when interdialytic fluid gains are large, treatment time is short, or vascular compliance is reduced. As venous return falls, preload declines, LV filling becomes more dependent on diastolic function, and stroke volume may drop, especially in patients with LV hypertrophy, myocardial fibrosis, or impaired relaxation, which are common in ESRD [50–52]. Intradialytic hypotension (IDH) is best understood as a mismatch between the rate of effective blood-volume reduction and the ability of the CV system to maintain cardiac output and systemic vascular resistance. IDH has been found to be multifactorial: beyond UF-driven hypovolemia, rapid osmotic/tonicity changes, impaired arteriolar constriction, autonomic dysfunction, and comorbid CVD, all contribute to hemodynamic fragility [50–52]. In a recent review, reduced effective blood volume and decreased plasma tonicity are highlighted as central physiological drivers that can undermine vascular refilling and vasomotor compensation during HD [51]. Afterload during HD is not static. In stable sessions, sympathetic activation and vasoconstriction can partially preserve blood pressure despite falling preload. In contrast, in IDH-prone individuals, peripheral vascular resistance may fail to rise appropriately (or may fall), so the same UF rate produces a larger drop in arterial pressure. Reviews of IDH consistently indicate the event as the end result of the interaction among UF rate, cardiac output, and arteriolar tone, an interaction that becomes especially unfavourable in older patients, those with diabetes, autonomic dysfunction, and significant cardiac structural disease [51, 52]. A key conceptual point for a "stress-test" framing is that standard HD repeatedly probes several reserve systems simultaneously: venous capacitance and plasma refill (preload reserve), myocardial ability to sustain output under reduced filling (pump reserve), and vasomotor capacity to defend perfusion pressure (afterload/autonomic reserve). When one or more of these reserves is limited, the hemodynamic phenotype (symptomatic IDH, silent hypoperfusion, post-dialysis fatigue) becomes more likely even at UF rates that appear acceptable by conventional thresholds [51, 52].

13.3.2 Microcirculatory and Coronary Effects

The coronary circulation is uniquely vulnerable during HD because myocardial oxygen delivery depends on both perfusion pressure and the ability of the microvasculature to dilate appropriately. Several lines of evidence support the idea that reduced myocardial blood flow (MBF) can occur during HD even without flow-limiting epicardial stenosis, consistent with a microcirculatory mechanism. The intradialytic PET study demonstrated an acute reduction in global and segmental MBF during HD and showed that the emergence of regional wall motion abnormalities (RWMAs), a functional signature of "myocardial stunning," co-localized with areas of reduced perfusion, despite the absence of angiographically significant coronary artery disease in the studied patients [12]. Subsequent work confirmed that HD-induced myocardial injury and stunning are clinically relevant phenomena associated with intradialytic hemodynamic stressors and adverse outcomes [1]. More recent intradialytic imaging studies continue to support this physiology. In an exploratory 2025 study using multimodal intradialytic assessment, dialysis-induced circulatory stress was associated with reduced myocardial perfusion and myocardial stunning in participants without CAD, with an apparent worsening after treatment end in those with coronary artery disease, suggesting that epicardial disease may amplify, but is not required for, the ischemic phenotype during HD [53]. Why can myocardial perfusion fall without major epicardial stenosis? A central explanation is that ESKD is associated with coronary microvascular dysfunction (CMD) and impaired flow reserve. CMD can be operationalized clinically through reduced coronary flow reserve (CFR) measured by echocardiographic Doppler, PET, or invasive physiology. In ESKD, impaired CFR has been documented compared with controls, supporting the presence of microvascular disease even before considering dialysis-specific stressors [54]. A broader 2022 systematic review and meta-analysis found significantly lower CFR in CKD than in non-CKD comparators, and importantly noted that this difference is observed even in studies excluding epicardial coronary artery disease, consistent with a microvascular rather than purely atherosclerotic explanation [55]. These chronic microvascular abnormalities matter because HD superimposes an acute reduction in perfusion pressure and circulating volume on a coronary circulation with limited vasodilatory reserve. In that setting, impaired coronary autoregulation, whether from endothelial dysfunction, vascular smooth muscle dysfunction, increased arterial stiffness, or uraemia-associated microvascular remodelling, can convert modest systemic changes into clinically meaningful reductions in subendocardial perfusion. The prognostic relevance of microvascular dysfunction in CKD is underscored by PET-based evidence that CFR is strongly associated with CV risk across CKD stages, suggesting that microvascular disease is a major pathway linking kidney disease to adverse cardiovascular outcomes [56]. Taken together, current evidence supports a coherent "microcirculatory vulnerability" model: CKD/ESKD is a CMD state with reduced flow reserve. HD transiently reduces effective circulating volume and perfusion, and the combination can produce intradialytic MBF reductions and myocardial stunning even when epicardial stenosis is not severe [12, 53, 55].

13.3.3 Concept of "Dialysis-Induced Multiorgan Ischemia"

The "dialysis-induced multiorgan ischemia" framework extends the myocardial stunning concept to other vascular beds and reframes HD as a systemic perfusion stress that can produce parallel, often subclinical, ischemic insults to multiple organs. McIntyre and colleagues summarized the evolving evidence for HD-related vascular injury, emphasizing that reductions in perfusion are not confined to the heart and that organ systems with high metabolic demand or limited autoregulatory capacity may be particularly vulnerable [16]. Earlier reviews similarly argued that intermittent HD can act as a disease modifier via repetitive circulatory stress, contributing to multiorgan injury superimposed on comorbidity [18].

Brain Cerebral perfusion changes during HD have been measured using multiple approaches. A prospective observational cohort study using transcranial Doppler in older HD patients found a decline in cerebral arterial mean flow velocity during dialysis and reported an association between cerebral blood flow variation and subsequent cognitive decline over follow-up, supporting a clinically meaningful brain-perfusion link, at least in vulnerable subgroups [57]. While cerebral autoregulation may buffer moderate changes, its lower limit and effectiveness can vary in HD populations, potentially allowing repetitive intradialytic hypoperfusion to contribute to cumulative injury [57].

Kidney (residual function). Although patients on maintenance HD have kidney failure, residual renal function (RRF) and residual perfusion can persist and are clinically important. Using imaging-based perfusion assessment, Marants et al. [58] showed an acute decrease in renal perfusion during HD. This observation supports a plausible pathway by which repeated intradialytic hypoperfusion could contribute to RRF decline, even if causality and effect size remain areas for ongoing research [58].

Gut–liver axis Splanchnic hypoperfusion is harder to capture directly in routine settings, but downstream physiological signatures have been described. HD was associated with altered hepatic perfusion dynamics and impaired flow-dependent hepatic function, alongside evidence consistent with increased endotoxemia, supporting the idea that circulatory stress during HD can influence gut-derived toxin handling through liver haemodynamics and clearance capacity [59]. These findings align with broader mechanistic models in which transient gut hypoperfusion and barrier dysfunction may promote systemic inflammation and vascular dysfunction, potentially feeding back into cardiovascular instability.

Multiorgan damage An important recent methodological advance has been the use of multiparametric MRI to assess organ-specific changes during dialysis within the same individuals. A randomized crossover trial comparing standard versus thermo-controlled HD used intradialytic cardiac, brain, and renal MRI to quantify physiological changes across organs, providing direct within-subject evidence that dialysis prescription (including temperature control) can influence organ perfusion and functional readouts during treatment [60]. Overall, the multiorgan ischemia concept is not a claim that every HD session causes clinically overt ischemic events; rather, it is a unifying, evidence-informed model in which repetitive, treatment-related reductions in perfusion, often clinically silent, may accumulate as microinjury in the heart, brain, gut-liver axis, and residual kidney. This model also clarifies why interventions that improve hemodynamic tolerability (e.g., prescription individualization, strategies that reduce circulatory stress) are being studied not merely for symptom control, but as potential organ-protective approaches [16, 18, 60].

13.4 Pathophysiology of Cardiac Stunning During Dialysis

13.4.1 Hemodynamic and Circulatory Drivers

Haemodialysis imposes a uniquely abrupt circulatory challenge: intravascular volume is removed over hours, while compensatory neurohumoral and microvascular responses are frequently blunted in ESKD. The most reproducible clinical drivers of dialysis-induced myocardial stunning are high ultrafiltration requirements (often reflecting large interdialytic weight gain) and intradialytic blood pressure (BP) instability. The review article describes this as treatment-related multiorgan ischemic stress, in which perfusion declines occur in parallel across vulnerable vascular beds, including the myocardium [16]. Ultrafiltration rate (UFR) matters not only because it can precipitate overt intradialytic hypotension, but also because it can cause subclinical circulatory stress (e.g., progressive reductions in stroke volume and tissue perfusion without meeting a strict BP threshold). In a pooled case-control analysis of >1000 HD sessions, the odds of IDH rose stepwise with higher UFR categories, with the authors concluding that UFR should be limited to ~12 mL/kg/h when feasible, and not exceed 16 mL/kg/h when higher removal is unavoidable [61]. Similarly, mechanistic imaging studies show that the severity of segmental contractile dysfunction during dialysis is proportional to ultrafiltration and BP reduction, supporting a dose-response relationship between circulatory stress and myocardial stunning [62]. Beyond symptoms, IDH has electrical consequences consistent with ischemia-linked myocardial vulnerability. In the Monitoring in Dialysis study (implantable loop recorders; 4720 sessions), IDH was common and associated with substantially higher rates of clinically significant arrhythmias during HD [63]. These observations reinforce a unifying model: recurrent hemodynamic stress episodes, sometimes clinically silent, promote repetitive subendocardial ischemia, contractile dysfunction, and an arrhythmogenic substrate.

13.4.2 Myocardial Supply-Demand Mismatch

Dialysis-induced myocardial stunning is best conceptualized as transient regional systolic dysfunction caused by a mismatch between myocardial oxygen supply and demand that develops during treatment and partially resolves after the stressor abates. During HD, myocardial oxygen supply can fall due to reduced preload, decreased stroke volume/cardiac output, lower diastolic perfusion pressure, haemoconcentration-related viscosity changes, and impaired microvascular vasodilation. At the same time, oxygen demand may rise (or fail to fall adequately) because of sympathetic activation, increases in heart rate, and heightened contractility, particularly when patients struggle to maintain BP. Structural heart disease common in ESKD amplifies this mismatch. Left ventricular hypertrophy (LVH) and myocardial fibrosis increase diastolic stiffness and elevate filling pressures, thereby reducing subendocardial perfusion reserve and narrowing the margin of safety when perfusion pressure drops. The 2024 JASN review on dialysis-induced multiorgan ischemia emphasizes that LVH, conduit artery stiffness, and microcirculatory dysfunction together reduce the ischemic threshold and predispose to dialysis-triggered ischemic injury [16]. In this setting, even modest reductions in perfusion can translate into regional wall motion or strain abnormalities during the dialysis "stress test."

13.4.3 Role of Coronary Artery Disease (CAD)

A key advance from intradialytic imaging is that dialysis-induced myocardial stunning does not require obstructive epicardial CAD, implicating coronary microvascular and vasoregulatory mechanisms as central contributors. The presence of CAD, however, plausibly lowers the threshold for ischemia and can add regional vulnerability. Recent studies using multiple complementary methods have begun to separate these effects. In an exploratory study, using coronary CT angiography with intradialytic CT perfusion and echocardiographic strain, reductions in myocardial perfusion and development of stunning were observed even in participants without identifiable CAD, while those with asymptomatic CAD showed additive segmental perfusion/contractile abnormalities during and after dialysis [53]. These data align with the broader concept that HD acts as a cardiovascular stressor that can provoke ischemia through perfusion pressure and microvascular reserve limitations, with epicardial stenoses acting as an additional, not obligatory, constraint.

13.4.4 Cellular and Molecular Mechanisms

At the tissue level, repeated dialysis-associated ischemic episodes are thought to behave like low-grade ischemia-reperfusion (I/R) injury, where restoration of flow after transient hypoperfusion paradoxically promotes oxidative and inflammatory injury. Canonical I/R biology includes bursts of ROS, mitochondrial dysfunction, and calcium handling disturbances that impair contractile recovery ("stunning") and can, over time, drive fibrosis and remodelling [64]. In ESKD, this biology is superimposed on a pro-oxidant, pro-inflammatory milieu. Oxidative stress and mitochondrial abnormalities are well described across CKD stages, including advanced disease, and are mechanistically linked to impaired energetics and heightened susceptibility to stress [65]. Importantly, HD itself has been associated with biologic signatures compatible with mitochondrial injury and apoptosis. In a clinical study, Raj and colleagues reported that haemodialysis induces mitochondrial dysfunction and apoptosis-related pathways, consistent with oxidant and inflammatory stress during treatment [66]. Bridging these cellular pathways to clinical stunning, the most defensible interpretation is mechanistic plausibility rather than single-pathway proof: repetitive, treatment-linked hypoperfusion episodes can produce transient regional dysfunction; repeated exposure may promote cumulative injury with structural consequences (fibrosis/remodelling) and progressive loss of contractile reserve. This trajectory is a central theme in modern overviews of dialysis-induced organ ischemia and its downstream morbidity [16].

13.4.5 Dialysis-Related Factors

Dialysate temperature Cooling strategies are among the best-supported dialysis-prescription approaches to reduce hemodynamic stress and stunning. In a randomized trial, individualized dialysate temperature improved intradialytic haemodynamics and reduced the burden of peak-stress regional wall motion abnormalities (a standard echocardiographic marker of stunning) [67]. More recently, a randomized trial using intradialytic cardiac/brain/renal MRI evaluated thermo-controlled HD versus standard 37 °C dialysis to quantify organ-specific effects of cooling-based strategies [60]. Together, these trials support the concept that temperature modulation can attenuate the circulatory stress that precipitates ischemic injury during HD.

Dialysate composition (bicarbonate, calcium, sodium) Composition can influence vascular tone, electrolytes, and myocardial excitability, thereby interacting with perfusion and contractile reserve. A randomized trial found that high dialysate bicarbonate (vs lower bicarbonate) was associated with alkalosis, hypocalcaemia, more pronounced hypokalaemia, and less favourable hemodynamic preservation (stroke volume/cardiac output) [68]. Although not designed primarily around stunning endpoints, the physiologic direction, reduced hemodynamic stability and electrolyte shifts, provides a credible pathway by which bicarbonate prescription could modulate ischemic risk. Dialysate calcium presents a nuanced trade-off: higher calcium can increase vascular tone and stabilize BP, yet may adversely affect myocardial performance in some settings. In a crossover physiologic study, higher dialysate calcium (1.75 mmol/L) was associated with worse global longitudinal strain during HD despite slightly better BP stability, suggesting that "better BP" does not necessarily equate to better myocardial energetics/perfusion [69]. For dialysate sodium, recent evidence syntheses emphasize uncertainty: lowering dialysate sodium can reduce interdialytic weight gain and BP, but may increase IDH risk and lower serum sodium [70]. Because IDH and high UFR are upstream drivers of ischemic stress, sodium strategies (including profiling) should be discussed as hemodynamic tools with potential downstream effects on stunning, rather than as proven anti-stunning therapies.

Modality (conventional HD vs HDF; high-flux vs low-flux) Data directly linking modality choice to acute stunning are mixed. In a randomized crossover trial using intradialytic cardiac MRI, hemodiafiltration (HDF) did not significantly differ from HD in the acute cardiovascular response; systolic function and myocardial perfusion decreased during both, and segmental dysfunction severity tracked with ultrafiltration and BP reduction [62]. Separate crossover data comparing predilution HDF and high-flux HD used echocardiography before/after mid-week sessions to evaluate intradialytic LV systolic function; such trials contribute important physiologic comparisons but, taken together, do not yet establish a consistent modality-dependent reduction in stunning across populations and prescriptions [71]. For membrane flux (high-flux vs low-flux), mechanistic plausibility exists via inflammatory/biocompatibility pathways, but robust evidence specifically demonstrating reductions in myocardial stunning remains limited; therefore, claims should remain appropriately circumscribed.

13.5 Epidemiology and Risk Factors

Dialysis-induced myocardial stunning, usually defined as new or worsening transient regional wall motion abnormalities (RWMAs) or segmental strain reductions that arise during HD and improve (at least partially) after treatment, is common, although reported prevalence varies widely because studies differ in definitions, imaging approaches (visual RWMA scoring vs speckle-tracking strain), and patient selection. In a well-characterized observational study of 70 prevalent HD patients, 64% met a predefined criterion for significant intradialytic RWMAs (>20% reduction in wall motion in >2 regions) [1]. In contrast, a smaller cohort using a different protocol (40 patients; 79 sessions) reported segmental worsening in ~20% of participants, highlighting the sensitivity of prevalence estimates to methodology and case-mix [72]. Contemporary reviews emphasize that this phenomenon is not rare and is clinically relevant because recurrent episodes plausibly contribute to longer-term structural and functional cardiac injury [16].

Patient-Related Risk Factors

Patient susceptibility appears to reflect both cardiac substrate (reduced ischemic tolerance) and limited hemodynamic reserve. Consistent determinants reported in observational work include:

- Older age and higher comorbidity burden (e.g., diabetes, vascular disease) [1].
- Heart failure phenotype/reduced cardiac reserve: In one cohort, the history of clinical HF was associated with a higher risk of intradialytic segmental wall motion worsening [72].
- Structural/functional changes frequent in ESKD (LV hypertrophy, diastolic dysfunction, microvascular dysfunction) are widely considered permissive factors that lower the threshold at which dialysis-related circulatory stress translates into regional ischemia and transient dysfunction [16].

Because dialysis-induced stunning can occur even in the absence of obstructive epicardial CAD, patient risk should not be framed solely around angiographic stenosis; rather, global vascular disease, microcirculatory impairment, and myocardial remodelling likely determine vulnerability [53].

Treatment-Related Risk Factors

Across studies, the strongest and most consistent treatment-level drivers are those that intensify intradialytic circulatory stress:

- High ultrafiltration requirement and aggressive fluid removal (often reflecting large interdialytic weight gain). In the 70-patient cohort above, ultrafiltration volume was independently associated with the presence of significant intradialytic RWMAs [1]. At the population level, a high proportion of sessions with UFR >13 mL/kg/h is common and is associated with higher mortality, underscoring that "how fast" fluid is removed matters [73, 74].
- Intradialytic hypotension (IDH) / BP instability, including repetitive "subthreshold" hypoperfusion. In the same observational study, intradialytic BP reductions were independent determinants of myocardial stunning [1]. IDH remains frequent in routine practice, although incidence varies substantially with the definition used; recent reviews continue to emphasize its multifactorial nature and its association with adverse outcomes [52, 75].
- Short treatment time (and, by extension, high UFR for a given fluid gain). Cohort analyses show that shorter session duration is associated with a higher likelihood of exceeding high-UFR thresholds [73].
- Dialysate temperature ("hot dialysate") and thermal balance. Meta-analytic and narrative syntheses published recently support that lower dialysate temperature reduces IDH risk and improves hemodynamic stability, with potential myocardial protection in selected patients (while tolerability remains an important trade-off) [60, 76, 77].

Clinically, these factors often cluster: large interdialytic gains → shorter available treatment time → high UFR → BP instability → repetitive hypoperfusion episodes, creating a reproducible pathway toward recurrent myocardial ischemia/stunning in vulnerable patients [1, 16].

Genetic and Biomarker Correlates

Genetics. Robust, replicated genetic determinants of dialysis-induced myocardial stunning have not been established. Evidence remains limited to candidate-gene associations; for example, a study reported that HIF-1α polymorphisms were associated with IDH (and acute myocardial infarction) in HD patients, but this should be interpreted cautiously as an exploratory signal requiring replication in contemporary, multiethnic cohorts [78].

Cardiac biomarkers. High-sensitivity troponins and natriuretic peptides are frequently elevated in ESKD, yet they retain prognostic information when interpreted longitudinally and in context. In a large prospective HD cohort, predialysis cTnI and NT-proBNP were associated with subsequent mortality, supporting their role as risk-stratification biomarkers rather than simple "false positives" [79]. NT-proBNP remains consistently linked to adverse outcomes in HD populations in more recent analyses as well [80]. Troponin T has been incorporated directly into risk models: in the 70-patient echocardiography study, cTnT was an independent determinant of intradialytic RWMAs, and the combination of stunning plus higher cTnT identified a group with particularly poor outcomes [1].

Novel biomarkers. Emerging candidates (e.g., soluble ST2, galectin-3, and proteomic risk scores) show associations with mortality and cardiovascular risk in dialysis cohorts and meta-analyses, but they are not yet specific for dialysis-induced stunning and should currently be viewed as adjunctive risk markers rather than mechanistic surrogates [81, 82].

13.6 Diagnostic Assessment

13.6.1 Echocardiography During Dialysis

In routine clinical research and in many mechanistic studies, serial transthoracic echocardiography performed before, during, and shortly after haemodialysis remains the pragmatic cornerstone for identifying dialysis-associated myocardial stunning. Stunning is typically captured as new or worsening RWMAs at peak intradialytic stress, increasingly complemented by speckle-tracking strain (e.g., global longitudinal strain) to detect more subtle, "preclinical" systolic impairment. These echocardiographic phenotypes are temporally linked to intradialytic circulatory stress and are commonly interpreted as transient ischemic dysfunction rather than fixed scar, particularly when reversibility is demonstrated across the session [83, 84]. A clinically useful feature of echocardiography is its ability to be paired with contemporaneous hemodynamic data (UFR, BP trajectories), while limitations include operator dependence, variable acoustic windows in ESKD, and sensitivity to the precise timing of image acquisition relative to nadir perfusion [83, 84].

13.6.2 Advanced Imaging Modalities

Advanced imaging has clarified that intradialytic dysfunction often reflects impaired myocardial perfusion and microvascular reserve, even without obstructive epicardial CAD. PET has been used to quantify intradialytic myocardial blood flow and demonstrated acute reductions during HD with concomitant functional consequences [16, 85]. Intradialytic cardiac magnetic resonance (CMR) provides high-fidelity assessment of volumes, function, and (in selected protocols) perfusion within the dialysis session, and has been used in randomized and crossover studies to compare treatment prescriptions and modalities (e.g., HD vs HDF; thermo-controlled vs standard dialysis) [60, 62]. More recently, intradialytic CT perfusion combined with coronary imaging has been applied as an exploratory approach to relate dialysis-induced circulatory stress to perfusion deficits and stunning, including in individuals without CAD [53]. Despite their mechanistic value, PET/CMR/CT remain resource-intensive and are best viewed as reference tools for phenotype definition and intervention trials rather than routine bedside diagnostics [16, 53, 62].

13.6.3 Biomarkers of Cardiac Injury

Cardiac troponins are frequently chronically elevated in ESKD, yet they still convey clinically meaningful information when interpreted against an individual baseline and the clinical context. Importantly, troponin T has been directly linked to dialysis-induced stunning: in a prospective study, higher troponin T concentrations were associated with the presence and severity of intradialytic RWMAs, supporting its role as a correlate of repetitive myocardial injury in this setting [84]. Because dialysis can influence circulating biomarker concentrations (via clearance, haemoconcentration, and biologic release), sampling time matters; recent work highlights that hs-cTnT may rise across a single HD session in some circumstances, underscoring the need for standardized timing when using serial measurements [86]. From a risk-stratification perspective, longitudinal ("trajectory") approaches may outperform single measurements: serial hs-cTnI patterns have been reported to independently predict major adverse cardiovascular events in maintenance HD cohorts [87]. Natriuretic peptides (BNP/NT-proBNP) remain valuable markers of volume/pressure load and prognosis in dialysis populations, but they are not specific for intradialytic ischemia or stunning; they are best used to contextualize hemodynamic stress (e.g., chronic congestion, cardiac strain) rather than to diagnose stunning per se [88, 89]. Overall, current reviews emphasize a combined strategy: phenotype stunning with imaging (often echocardiography), and use biomarkers (troponins, natriuretic peptides) as complementary indicators of myocardial injury and risk while recognizing assay-, timing-, and ESKD-specific interpretive caveats [90].

13.7 Clinical Consequences

13.7.1 Acute Manifestations

Dialysis-induced myocardial stunning spans a clinical spectrum from overt intradialytic symptoms to silent, imaging-only ischemic dysfunction. During the session, patients may develop chest discomfort, dyspnoea, nausea, cramps, or fatigue in parallel with blood pressure instability, and may experience clinically important arrhythmias, particularly in the setting of IDH and rapid volume removal [16, 63]. Importantly, several intradialytic echocardiography cohorts demonstrate that new RWMAs frequently occur without angina or other ischemic symptoms, consistent with "silent ischemia" in a population with autonomic dysfunction and altered pain perception [16, 91].

13.7.2 Chronic Structural and Functional Remodelling

The principal concern is cumulative injury: repeated, transient ischemic dysfunction may contribute to progressive loss of contractile reserve and transition toward persistent LV dysfunction and heart failure. In a longitudinal study of HD patients with demonstrable intradialytic ischemic dysfunction, repetitive stunning was associated with subsequent reductions in global and segmental systolic function over time, supporting a clinically meaningful remodelling trajectory [1]. Contemporary reviews reinforce this interpretation, framing dialysis as a recurrent circulatory stressor capable of driving cardiac injury and maladaptive remodelling in susceptible patients [16, 18].

13.7.3 Arrhythmias and Sudden Cardiac Death

Intradialytic ischemia and hemodynamic stress plausibly promote arrhythmogenesis via ischemia-related repolarization instability, electrolyte shifts, and autonomic activation. In the Monitoring in Dialysis study, IDH episodes were associated with a higher rate of clinically significant arrhythmias during HD sessions, underscoring the coupling between hemodynamic instability and electrical vulnerability [50, 63]. Broader evidence from long-term rhythm monitoring (implantable loop recorders) confirms a substantial arrhythmia burden in HD populations, though the precise terminal rhythms in sudden death vary and remain an area of ongoing investigation [92, 93]. The early dialysis period is a particularly high cardiovascular risk window: in the AROii incident HD cohort, cardiovascular event rates were highest soon after initiation [94].

13.7.4 Prognostic Impact

Across observational studies, intradialytic myocardial stunning is consistently associated with worse prognosis, including higher mortality and earlier cardiovascular events. In a prospective cohort of 105 HD patients undergoing serial intradialytic echocardiography, development of haemodialysis-induced regional LV systolic dysfunction was associated with increased subsequent mortality risk [91, 95]. Earlier mechanistic work similarly linked dialysis-induced cardiac injury phenotypes to adverse outcomes and to longer-term systolic impairment [1]. Collectively, these data support treating repeated intradialytic ischemic dysfunction not merely as a physiological curiosity, but as a clinically meaningful risk marker that identifies patients in whom dialysis prescription and hemodynamic protection strategies may be particularly important [16, 18].

13.8 Practical Clinical Approach

13.8.1 Identifying Patients at Risk

A practical approach starts by recognizing that dialysis-induced myocardial stunning is most likely when limited cardiovascular reserve is repeatedly exposed to high intradialytic circulatory stress. "Red flags" include:

- Dialysis-treatment red flags: frequent intradialytic hypotension (IDH), large interdialytic weight gains, short treatment time, and high ultrafiltration rate (UFR), particularly when UFR repeatedly exceeds commonly used risk thresholds (e.g., >10–13 mL/kg/h) that have been associated with higher mortality in observational cohorts [74, 96, 97].
- Clinical red flags: exertional dyspnoea, post-dialysis fatigue/out-of-proportion recovery time, recurrent intradialytic chest symptoms or "air hunger," and peridialytic palpitations/syncope. (Absence of symptoms does not exclude stunning) [16, 91].
- Cardiac substrate red flags (baseline echo): LV hypertrophy, diastolic dysfunction, reduced EF, high filling pressures/LA dilation, features that reduce ischemic tolerance during rapid preload reduction [16, 91].

Risk stratification is most informative when dialysis session data (UFR, BP nadirs/variability, temperature) are integrated with cardiac testing and biomarkers, consistent with KDIGO's emphasis on systematic volume/BP assessment and individualized prescription [98].

Biomarkers for risk-contextualization. Predialysis troponin T has been shown to correlate with the presence and severity of dialysis-induced stunning and can help identify a higher-risk phenotype when interpreted longitudinally (rather than as an isolated "positive") [84]. Natriuretic peptides (BNP/NT-proBNP) are useful for volume/pressure load and prognosis, but are not specific for intradialytic ischemia [80, 99].

13.8.2 Stepwise Evaluation of Suspected Cardiac Stunning

A pragmatic evaluation can be staged:

- At-chair assessment during/after symptoms or recurrent IDH: symptom review, focused exam (volume status), review of interdialytic weight gain and achieved UFR, and a 12-lead ECG when symptoms or arrhythmia are suspected [51, 98].
- Troponin strategy: obtain troponin when acute coronary syndrome is clinically suspected, but interpret against patient-specific baselines; troponin changes can occur across a session and timing should be standardized if used serially [84, 86, 91].

- Indications for intradialytic echocardiography: recurrent IDH with cardiopulmonary symptoms, unexplained decline in functional capacity, rising troponin trend without a clear alternative explanation, or high-risk dialysis patterns (persistently high UFR/short sessions) plus significant cardiac substrate. Intradialytic echo is the most practical method to document new regional dysfunction (RWMAs/strain changes) during the session [1, 91].
- When to consider advanced imaging (selected cases): if diagnosis remains uncertain, if coronary anatomy/perfusion clarification would change management, or in research/complex phenotyping, e.g., intradialytic CMR protocols that quantify functional/perfusion changes or intradialytic CT-perfusion approaches in specialized centres [16, 60, 62].

13.8.3 Algorithm for Management

Most contemporary frameworks prioritize reducing intradialytic circulatory stress first, then layering adjunctive therapies. A stepwise approach consistent with published algorithms/reviews is:

Step 1: Modify the dialysis prescription (first-line).

- Reduce circulatory stress by addressing UFR and treatment time (extend session duration or add treatments to lower UFR), reinforce sodium/fluid management to limit interdialytic gains, and reassess target weight systematically [97, 98].
- Address IDH-prone prescriptions: consider cooler/individualized dialysate temperature strategies (shown in trials to improve hemodynamic stability and reduce stunning or its progression) [60, 67, 100].

Step 2: Review medications that impair compensatory responses.

Reassess antihypertensive class and timing in IDH-prone patients; recent analyses/reviews highlight that drug class may influence IDH risk and emphasize individualized selection rather than one-size-fits-all withholding [101–103].

Step 3: Consider adjuncts for refractory IDH/stress physiology.

Midodrine may be considered in selected patients with resistant IDH, acknowledging that evidence quality varies and practice should be individualized [52, 104, 105].

Step 4: Consider modality and supportive strategies.

- If recurrent stunning persists despite optimization, consider whether an alternative regimen/modality is feasible; however, mechanistic CMR data show that acute cardiovascular stress can occur in both HD and HDF, so modality change should be framed as individualized rather than uniformly protective [62].

- Intradialytic exercise (IDE) is an emerging adjunct: randomized/controlled studies report improvements in regional myocardial mechanics and reductions in HD-induced stunning signals, supporting referral to structured IDE where available and appropriate [21, 106, 107].

This hierarchy aligns with modern reviews that place dialysis-induced stunning within a broader "multiorgan ischemia" paradigm and prioritize hemodynamic protection as a modifiable target [16, 108].

13.8.4 Multidisciplinary Care

Optimal implementation is multidisciplinary:

- Nephrologist: leads prescription modification (UFR/time, temperature, sodium/UF strategy), volume-targeting, and longitudinal biomarker interpretation [51, 98].
- Cardiologist: evaluates competing diagnoses (CAD/valvular disease/HF), guides antianginal/HF therapy compatible with dialysis haemodynamics, and assists with arrhythmia risk assessment [16, 91].
- Exercise physiologist/rehabilitation team: structures IDE programs shown to improve cardiac mechanics/stunning phenotypes in trials [106, 107].
- Dialysis nursing team: critical for real-time BP trend recognition, symptom capture, protocolized responses to IDH, and adherence support for fluid/sodium goals [51, 98].

13.9 Future Directions and Research Gaps

13.9.1 Need for Standardized Definitions and Outcomes

Progress is limited by heterogeneous case definitions of intradialytic myocardial stunning (visual RWMAs vs strain-based criteria; differing segment counts and timing of acquisition). Many contemporary protocols define stunning using segmental longitudinal strain decrements (often ≥20% from baseline) and require involvement of multiple LV segments, but implementation varies across studies and settings [21, 62, 109]. A near-term priority is a harmonized, consensus definition with a core outcome set that aligns intradialytic imaging endpoints (RWMAs/strain), perfusion measures (where available), and patient-centred outcomes, as emphasized in recent syntheses of dialysis-induced vascular injury and multiorgan ischemia [16].

13.9.2 Novel Monitoring and Imaging Technologies

Wearable monitoring is moving from proof-of-concept to real-world evaluation. Recent studies in HD populations support the feasibility of continuous rhythm surveillance using wearable ECG recorders, enabling detection of atrial fibrillation and ectopy outside brief in-unit snapshots [110, 111]. The research gap is linking wearable-derived hemodynamic/rhythm signatures to validated intradialytic ischemia/stunning phenotypes, and then to actionable prescription changes. On the imaging side, wider use of strain (including emerging indices such as myocardial work) improves sensitivity for subtle regional dysfunction, but requires standardization and quality control [62, 112]. Mechanistically, intradialytic CMR has proven uniquely informative for simultaneous assessment of volumes, function, and (in selected protocols) perfusion during treatment [60, 62]. Looking ahead, hybrid PET/CMR platforms by combining quantitative myocardial blood flow/coronary flow reserve with tissue/functional assessment, offer a compelling route to quantify ischemic burden and microvascular reserve, although dialysis-specific PET/CMR studies remain sparse [113, 114].

13.9.3 Interventional Trials

Most interventional evidence still centres on surrogate endpoints (BP stability, RWMAs/strain, MRI metrics) rather than hard cardiovascular outcomes. Trials support the biologic plausibility of hemodynamic protection:

- Dialysate cooling/thermo-control: individualized dialysate temperature improved intradialytic haemodynamics and reduced stunning burden in a controlled trial, and a more recent randomized crossover trial used intradialytic multiorgan MRI to quantify organ-specific effects of thermo-controlled HD [60, 67].
- More frequent HD schedules: observational comparisons show less dialysis-induced stunning with frequent regimens versus conventional HD [17].
- HDF vs HD: intradialytic CMR crossover data indicate that acute cardiac stress and perfusion/functional declines can occur with both modalities, underscoring the need for larger trials and careful phenotype selection [62].
- Intradialytic exercise (IDE): controlled trials and recent pilot data suggest IDE can improve LV remodelling and reduce stunning signals; a newly published randomized cycling trial further tests this strategy using standardized strain-based RWMA definitions [21, 107, 115].

A major gap is the absence (or scarcity) of adequately powered RCTs testing UFR limits, extended treatment time, and integrated hemodynamic strategies against hard endpoints (heart failure hospitalization, sudden death, cardiovascular mortality), rather than imaging surrogates alone [97, 116].

13.9.4 Translational Science Opportunities

Dialysis-induced stunning offers a tractable human model of repetitive low-grade ischemia-reperfusion stress superimposed on CKD-related microvascular dysfunction. Key opportunities include:

- Direct mechanistic studies of coronary microvascular dysfunction as a determinant of ischemic threshold (supported clinically by CAD-not-required stunning phenotypes and microvascular case evidence) [53, 117]
- Integrative work linking intradialytic perfusion/strain changes to oxidative stress, mitochondrial injury pathways, and fibrotic remodelling, ideally using longitudinal imaging plus molecular phenotyping to move beyond association [16, 118, 119]

In sum, the field now needs standardized definitions and endpoints, scalable monitoring that can be deployed around routine dialysis, and trials designed to test whether reducing intradialytic ischemic burden translates into fewer heart failure events and sudden death in the highest-risk phenotypes.

13.10 Summary and Key Take-Home Messages

HD can be viewed as a recurrent, time-compressed cardiovascular stress test in which rapid reductions in effective circulating volume and perfusion pressure interact with impaired vascular and coronary reserve typical of ESKD. The resulting phenotype, dialysis-induced myocardial ischemia with transient regional dysfunction ("stunning"), is increasingly framed within a broader paradigm of dialysis-induced multiorgan ischemia, reflecting parallel vulnerability of other beds (e.g., brain) during intradialytic circulatory stress [16].

Key Messages

- Circulatory stress is the dominant proximal driver. High ultrafiltration demands, short session time, and blood pressure instability promote episodes of overt IDH and "silent" hypoperfusion. Modern IDH reviews highlight reduced effective blood volume and impaired compensatory responses as central mechanisms [51].
- High UFR is consistently linked to harm in observational datasets. Faster fluid removal has been associated with increased mortality risk across large cohorts (not proof of causality, but clinically persuasive for risk minimization) [96, 97].
- Stunning can occur without obstructive CAD. Intradialytic imaging studies demonstrate reductions in myocardial perfusion and development of stunning even in patients without coronary artery disease, supporting a major role for microvascular dysfunction and limited autoregulatory reserve in ESKD [53].
- The phenomenon is prognostically meaningful. In a prospective intradialytic echocardiography cohort, HD-induced regional LV systolic dysfunction was

independently associated with higher mortality, supporting its use as a high-risk phenotype rather than an incidental finding [91].
- Electrical instability matters. IDH is associated with a higher rate of significant arrhythmias during HD in implantable monitoring data, aligning with a mechanistic link among hypoperfusion, autonomic activation, electrolyte shifts, and arrhythmogenesis [63].
- Interventions that reduce hemodynamic stress are the most actionable today. Individualized dialysate cooling improved intradialytic haemodynamics and reduced stunning burden in a controlled trial, and in incident HD patients a randomized trial suggested cooler dialysate was well tolerated and slowed progression of HD-associated cardiomyopathy [67, 100].
- Biomarkers support risk-contextualization, not standalone diagnosis. Troponins and natriuretic peptides are frequently elevated in ESKD; their greatest value is in serial, patient-specific interpretation alongside dialysis metrics and imaging, rather than as single "rule-in/rule-out" tests [51, 91].

Practical take-home: the most defensible clinical strategy is to identify the high-risk hemodynamic pattern (high UFR, repeated BP instability), confirm the phenotype when feasible (intradialytic echo/strain), and then prioritize prescription changes that reduce intradialytic circulatory stress, while coordinating nephrology–cardiology care for coexisting CAD/HF and arrhythmia risk.

References

1. Burton JO, Jefferies HJ, Selby NM, McIntyre CW. Hemodialysis-induced cardiac injury: determinants and associated outcomes. Clin J Am Soc Nephrol. 2009;4:914–20. https://doi.org/10.2215/cjn.03900808.
2. Kiuchi MG, Ho JK, Nolde JM, Gavidia LML, Carnagarin R, Matthews VB, Schlaich MP. Sympathetic activation in hypertensive chronic kidney disease—a stimulus for cardiac arrhythmias and sudden cardiac death? Front Physiol. 2020;10–2019 https://doi.org/10.3389/fphys.2019.01546.
3. Saravanan P, Davidson NC. Risk assessment for sudden cardiac death in dialysis patients. Circ Arrhythm Electrophysiol. 2010;3:553–9. https://doi.org/10.1161/CIRCEP.110.937888.
4. Makar MS, Pun PH. Sudden cardiac death among hemodialysis patients. Am J Kidney Dis. 2017;69:684–95. https://doi.org/10.1053/j.ajkd.2016.12.006.
5. Rzeszotarski J, Grzelakowski P, Manitius J, Naruszewicz R. Initiation of hemodialysis and sudden cardiac death — a constant challenge on the threshold of new therapy. Renal Dis Transpl Forum. 2023;16:14–20. https://doi.org/10.5603/RDTF.2023.0008.
6. Sarnak MJ, Foley RN. Cardiovascular mortality in the general population versus dialysis: a glass half full or empty? Am J Kidney Dis. 2011;58:4–6. https://doi.org/10.1053/j.ajkd.2011.04.004.
7. Rhee CM, Chou JA, Kalantar-Zadeh K. Dialysis prescription and sudden death. Semin Nephrol. 2018;38:570–81. https://doi.org/10.1016/j.semnephrol.2018.08.003.
8. Kloner RA. Stunned and hibernating myocardium: where are we nearly 4 decades later? J Am Heart Assoc. 2020;9:e015502. https://doi.org/10.1161/JAHA.119.015502.
9. Kim SJ, Depre C, Vatner SF. Novel mechanisms mediating stunned myocardium. Heart Fail Rev. 2003;8:143–53. https://doi.org/10.1023/a:1023040718319.

10. Bolli R. Myocardial 'stunning' in man. Circulation. 1992;86:1671–91. https://doi.org/10.1161/01.CIR.86.6.1671.
11. Rutkowski B, Storoniak H, Rutkowski P. Dialysate cooling - simple and safe prevention method of the cardiovascular disturbances development in dialysed patients. Forum Nefrologiczne. 2016;9:155–9.
12. McIntyre CW, Burton JO, Selby NM, Leccisotti L, Korsheed S, Baker CS, Camici PG. Hemodialysis-induced cardiac dysfunction is associated with an acute reduction in global and segmental myocardial blood flow. Clin J Am Soc Nephrol. 2008;3:19–26. https://doi.org/10.2215/cjn.03170707.
13. Breidthardt T, McIntyre C. Dialysis-induced myocardial stunning: the other side of the cardiorenal syndrome. Rev Cardiovasc Med. 2011;12:13–20. https://doi.org/10.3909/ricm0585.
14. Stefánsson BV, Brunelli SM, Cabrera C, Rosenbaum D, Anum E, Ramakrishnan K, Jensen DE, Stålhammar NO. Intradialytic hypotension and risk of cardiovascular disease. Clin J Am Soc Nephrol. 2014;9:2124–32. https://doi.org/10.2215/cjn.02680314.
15. Zuidema MY, Dellsperger KC. Myocardial stunning with hemodialysis: clinical challenges of the cardiorenal patient. Cardiorenal Med. 2012;2:125–33. https://doi.org/10.1159/000337476.
16. McIntyre CW. Update on hemodialysis-induced multiorgan ischemia: brains and beyond. J Am Soc Nephrol. 2024;35:653–64. https://doi.org/10.1681/asn.0000000000000299.
17. Jefferies HJ, Virk B, Schiller B, Moran J, McIntyre CW. Frequent hemodialysis schedules are associated with reduced levels of dialysis-induced cardiac injury (myocardial stunning). Clin J Am Soc Nephrol. 2011;6:1326–32. https://doi.org/10.2215/cjn.05200610.
18. Canaud B, Kooman JP, Selby NM, Taal MW, Francis S, Maierhofer A, Kopperschmidt P, Collins A, Kotanko P. Dialysis-induced cardiovascular and multiorgan morbidity. Kidney Int Rep. 2020;5:1856–69. https://doi.org/10.1016/j.ekir.2020.08.031.
19. Giannaki CD, Grigoriou SS, George K, Karatzaferi C, Zigoulis P, Lavdas E, Chaniotis D, Stefanidis I, Sakkas GK. Nine months of hybrid intradialytic exercise training improves ejection fraction and cardiac autonomic nervous system activity. Sports (Basel). 2023;11 https://doi.org/10.3390/sports11040079.
20. Verrelli D, Sharma A, Alexiuk J, Tays Q, Rossum K, Sharma M, Ford E, Iansavitchene A, Al-Jaishi AA, Whitlock R, et al. Effect of intradialytic exercise on cardiovascular outcomes in maintenance hemodialysis: a systematic review and meta-analysis. Kidney360. 2024;5:390–413. https://doi.org/10.34067/kid.0000000000000361.
21. Penny JD, Salerno FR, Brar R, Garcia E, Rossum K, McIntyre CW, Bohm CJ. Intradialytic exercise preconditioning: an exploratory study on the effect on myocardial stunning. Nephrol Dial Transplant. 2019;34:1917–23. https://doi.org/10.1093/ndt/gfy376.
22. Graham-Brown MPM, March DS, Young R, Highton PJ, Young HML, Churchward DR, Dungey M, Stensel DJ, Bishop NC, Brunskill NJ, et al. A randomized controlled trial to investigate the effects of intra-dialytic cycling on left ventricular mass. Kidney Int. 2021;99:1478–86. https://doi.org/10.1016/j.kint.2021.02.027.
23. Hur LYJ. Exploration of the pathophysiological mechanisms underlying hemodialysis associated cardiac ischemic injury, vol. 8987. Electronic Thesis and Dissertation Repository; 2022. https://ir.lib.uwo.ca/etd/8987
24. Shawky SM, Khalifa MMM, Amin KM, Hassan MS. Correlation between interdialytic weight gain, left ventricular hypertrophy and FGF- 23 in prevalent hemodialysis patients. J Clin Nephrol. 2020;4:036–43. https://doi.org/10.29328/journal.jcn.1001057.
25. Ahmadmehrabi S, Tang WHW. Hemodialysis-induced cardiovascular disease. Semin Dial. 2018;31:258–67.
26. Kloner RA. Stunned and hibernating myocardium: where are we nearly 4 decades later? J Am Heart Assoc. 2020;9:e015502. https://doi.org/10.1161/jaha.119.015502.
27. Yadav R, Abubakar AK, Mishra R, Gupta S, Maurya NK, Kashyap VK, Rustagi S, Singh DP, Kumar S. Exploring the interplay between kidney dysfunction and cardiovascular disease. Med Sci. 2025;13:80.

28. Braunwald E, Kloner RA. The stunned myocardium: prolonged, postischemic ventricular dysfunction. Circulation. 1982;66:1146–9. https://doi.org/10.1161/01.cir.66.6.1146.
29. Al-Awar A, Khan AW, Hussain S. Myocardial stunning: mechanisms, molecular insights, and gaps in knowledge. Biosci Rep. 2025;45 https://doi.org/10.1042/bsr20253410.
30. Heusch G, Schulz R. Perfusion-contraction match and mismatch. Basic Res Cardiol. 2001;96:1–10. https://doi.org/10.1007/s003950170072.
31. Vaidya Y, Cavanaugh SM, Dhamoon AS. Myocardial stunning and hibernation. In: StatPearls. Treasure Island (FL): StatPearls Publishing; 2025.
32. Le DE, Alkayed NJ, Cao Z, Chattergoon NN, Garcia-Jaramillo M, Thornburg K, Kaul S. Metabolomics of repetitive myocardial stunning in chronic multivessel coronary artery stenosis: effect of non-selective and selective β1-receptor blockers. J Physiol. 2024;602:3423–48. https://doi.org/10.1113/jp285720.
33. Kalogeris T, Baines CP, Krenz M, Korthuis RJ. Cell biology of ischemia/reperfusion injury. Int Rev Cell Mol Biol. 2012;298:229–317. https://doi.org/10.1016/b978-0-12-394309-5.00006-7.
34. Hausenloy DJ, Yellon DM. Myocardial ischemia-reperfusion injury: a neglected therapeutic target. J Clin Invest. 2013;123:92–100. https://doi.org/10.1172/jci62874.
35. Hausenloy DJ, Yellon DM. Ischaemic conditioning and reperfusion injury. Nat Rev Cardiol. 2016;13:193–209. https://doi.org/10.1038/nrcardio.2016.5.
36. Avkiran M, Marber MS. Na(+)/H(+) exchange inhibitors for cardioprotective therapy: progress, problems and prospects. J Am Coll Cardiol. 2002;39:747–53. https://doi.org/10.1016/s0735-1097(02)01693-5.
37. Chouchani ET, Pell VR, Gaude E, Aksentijević D, Sundier SY, Robb EL, Logan A, Nadtochiy SM, Ord ENJ, Smith AC, et al. Ischaemic accumulation of succinate controls reperfusion injury through mitochondrial ROS. Nature. 2014;515:431–5. https://doi.org/10.1038/nature13909.
38. Pell VR, Chouchani ET, Frezza C, Murphy MP, Krieg T. Succinate metabolism: a new therapeutic target for myocardial reperfusion injury. Cardiovasc Res. 2016;111:134–41. https://doi.org/10.1093/cvr/cvw100.
39. Chouchani ET, Pell VR, James AM, Work LM, Saeb-Parsy K, Frezza C, Krieg T, Murphy MP. A unifying mechanism for mitochondrial superoxide production during ischemia-reperfusion injury. Cell Metab. 2016;23:254–63. https://doi.org/10.1016/j.cmet.2015.12.009.
40. Bao Y, Hu C, Wang B, Liu X, Wu Q, Xu D, Shi Z, Sun C. Mitochondrial reverse electron transport: mechanisms, pathophysiological roles, and therapeutic potential. Biology (Basel). 2025;14 https://doi.org/10.3390/biology14091140.
41. Heusch G, Andreadou I, Bell R, Bertero E, Botker HE, Davidson SM, Downey J, Eaton P, Ferdinandy P, Gersh BJ, et al. Health position paper and redox perspectives on reactive oxygen species as signals and targets of cardioprotection. Redox Biol. 2023;67:102894. https://doi.org/10.1016/j.redox.2023.102894.
42. Cipriano A, Viviano M, Feoli A, Milite C, Sarno G, Castellano S, Sbardella G. NADPH oxidases: from molecular mechanisms to current inhibitors. J Med Chem. 2023;66:11632–55. https://doi.org/10.1021/acs.jmedchem.3c00770.
43. Kumar V, Kleffmann T, Hampton MB, Cannell MB, Winterbourn CC. Redox proteomics of thiol proteins in mouse heart during ischemia/reperfusion using ICAT reagents and mass spectrometry. Free Radic Biol Med. 2013;58:109–17. https://doi.org/10.1016/j.freeradbiomed.2013.01.021.
44. Bernardi P, Gerle C, Halestrap AP, Jonas EA, Karch J, Mnatsakanyan N, Pavlov E, Sheu S-S, Soukas AA. Identity, structure, and function of the mitochondrial permeability transition pore: controversies, consensus, recent advances, and future directions. Cell Death Differ. 2023;30:1869–85. https://doi.org/10.1038/s41418-023-01187-0.
45. Morciano G, Pinton P. Modulation of mitochondrial permeability transition pores in reperfusion injury: mechanisms and therapeutic approaches. Eur J Clin Investig. 2025;55:e14331. https://doi.org/10.1111/eci.14331.

46. Bertero E, Popoiu TA, Maack C. Mitochondrial calcium in cardiac ischemia/reperfusion injury and cardioprotection. Basic Res Cardiol. 2024;119:569–85. https://doi.org/10.1007/s00395-024-01060-2.
47. Murphy E, Eisner DA. How does mitochondrial Ca2+ change during ischemia and reperfusion? Implications for activation of the permeability transition pore. J Gen Physiol. 2025;157 https://doi.org/10.1085/jgp.202313520.
48. Bolli R, Marbán E. Molecular and cellular mechanisms of myocardial stunning. Physiol Rev. 1999;79:609–34. https://doi.org/10.1152/physrev.1999.79.2.609.
49. Gao WD, Atar D, Liu Y, Perez NG, Murphy AM, Marban E. Role of troponin I proteolysis in the pathogenesis of stunned myocardium. Circ Res. 1997;80:393–9.
50. Kanbay M, Ertuglu LA, Afsar B, Ozdogan E, Siriopol D, Covic A, Basile C, Ortiz A. An update review of intradialytic hypotension: concept, risk factors, clinical implications and management. Clin Kidney J. 2020;13:981–93. https://doi.org/10.1093/ckj/sfaa078.
51. Habas E, Rayani A, Habas A, Farfar K, Habas E, Alarbi K, Habas A, Errayes E, Alfitori G. Intradialytic hypotension pathophysiology and therapy update: review and update. Blood Press. 2025:1–18. https://doi.org/10.1080/08037051.2025.2469260.
52. Haddiya I, Simanjuntak G, Ramdani S. Updates in the management of intradialytic hypotension: emerging strategies and innovations. World J Nephrol. 2025;14:109168. https://doi.org/10.5527/wjn.v14.i4.109168.
53. Hur L, Islam A, Penny JD, Dorie J, McIntyre CW. Coronary artery disease and intradialytic myocardial ischemia in hemodialysis: an exploratory study using intradialytic imaging. Kidney Med. 2025;7:101126. https://doi.org/10.1016/j.xkme.2025.101126.
54. Bozbas H, Pirat B, Demirtas S, Simşek V, Yildirir A, Sade E, Sayin B, Sezer S, Karakayali H, Muderrisoglu H. Evaluation of coronary microvascular function in patients with end-stage renal disease, and renal allograft recipients. Atherosclerosis. 2009;202:498–504. https://doi.org/10.1016/j.atherosclerosis.2008.04.043.
55. Jain V, Gupta K, Bhatia K, Rajapreyar I, Singh A, Zhou W, Klein A, Nanda NC, Prabhu SD, Bajaj NS. Coronary flow abnormalities in chronic kidney disease: a systematic review and meta-analysis. Echocardiography. 2022;39:1382–90. https://doi.org/10.1111/echo.15445.
56. Charytan DM, Skali H, Shah NR, Veeranna V, Cheezum MK, Taqueti VR, Kato T, Bibbo CR, Hainer J, Dorbala S, et al. Coronary flow reserve is predictive of the risk of cardiovascular death regardless of chronic kidney disease stage. Kidney Int. 2018;93:501–9. https://doi.org/10.1016/j.kint.2017.07.025.
57. Guo Y, Cui W, Ye P, Luo Y. Association between cerebral blood flow variation and cognitive decline in older patients undergoing hemodialysis. Front Aging Neurosci. 2024;16:1457675. https://doi.org/10.3389/fnagi.2024.1457675.
58. Marants R, Qirjazi E, Grant CJ, Lee TY, McIntyre CW. Renal perfusion during hemodialysis: intradialytic blood flow decline and effects of dialysate cooling. J Am Soc Nephrol. 2019;30:1086–95. https://doi.org/10.1681/asn.2018121194.
59. Marants R, Qirjazi E, Lai KB, Szeto CC, Li PKT, Li F, Lee TY, McIntyre CW. Exploring the link between hepatic perfusion and endotoxemia in hemodialysis. Kidney Int Rep. 2021;6:1336–45. https://doi.org/10.1016/j.ekir.2021.02.008.
60. Gullapudi VRL, Cox EF, Buchanan CE, Canaud B, White K, Taal MW, Selby NM, Francis ST. Randomized trial comparing standard versus thermocontrolled haemodialysis using intradialytic cardiac, brain and renal magnetic resonance imaging. Nephrol Dial Transplant. 2024;39:233–41. https://doi.org/10.1093/ndt/gfad150.
61. Thongdee C, Phinyo P, Patumanond J, Satirapoj B, Spilles N, Laonapaporn B, Tantiyavarong P, Tasanarong A. Ultrafiltration rates and intradialytic hypotension: a case-control sampling of pooled haemodialysis data. J Ren Care. 2021;47:34–42. https://doi.org/10.1111/jorc.12340.
62. Buchanan C, Mohammed A, Cox E, Köhler K, Canaud B, Taal MW, Selby NM, Francis S, McIntyre CW. Intradialytic cardiac magnetic resonance imaging to assess cardiovascular responses in a short-term trial of hemodiafiltration and hemodialysis. J Am Soc Nephrol. 2017;28:1269–77. https://doi.org/10.1681/asn.2016060686.

63. Mc Causland FR, Tumlin JA, Roy-Chaudhury P, Koplan BA, Costea AI, Kher V, Williamson D, Pokhariyal S, Charytan DM. Intradialytic hypotension and cardiac arrhythmias in patients undergoing maintenance hemodialysis: results from the monitoring in dialysis study. Clin J Am Soc Nephrol. 2020;15:805–12. https://doi.org/10.2215/cjn.06810619.
64. Frank A, Bonney M, Bonney S, Weitzel L, Koeppen M, Eckle T. Myocardial ischemia reperfusion injury: from basic science to clinical bedside. Semin Cardiothorac Vasc Anesth. 2012;16:123–32. https://doi.org/10.1177/1089253211436350.
65. Ho HJ, Shirakawa H. Oxidative stress and mitochondrial dysfunction in chronic kidney disease. Cells. 2022;12 https://doi.org/10.3390/cells12010088.
66. Raj DS, Boivin MA, Dominic EA, Boyd A, Roy PK, Rihani T, Tzamaloukas AH, Shah VO, Moseley P. Haemodialysis induces mitochondrial dysfunction and apoptosis. Eur J Clin Investig. 2007;37:971–7. https://doi.org/10.1111/j.1365-2362.2007.01886.x.
67. Jefferies HJ, Burton JO, McIntyre CW. Individualised dialysate temperature improves intradialytic haemodynamics and abrogates haemodialysis-induced myocardial stunning, without compromising tolerability. Blood Purif. 2011;32:63–8. https://doi.org/10.1159/000324199.
68. Jensen JSK, Jørgensen IH, Buus NH, Jensen JD, Peters CD. Hemodynamic effects of low versus high dialysate bicarbonate concentration in hemodialysis patients. Hemodial Int. 2024;28:290–303. https://doi.org/10.1111/hdi.13162.
69. Silva VB, Macedo TA, Braga TMS, Silva BC, Graciolli FG, Dominguez WV, Drager LF, Moysés RM, Elias RM. High dialysate calcium concentration is associated with worsening left ventricular function. Sci Rep. 2019;9:2386. https://doi.org/10.1038/s41598-019-38887-y.
70. Marshall MR, Wang MY, Vandal AC, Dunlop JL. Low dialysate sodium levels for chronic haemodialysis. Cochrane Database Syst Rev. 2024;11:Cd011204. https://doi.org/10.1002/14651858.CD011204.pub3.
71. Li Y, Fu M, Yang C, Li S, Li Z, Ma J, Lin T, Wen F, Xu L, Ye Z, et al. Effects of predilution hemodiafiltration-induced intradialytic left ventricular systolic dysfunction compared to high-flux hemodialysis. Int Urol Nephrol. 2022;54:2653–62. https://doi.org/10.1007/s11255-022-03177-6.
72. Dubin RF, Beatty AL, Teerlink JR, Schiller NB, Bolger AF, Alokozai D, Peralta CA, Johansen KL. Determinants of hemodialysis-induced segmental wall motion abnormalities. Hemodial Int. 2014;18:396–405. https://doi.org/10.1111/hdi.12111.
73. Navarrete JE, Rajabalan A, Cobb J, Lea JP. Proportion of hemodialysis treatments with high ultrafiltration rate and the association with mortality. Kidney360. 2022;3:1359–66. https://doi.org/10.34067/kid.0001322022.
74. Raimann JG, Wang Y, Mermelstein A, Kotanko P, Daugirdas JT. Ultrafiltration rate thresholds associated with increased mortality risk in hemodialysis, unscaled or scaled to body size. Kidney Int Rep. 2022;7:1585–93. https://doi.org/10.1016/j.ekir.2022.04.079.
75. Wu Y, Lu J, Wang T, Zhu X, Xue J, You L. Association of frequent intradialytic hypotension with the clinical outcomes of patients on hemodialysis: a prospective cohort study. Ren Fail. 2024;46:2296612. https://doi.org/10.1080/0886022x.2023.2296612.
76. Tan TW, Tan HL, Lin WS, Chung YC. Effects of low dialysate temperature on intradialytic hypotension and dialysis adequacy in chronic hemodialysis: a systematic review and meta-analysis. Semin Dial. 2025;38:303–15. https://doi.org/10.1111/sdi.70010.
77. D'Elia L, Di Vico D, Otranto G, Villani A, Di Lullo L, Bellasi A, Barbera V. Does low-temperature dialysis still represent an advantage?: a narrative review from the last decade. Int Urol Nephrol. 2025; https://doi.org/10.1007/s11255-025-04850-2.
78. Zheng ZL, Hwang YH, Kim SK, Kim S, Son MJ, Ro H, Sung SA, Lee HH, Chung WK, Joo KW, et al. Genetic polymorphisms of hypoxia-inducible factor-1 alpha and cardiovascular disease in hemodialysis patients. Nephron Clin Pract. 2009;113:c104–11. https://doi.org/10.1159/000228542.
79. Eriguchi M, Tsuruya K, Lopes M, Bieber B, McCullough K, Pecoits-Filho R, Robinson B, Pisoni R, Kanda E, Iseki K, et al. Routinely measured cardiac troponin I and N-terminal pro-

B-type natriuretic peptide as predictors of mortality in haemodialysis patients. ESC Heart Fail. 2022;9:1138–51. https://doi.org/10.1002/ehf2.13784.
80. Chen C, Hsu YC, Chou KW, Chang KS, Hsu YH, Chiu WH, Lee CW, Yang PS, Chang WH, Huang YK, et al. NT-proBNP point-of-care testing for predicting mortality in end-stage renal disease: a survival analysis. Heliyon. 2024;10:e30581. https://doi.org/10.1016/j.heliyon.2024.e30581.
81. Bellos I, Marinaki S, Lagiou P, Benetou V. Association of soluble suppression of tumorigenicity 2 with mortality and adverse outcomes in chronic kidney disease: a systematic review and meta-analysis. Clin Exp Nephrol. 2024;28:988–1003. https://doi.org/10.1007/s10157-024-02506-6.
82. Ren Y, Segal MR, Shafi T, Pico AR, Shin M-G, Traglia M, Li H, Rosas SE, Choles HR, Rao PS, et al. Risk factors for mortality in patients with kidney failure on hemodialysis identified by proteomic analysis of CRIC and PACE studies. Nat Commun. 2025;16:11689. https://doi.org/10.1038/s41467-025-66763-z.
83. Selby NM, McIntyre CW. The acute cardiac effects of dialysis. Semin Dial. 2007;20:220–8. https://doi.org/10.1111/j.1525-139X.2007.00281.x.
84. Breidthardt T, Burton JO, Odudu A, Eldehni MT, Jefferies HJ, McIntyre CW. Troponin T for the detection of dialysis-induced myocardial stunning in hemodialysis patients. Clin J Am Soc Nephrol. 2012;7:1285–92. https://doi.org/10.2215/cjn.00460112.
85. Dasselaar JJ, Slart RH, Knip M, Pruim J, Tio RA, McIntyre CW, de Jong PE, Franssen CF. Haemodialysis is associated with a pronounced fall in myocardial perfusion. Nephrol Dial Transplant. 2009;24:604–10. https://doi.org/10.1093/ndt/gfn501.
86. Tinawi M, Bastani B. Effect of hemodialysis on high-sensitivity cardiac troponin T levels in patients with hypervolemia. Front Nephrol. 2025;5:1717448. https://doi.org/10.3389/fneph.2025.1717448.
87. Wu Y, Li F, Fu Q, Wang Y, Wang J, Chen X, Wu T, Chen Q, Zhang N, Zhu D, et al. Serial high-sensitivity cardiac troponin I trajectories predict cardiovascular events in hemodialysis patients. Clin Kidney J. 2025;18:sfaf294. https://doi.org/10.1093/ckj/sfaf294.
88. Rossignol P, Duarte K, Bresso E, Åsberg A, Devignes MD, Eriksson N, Girerd N, Glerup R, Jardine AG, Holdaas H, et al. NT-proBNP and stem cell factor plasma concentrations are independently associated with cardiovascular outcomes in end-stage renal disease hemodialysis patients. Eur Heart J Open. 2022;2 https://doi.org/10.1093/ehjopen/oeac069.
89. Ooi SH, Ng KP, Hasan MSB, Lau WP, Tah PC, Lim KW. Clinical utility of NTproBNP as a fluid assessment and prognostic tool in PD patients. Sci Rep. 2025;15:32819. https://doi.org/10.1038/s41598-025-17785-6.
90. Murphy D, Banerjee D. Cardiac troponins in kidney disease. Eur Cardiol. 2025;20:e22. https://doi.org/10.15420/ecr.2024.51.
91. Assa S, Hummel YM, Voors AA, Kuipers J, Westerhuis R, de Jong PE, Franssen CF. Hemodialysis-induced regional left ventricular systolic dysfunction: prevalence, patient and dialysis treatment-related factors, and prognostic significance. Clin J Am Soc Nephrol. 2012;7:1615–23. https://doi.org/10.2215/cjn.00850112.
92. Roberts PR, Zachariah D, Morgan JM, Yue AM, Greenwood EF, Phillips PC, Kalra PA, Green D, Lewis RJ, Kalra PR. Monitoring of arrhythmia and sudden death in a hemodialysis population: the CRASH-ILR study. PLoS One. 2017;12:e0188713. https://doi.org/10.1371/journal.pone.0188713.
93. Roberts PR, Stromberg K, Johnson LC, Wiles BM, Mavrakanas TA, Charytan DM. A systematic review of the incidence of arrhythmias in hemodialysis patients undergoing long-term monitoring with implantable loop recorders. Kidney Int Rep. 2021;6:56–65. https://doi.org/10.1016/j.ekir.2020.10.020.
94. Eckardt KU, Gillespie IA, Kronenberg F, Richards S, Stenvinkel P, Anker SD, Wheeler DC, de Francisco AL, Marcelli D, Froissart M, et al. High cardiovascular event rates occur within the first weeks of starting hemodialysis. Kidney Int. 2015;88:1117–25. https://doi.org/10.1038/ki.2015.117.

95. Chirakarnjanakorn S, Navaneethan SD, Francis GS, Tang WH. Cardiovascular impact in patients undergoing maintenance hemodialysis: clinical management considerations. Int J Cardiol. 2017;232:12–23. https://doi.org/10.1016/j.ijcard.2017.01.015.
96. Flythe JE, Kimmel SE, Brunelli SM. Rapid fluid removal during dialysis is associated with cardiovascular morbidity and mortality. Kidney Int. 2011;79:250–7. https://doi.org/10.1038/ki.2010.383.
97. Assimon MM, Wenger JB, Wang L, Flythe JE. Ultrafiltration rate and mortality in maintenance hemodialysis patients. Am J Kidney Dis. 2016;68:911–22. https://doi.org/10.1053/j.ajkd.2016.06.020.
98. Flythe JE, Chang TI, Gallagher MP, Lindley E, Madero M, Sarafidis PA, Unruh ML, Wang AY, Weiner DE, Cheung M, et al. Blood pressure and volume management in dialysis: conclusions from a kidney disease: improving global outcomes (KDIGO) controversies conference. Kidney Int. 2020;97:861–76. https://doi.org/10.1016/j.kint.2020.01.046.
99. Paniagua R, Ventura M-d-J, Ávila-Díaz M, Hinojosa-Heredia H, Méndez-Durán A, Cueto-Manzano A, Cisneros A, Ramos A, Madonia-Juseino C, Belio-Caro F, et al. NT-proBNP, fluid volume overload and dialysis modality are independent predictors of mortality in ESRD patients. Nephrol Dial Transplant. 2009;25:551–7. https://doi.org/10.1093/ndt/gfp395.
100. Odudu A, Eldehni MT, McCann GP, McIntyre CW. Randomized controlled trial of individualized dialysate cooling for cardiac protection in hemodialysis patients. Clin J Am Soc Nephrol. 2015;10:1408–17. https://doi.org/10.2215/cjn.00200115.
101. Zoccali C, Tripepi G, Mallamaci F, Usvyat LS, Maddux FW, Stuard S. Choosing the right antihypertensive drug to avoid intradialytic hypotension. Clin Kidney J. 2025;18:ii47–ii54. https://doi.org/10.1093/ckj/sfaf315.
102. Zoccali C, Tripepi G, Carioni P, Fu EL, Dekker F, Stel V, Jager KJ, Mallamaci F, Hymes JL, Maddux FW, et al. Antihypertensive drug treatment and the risk for intrahemodialysis hypotension. Clin J Am Soc Nephrol. 2024;19:1310–8. https://doi.org/10.2215/cjn.0000000000000521.
103. Wang KM, Sirich TL, Chang TI. Timing of blood pressure medications and intradialytic hypotension. Semin Dial. 2019;32:201–4. https://doi.org/10.1111/sdi.12777.
104. Xiao D, Nguyen T. Midodrine for intradialytic hypotension. Nephrol Nurs J. 2024;51:549–52.
105. House AA, McIntyre CW. Midodrine is an effective therapy for resistant intradialytic hypotension: PRO. Kidney360. 2023;4:299–301. https://doi.org/10.34067/kid.0007432021.
106. Josse M, Patrier L, Isnard M, Turc-Baron C, Grandperrin A, Nottin S, Mandigout S, Cristol JP, Maufrais C, Obert P. Cardioprotective effect of acute intradialytic exercise: a comprehensive speckle-tracking echocardiography analysis. J Am Soc Nephrol. 2023;34:1445–55. https://doi.org/10.1681/asn.0000000000000149.
107. Josse M, Patrier L, Cristol JP, Isnard M, Grandperrin A, Turc-Baron C, Nottin S, Mandigout S, Maufrais C, Obert P. Effect of intradialytic exercise training on hemodialysis-induced myocardial stunning: a pilot-controlled trial. Clin Kidney J. 2025;18:sfae352. https://doi.org/10.1093/ckj/sfae352.
108. Dorairajan S, Chockalingam A, Misra M. Myocardial stunning in hemodialysis: what is the overall message? Hemodial Int. 2010;14:447–50. https://doi.org/10.1111/j.1542-4758.2010.00495.x.
109. Berrichi H, Bekkaoui S, Oujidi Y, Laaribi I, Bkiyar H, Housni B. Assessing myocardial stunning during continuous renal replacement therapy in critically ill patients. Int J Crit Illn Inj Sci. 2025;15:57–65. https://doi.org/10.4103/ijciis.ijciis_95_24.
110. Yu SB, Huang LX, Ma HC, Yan TY, Qi M, Chen DZ, Liu GL, Zhu ZZ, Fu P, Zeng XX. Real-world evaluation of arrhythmias detection in hemodialysis patients using wearable electrocardiogram monitor: a two-phase multicenter observational study. BMC Nephrol. 2025;26:563. https://doi.org/10.1186/s12882-025-04489-2.
111. Gaoudam N, Sakhamudi SK, Kamal B, Addla N, Reddy EP, Ambala M, Lavanya K, Palaparthi EC, Bhattam A, Periasamy P, et al. Wearable devices and AI-driven remote moni-

toring in cardiovascular medicine: a narrative review. Cureus. 2025;17:e90208. https://doi.org/10.7759/cureus.90208.
112. Frişan AC, Mornoş C, Lazăr MA, Şoşdean R, Crişan S, Ionac I, Luca CT. Echocardiographic myocardial work: a novel method to assess left ventricular function in patients with coronary artery disease and diabetes mellitus. Medicina (Kaunas). 2024;60 https://doi.org/10.3390/medicina60020199.
113. Veneziano FA, Gioia FA, Gentile F. Hybrid PET/CT and PET/MR in coronary artery disease: an update for clinicians, with insights into AI-guided integration. J Cardiovasc Dev Dis. 2025;12 https://doi.org/10.3390/jcdd12090338.
114. Huck DM, Weber B, Schreiber B, Pandav J, Parks S, Hainer J, Brown JM, Divakaran S, Blankstein R, Dorbala S, et al. Comparative effectiveness of PET and SPECT MPI for predicting cardiovascular events after kidney transplant. Circ Cardiovasc Imaging. 2024;17:e015858. https://doi.org/10.1161/CIRCIMAGING.123.015858.
115. Bennett PN, Penny JD, McIntyre CW, Vanderlinden J, Borkum MS, Castillo G, Collister D, Corradetti B, Duhamel TA, Farion H, et al. Randomized controlled trial of intradialytic cycling as kidney exercise rehabilitation for cardiac stunning in hemodialysis (TICKERS_HD): a clinical research protocol. Can J Kidney Health Dis. 2026;13:20543581251391112. https://doi.org/10.1177/20543581251391112.
116. Canney M, Clark EG. Risk-based thresholds for hemodialysis ultrafiltration rates: a warning signal or a call to action? Clin J Am Soc Nephrol. 2023;18:693–5. https://doi.org/10.2215/cjn.0000000000000181.
117. Yokoi M, Ito T, Suzuki W, Yamamoto J, Nakayama T, Ichihashi T, Kikuchi S, Kitada S, Goto T, Seo Y. Hemodialysis-induced myocardial stunning with no obstructive coronary artery disease: pathophysiological significance of coronary microvascular dysfunction. Intern Med. 2024;63:2023–6. https://doi.org/10.2169/internalmedicine.2388-23.
118. Goto J, Ott M, Stegmayr B. Myocardial markers are highly altered by higher rates of fluid removal during hemodialysis. Hemodial Int. 2024;28:17–23. https://doi.org/10.1111/hdi.13124.
119. Hart A, Johansen KL. Cardiovascular protection and mounting evidence for the benefits of intradialytic exercise. Nephrol Dial Transplant. 2019;34:1816–8. https://doi.org/10.1093/ndt/gfz038.

Chapter 14
Anemia and Iron Deficiency in Cardio-Renal Syndromes

Ioannis Kontogiorgos, Stefanos Roumeliotis, Athanasios Roumeliotis, and Vassilios Liakopoulos

14.1 Introduction

Heart failure (HF) is a multifactorial clinical syndrome associated with poor outcomes worldwide. Large-scale epidemiological studies have demonstrated that HF affects 1.9–2.8% of the adult population, while individuals over 65 years of age experience a four-fold higher prevalence, increasing the lifetime risk of HF to 24% [1]. HF has a significant impact on patient life expectancy, with the 1-year mortality rate estimated at 6–10% for patients with chronic HF across different registries [2]. Chronic kidney disease (CKD) is also recognized as a disease with continuously rising prevalence and incidence worldwide. Currently, the global prevalence of CKD is approximately 11%, while the disease remains highly underdiagnosed, with approximately 80–95% of patients being unaware of their condition [3, 4]. Progressive loss of kidney function gradually increases the risk of hospitalizations, cardiovascular and all-cause mortality in these patients; notably, patients at CKD stage 3a exhibit a 1.2-fold risk for all-cause mortality, whereas in stage 5 this risk rises to 5.9 [5]. Moreover, patients with early CKD are at a greater risk of developing a fatal cardiovascular event than progressing to end-stage kidney disease (ESKD) requiring dialysis.

CKD and HF frequently coexist, as CKD develops in approximately 40% of patients with HF with reduced ejection fraction (HFrEF), while conversely, 30% of patients with HFrEF experience CKD during their lifetime [6]. Furthermore, among hospitalized patients diagnosed with HF, acute decline of kidney function is a frequent complication (33.7% of patients), which makes the therapeutic management of these patients more challenging and worsens the prognosis [7]. Similarly, in patients with cardiorenal syndrome (CRS), kidney function impairment not only

I. Kontogiorgos · S. Roumeliotis (✉) · A. Roumeliotis · V. Liakopoulos
2nd Department of Nephrology, AHEPA Hospital, Aristotle University of Thessaloniki, Thessaloniki, Greece

A. Covic, A. Burlacu (eds.), *Renal Dysfunction in Cardiovascular Pathologies*,
https://doi.org/10.1007/978-3-032-25434-4_14

complicates the management of patients with HF and CKD but is also associated with adverse clinical outcomes, including mortality. Every 10 ml/min decrease in eGFR has been linked to a 7% increase in mortality risk [8].

Anemia develops in patients with both HF and CKD and is a strong risk factor for the progression of both cardiovascular disease (CVD) and CKD [9]. The close and strong association among CKD, HF and anemia has led to the introduction of the term cardiorenal anemia syndrome (CRAS), highlighting anemia as a pivotal player in the development and progression of CRS [10]. The prevalence of anemia increases with both declining kidney and worsening cardiac function, representing not only a factor that aggravates these clinical conditions but also a complication of their progression and a major therapeutic target [11]. Moreover, the coexistence of anemia and CRS is associated with worse outcomes and an increased risk of all-cause mortality [11, 12].

Multiple pathophysiological mechanisms often underlie both HF and CKD, including iron deficiency (ID), decreased erythropoietin production and/or resistance to its action, and oxidative stress, which contribute to the development of anemia in patients with CRS [13]. ID is highly prevalent in both HF and CKD and is linked to adverse outcomes, including mortality, representing an even stronger prognostic factor than anemia per se [6]. Since currently there are no consensus or specific guidelines for the management of CRAS, in daily clinical practice, therapeutic approaches targeting different pathophysiological mechanisms are used for anemia treatment in these patients. Herein, we present the underlying mechanisms leading to CRAS, the diagnostic approach, and the current therapeutic options.

14.2 Epidemiology of Anemia in Cardiorenal Syndromes

According to the World Health Organization (WHO), anemia is defined as a hemoglobin (Hb) concentration of < 13 g/dl in men and < 12 g/dl in women [14]. As previously mentioned, anemia is a particularly common finding in patients with HF and CKD. Among patients with HF, the prevalence of anemia ranges from 30% in stable patients to 50% in hospitalized patients, while the occurrence of anemia does not appear to vary in different values of left ventricular ejection fraction [15]. In patients with CKD, anemia is also common (two-fold higher prevalence compared to the general population), and increases further as kidney function deteriorates, reaching 53% in ESKD [16]. In addition, ID, a leading cause of anemia, is also highly prevalent among patients with HF and CKD. In patients with chronic HF, the prevalence of ID may reach 68%, and it appears to be more common among females and in patients with HF with preserved ejection fraction [17]. The prevalence of ID also appears to be high among patients with CKD, with rates reaching 47% [18].

The epidemiology of CRAS remains challenging to determine accurately, as the syndrome by definition comprises three components (HF, CKD, anemia), which show considerable heterogeneity in their definitions and diagnostic criteria across studies. Most studies define CRAS as the coexistence of HF, CKD with an eGFR < 60 ml/min/1.73 m^2, and Hb levels < 13 g/dl for males and < 12 g/dl for females. Based on the above criteria, anemia is particularly common in patients with CRS. In a study including 423 patients with HF and CKD the prevalence of anemia was 47.5% while it became more prevalent as kidney function declined, reaching almost 80% in patients with an eGFR < 30 ml/min/1.73m^2 [19]. In another study with 748 patients with HF, the prevalence of CRAS was found to be 30%. Interestingly, 49% of patients met the criteria for CRS, with the prevalence of anemia reaching 61% in this subgroup [12]. Therefore, it became evident that large epidemiological studies focusing exclusively on patients with CRS are needed for an accurate determination of anemia prevalence in this population.

14.3 Pathophysiology of Anemia in Cardiorenal Syndromes

Anemia in patients with CRS is both a frequent manifestation and a major contributor to disease progression. Both CKD and HF can lead to fluid overload and anemia. Conversely, anemia per se is considered a major cause of kidney function deterioration and HF decompensation through the development of tissue hypoxia and peripheral vasodilation [13]. Although the pathophysiology of CRAS has not been fully understood, multiple mechanisms, often shared by CKD and HF, interact and play a pivotal role in the development and persistence of anemia in patients with CRS (Fig. 14.1).

Disturbances in both the production and function of erythropoietin (EPO) represent a key mechanism underlying anemia in patients with CRS. Patients with HF often have elevated EPO levels, which not only correlate poorly with Hb levels but

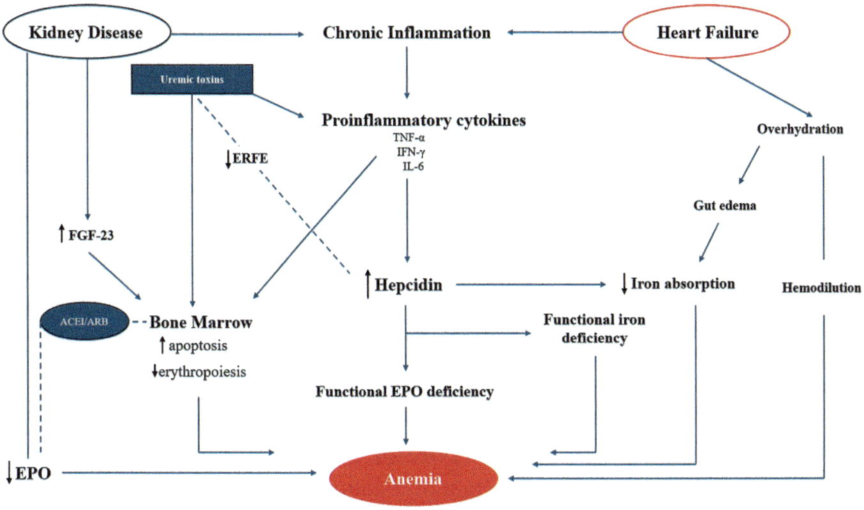

Fig. 14.1 Pathophysiology of CRAS

also seem to have adverse prognostic significance [20]. Chronic HF is characterized by systemic inflammation, which affects bone marrow and leads to EPO resistance and impaired erythropoiesis, resulting in an adaptive increase in circulating EPO levels [21]. However, the coexistence of CKD and HF appears to further complicate the pathophysiology of anemia in patients with CRS. In patients with CKD, EPO levels are low (relatively to the degree of anemia). Reduced EPO production begins in the early stages of CKD and is more pronounced when eGFR declines below 30 ml/min/1.73m^2 [22]. In CKD, renal blood flow is decreased, resulting in lower oxygen delivery and relative renal hypoxia. An important adaptive mechanism is the reduced oxygen consumption by the renal parenchyma, which helps maintain a normal tissue oxygen gradient, resulting in inadequate activation of the EPO gene [23]. However, CRAS appears to be derived mainly from a functional EPO deficiency or resistance rather than an absolute deficiency. Both CKD and HF are considered chronic inflammatory conditions, characterized by an abnormal inflammatory response that eventually leads to the release of proinflammatory cytokines and oxidative stress [16, 24]. Inflammatory cytokines (e.g., TNF-α, IL-6, IFN-γ) act directly on the bone marrow, leading to reduced response of hematopoietic progenitor cells to EPO [25]. Furthermore, accumulating evidence suggests that inflammatory cytokines induce apoptosis of erythroid progenitor cells and promote the production of peptides that act as inhibitors of EPO receptors, thereby contributing to the development of CRAS [25, 26].

One of the main factors contributing to the development of CRAS is ID. However, complete depletion of iron stores is not always required, as patients with CRAS and chronic inflammation often develop functional ID. In patients with CRS, absolute iron deficiency results from impaired iron absorption due to gut edema, chronic subclinical bleeding, or inadequate dietary intake [27]. However, functional ID appears to play a more important role in patients with CRS. Iron is released from body iron stores to the circulation via ferroportin, binds to transferrin, and is subsequently delivered to target cells through transferrin receptors [28]. Hepcidin is considered the main regulator of iron homeostasis by inhibiting the release of iron from both macrophages and intestinal enterocytes. Hepcidin reduces duodenal iron absorption by suppressing apical divalent metal transporter-1 (DMT-1) expression in enterocytes and regulates iron storage by inducing ferroportin internalization and degradation, limiting iron release from iron stores [28]. Hepcidin synthesis is increased in response to iron excess and inflammatory stimuli, whereas it is downregulated under conditions of iron deficiency, hypoxia, or enhanced erythropoietic activity [29]. The release of proinflammatory cytokines increases hepcidin levels, leading to reduced iron absorption, limited availability of stored iron, and eventually anemia [13, 30].

Chronic inflammation also has multiple effects on the bone marrow, resulting in the development of anemia. Proinflammatory cytokines, such as TNF-α, act directly on the bone marrow, interfering with erythroid differentiation, impairing erythroid progenitors, and suppressing production of mature RBCs [31]. Chronic inflammation not only leads to EPO resistance but also induces apoptosis and cell death of early erythroid precursors, indicating an EPO-independent mechanism of anemia development [31]. The accumulation of uremic toxins is also related to bone marrow suppression and impaired erythropoiesis. Uremic toxins reduce the response of erythroblasts to EPO, resulting in decreased erythroferrone (ERFE) production. Under nonanemic conditions, ERFE regulates hepcidin secretion; elevated ERFE levels suppress hepcidin, thereby promoting the use of iron for erythropoiesis. In CKD, the decreased response to EPO leads to lower ERFE levels, which in turn increase hepcidin concentration, contributing to the development of CRAS [32].

Disorders of calcium and phosphate homeostasis represent another potential mechanism contributing to CRAS. Secondary hyperparathyroidism reduces EPO production and shortens red blood cell lifespan [33]. Moreover, fibroblast growth factor 23 (FGF-23) directly suppresses EPO production as well as erythropoiesis in the bone marrow, mainly by interfering with hematopoietic stem cell differentiation [34]. FGF-23 leads to the release of proinflammatory cytokines, while chronic inflammation in turn increases FGF-23 levels [34]. This interaction contributes to the development of inflammation-driven anemia, as previously described.

The use of angiotensin-converting enzyme inhibitors (ACEIs) and angiotensin II receptor blockers (ARBs), two drug classes that are commonly prescribed in patients with CKD and HF, has also been associated with CRAS. ACEIs may directly affect EPO production by reducing the synthesis of angiotensin II [35]. In addition, ACEIs have been shown to act directly on bone marrow hematopoiesis by decreasing the degradation of various inhibitors of hemopoietic stem cell proliferation [35, 36]. Several comorbidities in patients with CRS might also contribute to the development of anemia. Diabetes mellitus, the most common cause of CKD, can lead to anemia through impaired EPO production (as a result of diabetic nephropathy or interstitial fibrosis) or through reduced response secondary to glycation of EPO receptors [37]. Moreover, diabetes is characterized by chronic inflammation, which, as discussed above, is a key factor in the development of anemia.

14.4 Diagnosis of Anemia and ID in Cardiorenal Syndromes

As mentioned above, anemia is defined by Hb levels < 13 g/dl in males and < 12 g/dl in females, according to the WHO [14]. However, taking into consideration the multifactorial etiology of anemia in patients with CRS, a comprehensive evaluation should extend beyond Hb levels to include laboratory tests assessing iron metabolism and kidney function. Moreover, several limitations exist regarding the diagnosis and, more importantly, the treatment of CRAS, as there is a lack of specific guidelines for anemia in patients with CRS. Consequently, in everyday clinical practice, managing a patient with CRAS requires decisions based on the recommendations of CKD and HF anemia guidelines.

Routine screening for anemia in patients with HF is recommended by the European Society of Cardiology (ESC) and the American College of Cardiology Foundation, American Heart Association Task Force on Clinical Practice Guidelines, and Heart Failure Society of America [38, 39]. The diagnostic work-up of anemia should include not only Hb levels, but also reticulocyte count, serum ferritin, transferrin saturation (TSAT), as well as vitamin B12 and folate levels, in order to exclude other causes of anemia and absolute iron deficiency [13]. In patients without comorbidities, the diagnosis of ID can be easily established, since serum ferritin and TSAT levels serve as indicators of iron store status [21]. However, ferritin is an acute-phase protein that rises in inflammatory states and interferes with iron homeostasis, leading to the development of functional ID. Both HF and CKD are regarded as chronic inflammatory conditions, characterized by increased levels of cytokines (IL-1, IL-6, TNF-α), which modulate the inflammatory response and contribute to the development of functional ID. Therefore, the diagnosis of ID, absolute or functional, remains challenging in patients with CRS.

In the general adult population, ID is defined as a serum ferritin level < 15 μg/L, but in chronic inflammatory conditions a higher ferritin threshold is recommended to account for functional ID [6]. In chronic HF, ID is defined as a serum ferritin <100 μg/L or a serum ferritin 100 to 299 μg/L if TSAT is < 20% [38, 39]. However, this definition was adopted into practice without prior validation, mainly based on previous studies conducted in patients with CKD [40, 41]. When compared to the gold standard of bone marrow iron staining, it became clear that a considerable proportion of patients classified as iron-deficient by ferritin and TSAT criteria did not show ID on bone marrow examination [42]. Specifically, most patients with ferritin levels < 100 μg/L but TSAT > 20% lacked evidence of iron deficiency on bone marrow staining, leading to the introduction of the term isolated hypoferritimemia to describe this entity [42]. Furthermore, a large-scale observational study assessed the prognostic impact of ID in 4422 patients with HF and demonstrated that TSAT < 20% and serum iron ≤ 13 μmol/L, but not the current guideline criteria, were related to an increased 5-year mortality, whereas patients with isolated hypoferritinemia appeared to have a better prognosis [17]. This could be partly explained by the pathophysiology of iron metabolism in myocardial cells. Heart is considered a highly iron-dependent tissue, where transferrin binds through transferrin receptors, in order to maintain intracellular iron. In HF, the expression of transferrin receptors is suppressed due to neurohormonal activation and explains why reduced TSAT is associated with adverse outcomes even though anemia is not present [43]. Moreover, myocardial iron depletion contributes to cardiac remodelling, impaired contractile and diastolic dysfunction, which are exacerbated by low TSAT but can be improved with iron repletion [41, 44]. Therefore, in patients with HF it remains uncertain whether the diagnosis and management of ID should be based primarily on serum ferritin, as those with isolated hypoferritinemia may not experience additional benefit from further increasing TSAT.

In CKD, ID is defined as absolute when serum ferritin is < 100 μg/L and TSAT < 20%, while functional ID is present when serum ferritin is > 100 μg/L and TSAT is < 20% [6]. In contrast to the HF guidelines, the Kidney Disease: Improving Global Outcomes (KDIGO) work group guidelines (2012) recommend iron supplementation in patients with serum ferritin ≤ 500 μg/L and TSAT ≤ 30% [45]. However, emerging evidence suggests that the levels of serum ferritin lack sensitivity for detecting ID in patients with CKD, as they do not diagnose ID correctly compared with the gold standard of bone marrow iron staining [46]. As in HF, CKD is also characterized by chronic inflammation; therefore, the values of ferritin (which is an acute-phase reactant) should always be interpreted with caution [47]. Moreover, observational studies have shown that low TSAT is strongly related to increased mortality, irrespective of serum ferritin levels, indicating that functional ID is an important and underrecognized risk factor for poor outcomes [48, 49]. Taking the above into consideration, it becomes evident that new, more accurate and sensitive biomarkers are needed to assess iron status in patients with CRS.

The soluble transferrin receptor (sTfR) has been investigated as a potential marker of ID in both HF and CKD populations. The levels of sTfR increase early during ID, even before the development of anemia, making it a useful biomarker in the detection of tissue ID, even in the absence of systemic ID or anemia [50]. Elevated levels of sTfR have been shown to independently predict mortality in diabetic patients with coronary artery disease, comorbidities that are highly prevalent in patients with CRS [51]. In HF patients, elevated sTfR levels provide an accurate indication of depleted bone marrow iron stores and can identify individuals at increased risk of mortality [52]. Moreover, besides its association with hard outcomes, such as overall mortality, increased levels of sTfR have also been linked to impaired physical function and decreased QoL [53]. In CKD, the use of sTfR as a marker for assessing ID and anemia remains controversial. Previous studies conducted in ESKD patients undergoing hemodialysis have demonstrated that sTfR is a marker of erythropoiesis rather than ID [54, 55]. The sTfR index (ratio of sTfR to log-transformed serum ferritin), on the other hand, may be superior to sTfR and provide a better estimation of ID if combined with serum ferritin, TSAT and other anemia indices; still, it remains an unvalidated method in CKD patients [56]. Other biomarkers, such as hepcidin and plasma neutrophil gelatinase-associated lipocalin (NGAL) have been studied as potential ID markers but have failed to demonstrate a strong correlation with ID so far and remain of limited utility [57].

Large, well-designed studies and specific guidelines are needed to evaluate the diagnostic accuracy of different iron metabolism indices in patients with CRAS.

14.5 Implications of Anemia and ID in Cardiorenal Syndromes

Both anemia and ID are considered significant factors that independently affect morbidity and mortality in patients with CRS. A growing body of evidence from epidemiological studies and clinical trials highlights the prognostic importance of these conditions and supports their recognition as major therapeutic targets. Moreover, although QoL has not been specifically assessed in patients with CRAS, individuals with type II CRS seem to experience higher rates of depression, limitations in daily activities and reduced vitality when compared with patients with HF without kidney dysfunction [13]. Hospitalized patients at for HF with concomitant anemia and CKD have an increased risk for major adverse cardiovascular events and hospitalization compared with those without either condition (31.9% for patients with anemia and CKD, 18.5% for patients with only CKD, 13.5% for patients with only anemia, and 11.5% for patients with no anemia or CKD, $p < 0.001$) [58]. Similarly, patients with chronic HF and systolic dysfunction with CRAS have a 2.2-fold increased risk for all-cause mortality and urgent heart transplantation [19]. Comparable results have also been reported in prospective studies. In a prospective study of 748 patients with HF with a mean follow-up of 2.5 years, those with CRAS (30%) experienced a higher risk for all-cause mortality compared with patients with only HF (51% vs. 26%, $p < 0.001$) [12]. Another, more recent prospective study, explored the impact of CRAS on cardiac death, non-fatal myocardial infarction and rehospitalization in 303 hospitalized patients with HF [59]. Patients with CRAS (21%) had a higher risk for the composite primary outcome compared with those without anemia or CKD (27.5% vs. 10.7%, $p < 0.001$) [59]. Besides anemia, ID is also associated with adverse outcomes in patients with CRAS. A multicenter pooled cohort investigated the prognostic implications of ID in 1506 patients with chronic HF [60]. In multivariate analysis, ID emerged as an independent predictor of mortality (HR: 1.42, 95%CI: 1.14–1.77, $p = 0.002$), whereas patients with eGFR < 60 ml/min/1.73 m^2 had worse outcomes compared to those with preserved renal function [60]. The secondary analysis of the BIOSTAT-CHF study also provides important insights [61]. In this analysis, ID was present in 59.3% of the patients overall and in 69% of those with CKD, while it was more prevalent in patients with both anemia and CKD (77.5% vs. 59.3%, $p < 0.001$) [61]. After adjusting for anemia and CKD, ID was shown to be an independent predictor of all-cause mortality (HR: 1.30, 95% CI: 1.05–1.70, $p = 0.045$) [61].

14.6 Management of Anemia in Cardiorenal Syndromes

As mentioned earlier, there are no specific guidelines for CRAS, and its management requires a comprehensive approach that considers the dual nature of the disease, the stage of CKD and HF, and the iron status. The use of erythropoietin-stimulating agents (ESAs) and the administration of iron, either intravenously or per os, are the main therapeutic approaches in CKD-related anemia [45]. However, an international KDIGO consensus meeting on HF and CKD concluded that in the presence of anemia, ESAs do not provide benefit in the prevention or treatment of HF in this population, whereas iron administration was considered an appropriate option for patients with concurrent HF and CKD, improving anemia-related symptoms, exercise capacity, and even eGFR [62]. Moreover, the use of hypoxia-inducible factor prolyl hydroxylase inhibitors (HIF- PHIs) has been recognized as a promising therapeutic approach, while sodium-glucose co-transporter type 2 inhibitors (SGLT2is), a drug class with well-documented cardio- and renoprotective benefits, have also been shown to have a favorable effect on Hb levels [6, 35]. The therapeutic management of patients with concomitant anemia, HF, and CKD is therefore challenging. The following section will highlight the potential treatment options for CRAS.

14.6.1 Erythropoiesis-Stimulating Agents

Treatment with ESAs improves Hb levels and has been associated with favorable renal outcomes, as well as with cardiac remodeling, including reductions in left ventricular mass and wall thickness in patients with HF and CKD [63]. In HF, the combination of ESA therapy and intravenous iron has been shown to increase Hb levels, stabilize declining kidney function, and reduce the need for hospitalizations [11]. However, in a study including 2278 non-ID patients with systolic HF and mild-to-moderate anemia, the RED-HF trial, therapy with darbepoetin alfa failed to significantly lower the risk of all-cause mortality or first hospitalization for worsening HF, despite effectively raising Hb levels [64]. Moreover, patients on darbepoetin alfa experienced higher rates of thromboembolic adverse events, a finding that, in combination with the poor clinical outcomes of ESA treatment, did not support the use of ESAs in these patients [64]. A meta-analysis, which included 13 studies and 3172 patients with chronic HF under ESAs, demonstrated that ESA treatment did not improve all-cause mortality and rehospitalization but increased the risk of thromboembolic events [65]. Based on the aforementioned studies, the American and European HF guidelines do not recommend the use of ESAs in patients with anemia and HF [38, 39].

In patients with CKD, the KDIGO guidelines for anemia in CKD (2012) recommend maintaining Hb levels between 10 and 11.5 g/dl in those receiving ESA therapy [45]. This recommendation is based on evidence showing that in patients with CKD and anemia, targeting Hb levels above 11.5 g/dl with ESA therapy has not been shown to improve survival and may increase the risk of cardiovascular complications. A meta-analysis of 27 studies including 10,452 patients with CKD on ESA treatment showed that higher Hb levels are related to increased risk for adverse cardiovascular events, such as stroke, hypertension, and vascular access thrombosis [66]. As mentioned before, both HF and CKD are characterized by chronic inflammation, which contributes to resistance to erythropoietin and consequently leads to the need for higher ESA doses. However, a secondary analysis of the CHOIR trial, which included 1244 CKD patients treated with epoetin-alfa, demonstrated that higher ESA doses were associated with a high risk for adverse cardiovascular events, regardless of Hb levels [67]. Recent evidence suggests that fibroblast growth factor 23 (FGF23) may act as a potential mediator in the development of adverse outcomes. ESA administration increases C-terminal FGF23 levels, which have been associated with a higher risk of mortality in patients with CKD and HF [68].

As previously discussed, the KDIGO consensus meeting on HF and CKD indicated that ESAs offer no benefit for preventing or treating HF in anemic patients [62]. However, approximately 10% of patients with CRAS receive ESA therapy, while prior iron administration and impaired kidney function appear to be predictors for initiating ESA treatment [69]. In everyday clinical practice, ESA therapy in patients with CRAS should be individualized, given the absence of specific guidelines for the management of anemia in this population.

14.6.2 Iron Therapy

Iron therapy represents a major cornerstone in the management of anemia, both in patients with HF and in those with CKD. As already discussed, both absolute and functional IDs are considered one of the main causes of anemia in patients with CRS. However, beyond the challenges associated with establishing the diagnosis of ID in CRAS, its correction remains demanding.

A large body of evidence suggests that in patients with HF, correction of ID through intravenous iron supplementation is associated with improvements in symptoms, functional capacity, and QoL [70–74]. Nevertheless, regarding the effect on major clinical outcomes, such as mortality or HF-related hospitalizations, the results across studies have been inconsistent. The AFFIRM-HF trial included 1132 patients recently hospitalized for HF and diagnosed with ID, who were randomly assigned to receive either intravenous ferric carboxymaltose or placebo [73]. The study did not demonstrate a statistically significant difference in the composite endpoint of HF hospitalization or CV death during a 52-week follow-up period (rate ratio [RR]: 0.79, 95% CI: 0.62–1.01, $p = 0.059$) [73]. However, the study did show favorable effects of ferric carboxymaltose administration on the secondary composite endpoints, such as the first HF hospitalization or cardiovascular death (HR: 0.80, 95% CI: 0.66–0.98, $p = 0.030$) [73]. A subsequent study, the IRONMAN trial, enrolled 1137 patients with HF and ID who were randomized to receive either intravenous ferric derisomaltose or usual care, with the primary endpoint being recurrent HF hospitalizations and CV death [74]. Over a median follow-up period of 2.7 years, no statistically significant difference was observed between the two groups in the incidence of the primary outcome (rate ratio [RR]: 0.82, 95% CI: 0.66–1.02, p = 0.070) [74]. More comprehensive data were reported from the HEART-FID trial, the largest study to date in patients with HF and ID, which enrolled 3065 participants randomized to receive either intravenous ferric carboxymaltose or placebo [75]. The primary endpoint was a hierarchical composite of death, HF hospitalizations, or change in the 6-min walk distance test [75]. This study did not demonstrate a significant benefit of ferric carboxymaltose, with an unmatched win ratio for the primary composite endpoint of 1.10 (95% CI: 0.99–1.23) compared to placebo [75].

However, important evidence also emerges from 4 meta-analyses, which demonstrated that intravenous iron administration in patients with HF reduces the risk for first or recurrent HF hospitalizations, although no significant benefit, but rather a trend, was observed in reducing cardiovascular or all-cause mortality [76–79]. It is important to highlight that in the aforementioned studies, the beneficial effect of intravenous iron administration was observed both in patients with normal and reduced eGFR, thereby providing valuable insights into iron therapy in patients with CRAS. Moreover, it should be emphasized that all the aforementioned studies included patients with HFrEF, with the effects of iron administration in those with HFpEF remaining uncertain. Additionally, all trials investigated intravenous iron supplementation rather than oral iron, as oral formulations have been associated with poor clinical outcomes due to limited iron absorption in this patient population [80]. Taking all the above into consideration, both the AHA/ACC and ESC HF guidelines recommend intravenous iron administration in patients with HFrEF and ID, defined as serum ferritin < 100 μg/L or serum ferritin between 100 and 299 μg/L with a TSAT < 20% [38, 39].

In patients with CKD, the treatment of ID is a main pillar in the management of CKD-related anemia. Iron supplementation appears to improve Hb levels and other ID indices, enhance functional capacity and QoL, and reduce the need for ESA therapy [81–85]. Although large randomized clinical trials evaluating the impact of iron supplementation on hard endpoints, such as decline of kidney function, the need for dialysis, or mortality, are lacking, iron therapy appears to reduce the risk of hospitalization, dialysis initiation, and death [83]. Both oral and intravenous iron administration are effective and safe options for patients with CKD, although intravenous iron seems to achieve a better Hb response, without, however, showing any significant difference in mortality risk or adverse events [86, 87]. According to the current KDIGO anemia guidelines, iron supplementation is recommended only in anemic patients with serum ferritin ≤ 500 μg/L and TSAT < 20% in order to either raise Hb levels without initiating ESA therapy, or in patients already receiving ESAs, to enhance Hb response or allow for a reduction in ESA dosage [45]. However, the upcoming KDIGO guidelines on anemia management in CKD are expected to propose revised ferritin and TSAT thresholds for initiating iron therapy in patients with non-dialysis CKD; specifically, ferritin < 100 μg/l and TSAT < 40%, or ferritin ≥ 100 μg/l and < 300 μg/l and TSAT <25% [88].

Data regarding iron administration in patients with CRAS remain limited. A retrospective study evaluated the effect of intravenous iron therapy compared to ESA treatment in 81 patients with CRAS. The study demonstrated that intravenous iron administration resulted in a greater increase in Hb levels compared to the ESA group (2.17 vs. 1.24 g/dl, $p = 0.001$) [89]. In a subgroup analysis of the AFFIRM-HF trial (1132 patients with HF and ID randomized to receive either ferric carboxymaltose or placebo), it was found that 60% of participants had an eGFR < 60 ml/min/1.73 m^2 [90]. The results showed that, although patients with impaired kidney function exhibited overall higher event rates for all endpoints, no statistically significant difference was observed between the iron and placebo groups regarding efficacy and safety [90].

Based on the above, intravenous iron administration represents a safe and effective therapeutic option for patients with CRAS, aiming to increase Hb levels. However, its impact on cardiovascular and all-cause mortality remains to be clarified through large randomized clinical trials.

14.6.3 Hypoxia-Inducible Factor Prolyl Hydroxylase Inhibitors

Hypoxia-inducible factors (HIFs) are heterodimeric transcription factors primarily regulated by oxygen levels. HIFs activation leads to erythropoietin production, increases iron uptake by erythroblasts, and suppresses hepcidin synthesis, resulting in enhanced iron absorption and mobilization of stored iron from the reticuloendothelial system for erythropoiesis [91, 92]. Under normal oxygen levels, prolyl hydroxylase enzymes hydroxylate the oxygen-sensitive HIF-α subunit, leading to its degradation [93]. Oral HIF-PHIs mimic the effects of hypoxia on HIFs by inhibiting prolyl hydroxylation, thereby stimulating erythropoiesis [94].

HIF-PHIs increase Hb levels compared to ESAs in patients with pre-dialysis CKD [95–97]. However, there are safety concerns, as their use may be associated with a higher risk of major adverse cardiovascular events (MACE) and thromboembolic events [98, 99]. According to the recent KDIGO controversies conference conclusions, HIF-PHIs are considered non-inferior to ESAs in terms of efficacy for anemia correction, but regarding cardiovascular safety, they seem to be inferior to, or at best, comparable with ESAs [100]. Regarding patients with HF, available data are limited. In a retrospective study including 206 patients with CKD stages 3-5D and HF, roxadustat was shown to be effective in treating anemia without an increased risk for adverse outcomes, 2-year mortality, or rehospitalization [101]. In another recent randomized clinical trial, 21 patients with CRAS were randomly assigned to receive either daprodustat or standard therapy [102]. Patients in the daprodustat group showed an increase in Hb levels, a reduction in hepcidin levels, and an improvement in iron mobilization [102]. On the contrary, in a post hoc analysis of the ASCEND-D and ACEND-ND trials, which included 6836 patients with anemia and CKD on dialysis or not, daprodustat, compared to ESAs, was associated with a non-significant increase in HF hospitalizations [99]. Until further evidence becomes available regarding the use of HIF-PHIs in patients with CRAS, their use in this particular population remains controversial.

14.6.4 Sodium-Glucose Co-transporter Type 2 Inhibitors

Recent studies have demonstrated that SGLT2is increase hemoglobin levels in patients with HF and CKD [103–106]. This drug category appears to improve anemia through multiple mechanisms, many of which are still not fully understood. SGLT2is enhance iron absorption and increase its availability for erythropoiesis, elevate erythropoietin levels early after treatment initiation, and appear to reduce hepcidin levels [107, 108]. Regarding the effect of SGLT2is on erythropoietin production, they seem to reduce ATP consumption in proximal tubular epithelial cells by inhibiting Na^+/K^+-ATPase activity. This results in improved oxygen availability, prevention of erythropoietin-producing fibroblasts, prevention of their transformation into myofibroblasts, and eventually increased erythropoietin synthesis [108].

Moreover, SGLT2is have been shown to lower both hepcidin and ferritin levels. The reduction in ferritin levels may not indicate iron deficiency but rather reflects the role of ferritin as an inflammatory reactant and the anti-inflammatory effects of SGLT2is, which contribute to the reduction of chronic inflammation, a mechanism known as cytosolic iron repletion [109]. However, as previously believed, the reduction of ferritin levels may also suggest cytosolic iron depletion following the initiation of SGLT2is and the stimulation of erythropoietin production, leading to ID and adaptive decrease in hepcidin and ferritin levels [109, 110]. Distinguishing between iron repletion and depletion is important, as iron supplementation is not needed in cases of repletion but is necessary when depletion is present in order to correct ID. However, treatment with SGLT2is leads to an average increase in Hb levels of approximately 0.7 g/dl, and concomitant iron supplementation may carry potential risks of further Hb elevation and thromboembolic events [110]. In light of these findings, combination therapy with SGLT2is and iron should be reserved only for patients with severe ID, pending clinical trials that will further evaluate the outcomes and possible implications of this co-administration.

Declarations

Competing Interests The author(s) has no competing interests to declare that are relevant to the content of this manuscript.

Ethics Approval The author(s) declares that this manuscript does not include primary research with human participants.

The author(s) declares that this manuscript does not include primary studies involving animals.

References

1. Bozkurt B, Ahmad T, Alexander K, Baker WL, Bosak K, Breathett K, et al. HF STATS 2024: Heart Failure Epidemiology and Outcomes Statistics An Updated 2024 Report from the Heart Failure Society of America. J Card Fail. 2025;31(1):66–116.
2. Shahim B, Kapelios CJ, Savarese G, Lund LH. Global public health burden of heart failure: an updated review. Card Fail Rev. 2023;9:e11.
3. Jager KJ, Kovesdy C, Langham R, Rosenberg M, Jha V, Zoccali C. A single number for advocacy and communication-worldwide more than 850 million individuals have kidney diseases. Kidney Int. 2019;96(5):1048–50.
4. Luyckx VA, Tuttle KR, Abdellatif D, Correa-Rotter R, Fung WWS, Haris A, et al. Mind the gap in kidney care: translating what we know into what we do. Kidney Int Rep. 2024;9(6):1541–52.
5. Go AS, Chertow GM, Fan D, McCulloch CE, Hsu C, yuan. Chronic kidney disease and the risks of death, cardiovascular events, and hospitalization. N Engl J Med. 2004;351(13):1296–305.
6. Marques Vidas M, Portolés J, Cobo M, Gorriz JL, Nuñez J, Cases A. Anemia management in the cardiorenal patient: a nephrological perspective. J Am Heart Assoc. 2025;14(5):e037363.
7. Asbagh AG, Sadeghi MT, Ramazanilar P, Nateghian H. Worsening renal function in hospitalized patients with systolic heart failure: prevalence and risk factors. ESC Heart Fail. 2023;10(5):2837–42.

8. Smith GL, Lichtman JH, Bracken MB, Shlipak MG, Phillips CO, DiCapua P, et al. Renal impairment and outcomes in heart failure: systematic review and meta-analysis. J Am Coll Cardiol. 2006;47(10):1987–96.
9. Kim-Mitsuyama S, Soejima H, Yasuda O, Node K, Jinnouchi H, Yamamoto E, et al. Anemia is an independent risk factor for cardiovascular and renal events in hypertensive outpatients with well-controlled blood pressure: a subgroup analysis of the ATTEMPT-CVD randomized trial. Hypertens Res. 2019;42(6):883–91.
10. Silverberg DS, Wexler D, Blum M, Tchebiner J, Sheps D, Keren G, et al. The correction of anemia in severe resistant heart failure with erythropoietin and intravenous iron prevents the progression of both the heart and the renal failure and markedly reduces hospitalization. Clin Nephrol. 2002;58(Suppl 1):S37–45.
11. Silverberg DS, Wexler D, Blum M, Keren G, Sheps D, Leibovitch E, et al. The use of subcutaneous erythropoietin and intravenous iron for the treatment of the anemia of severe, resistant congestive heart failure improves cardiac and renal function and functional cardiac class, and markedly reduces hospitalizations. J Am Coll Cardiol. 2000;35(7):1737–44.
12. Lu KJ, Kearney LG, Hare DL, Ord M, Toia D, Jones E, et al. Cardiorenal anemia syndrome as a prognosticator for death in heart failure. Am J Cardiol. 2013;111(8):1187–91.
13. McCullough PA. Anemia of cardiorenal syndrome. Kidney Int Suppl. 2021;11(1):35–45.
14. Cappellini MD, Motta I. Anemia in clinical practice-definition and classification: does hemoglobin change with aging? Semin Hematol. 2015;52(4):261–9.
15. Anand IS, Gupta P. Anemia and iron deficiency in heart failure: current concepts and emerging therapies. Circulation. 2018;138(1):80–98.
16. Portolés J, Martín L, Broseta JJ, Cases A. Anemia in chronic kidney Disease: from pathophysiology and current treatments, to future agents. Front Med. 2021;8:642296.
17. Masini G, Graham FJ, Pellicori P, Cleland JGF, Cuthbert JJ, Kazmi S, et al. Criteria for iron deficiency in patients with heart failure. J Am Coll Cardiol. 2022;79(4):341–51.
18. Cacoub P, Choukroun G, Cohen-Solal A, Luporsi E, Peyrin-Biroulet L, Peoc'h K, et al. Towards a common definition for the diagnosis of iron deficiency in chronic inflammatory diseases. Nutrients. 2022;14(5):1039.
19. Scrutinio D, Passantino A, Santoro D, Catanzaro R. The cardiorenal anaemia syndrome in systolic heart failure: prevalence, clinical correlates, and long-term survival. Eur J Heart Fail. 2011;13(1):61–7.
20. Belonje AMS, Voors AA, van der Meer P, van Gilst WH, Jaarsma T, van Veldhuisen DJ. Endogenous erythropoietin and outcome in heart failure. Circulation. 2010;121(2):245–51.
21. Weiss G, Goodnough LT. Anemia of chronic disease. N Engl J Med. 2005;352(10):1011–23.
22. Fehr T, Ammann P, Garzoni D, Korte W, Fierz W, Rickli H, et al. Interpretation of erythropoietin levels in patients with various degrees of renal insufficiency and anemia. Kidney Int. 2004;66(3):1206–11.
23. Wenger RH, Hoogewijs D. Regulated oxygen sensing by protein hydroxylation in renal erythropoietin-producing cells. Am J Physiol Renal Physiol. 2010;298(6):F1287–96.
24. Bhangal R, Cancarevic I, Nassar M, Umar Z. Impact of erythropoietin therapy on cardiorenal syndrome: a systematic review with meta-analysis. World J Cardiol. 2023;15(5):273–83.
25. Ganz T. Anemia of inflammation. N Engl J Med. 2019;381(12):1148–57.
26. Macdougall IC, Cooper AC. Erythropoietin resistance: the role of inflammation and proinflammatory cytokines. Nephrol Dial Transplant. 2002;17(Suppl 11):39–43.
27. Lanser L, Poelzl G, Messner M, Ungericht M, Zaruba MM, Hirsch J, et al. Imbalance of iron availability and demand in patients with acute and chronic heart failure. J Am Heart Assoc. 2024;13(9):e032540.
28. van Swelm RPL, Wetzels JFM, Swinkels DW. The multifaceted role of iron in renal health and disease. Nat Rev Nephrol. 2020;16(2):77–98.
29. Nemeth E, Ganz T. Hepcidin and iron in health and Disease. Annu Rev Med. 2023;74:261–77.
30. van der Putten K, Braam B, Jie KE, Gaillard CAJM. Mechanisms of Disease: erythropoietin resistance in patients with both heart and kidney failure. Nat Clin Pract Nephrol. 2008;4(1):47–57.

31. Morceau F, Dicato M, Diederich M. Pro-inflammatory cytokine-mediated anemia: regarding molecular mechanisms of erythropoiesis. Mediat Inflamm. 2009;2009:405016.
32. Hamza E, Metzinger L, Metzinger-Le MV. Uremic toxins affect erythropoiesis during the course of chronic kidney disease: a review. Cells. 2020;9(9):2039.
33. Tanaka M, Komaba H, Fukagawa M. Emerging association between parathyroid hormone and anemia in hemodialysis patients. Ther Apher Dial. 2018;22(3):242–5.
34. Czaya B, Faul C. The role of fibroblast growth factor 23 in inflammation and anemia. Int J Mol Sci. 2019;20(17):4195.
35. Heng J, Li ZT, Yao DD, Li XY, Cui MX, Li ZL. Anemia in cardiorenal disease: from pathogenesis to treatment. Eur J Intern Med. 2025;143:106506.
36. van der Meer P, Lipsic E, Westenbrink BD, van de Wal RMA, Schoemaker RG, Vellenga E, et al. Levels of hematopoiesis inhibitor N-acetyl-seryl-aspartyl-lysyl-proline partially explain the occurrence of anemia in heart failure. Circulation. 2005;112(12):1743–7.
37. Deray G, Heurtier A, Grimaldi A, Launay Vacher V, Isnard BC. Anemia and diabetes. Am J Nephrol. 2004;24(5):522–6.
38. McDonagh TA, Metra M, Adamo M, Gardner RS, Baumbach A, Böhm M, et al. 2023 Focused Update of the 2021 ESC Guidelines for the diagnosis and treatment of acute and chronic heart failure. Eur Heart J. 2023;44(37):3627–39.
39. Heidenreich PA, Bozkurt B, Aguilar D, Allen LA, Byun JJ, Colvin MM, et al. 2022 AHA/ACC/HFSA Guideline for the Management of Heart Failure: A Report of the American College of Cardiology/American Heart Association Joint Committee on Clinical Practice Guidelines. Circulation. 2022;145(18):e895–1032.
40. Cheema B, Chokshi A, Orimoloye O, Ardehali H. Intravenous iron repletion for patients with heart failure and iron deficiency: JACC state-of-the-art review. J Am Coll Cardiol. 2024;83(25):2674–89.
41. Martens P, Tang WHW. Defining iron deficiency in heart failure: importance of transferrin saturation. Circ Heart Fail. 2024;17(4):e011440.
42. Grote Beverborg N, Klip IT, Meijers WC, Voors AA, Vegter EL, van der Wal HH, et al. Definition of iron deficiency based on the gold standard of bone marrow iron staining in heart failure patients. Circ Heart Fail. 2018;11(2):e004519.
43. Maeder MT, Khammy O, dos Remedios C, Kaye DM. Myocardial and systemic iron depletion in heart failure implications for anemia accompanying heart failure. J Am Coll Cardiol. 2011;58(5):474–80.
44. Martens P, Dupont M, Dauw J, Nijst P, Herbots L, Dendale P, et al. The effect of intravenous ferric carboxymaltose on cardiac reverse remodelling following cardiac resynchronization therapy-the IRON-CRT trial. Eur Heart J. 2021;42(48):4905–14.
45. Kidney Disease: Improving Global Outcomes (KDIGO) Anemia Work Group. KDIGO clinical practice guideline for anemia in chronic kidney Disease. Kidney Int Suppl. 2012;2:279–335.
46. Stancu S, Bârsan L, Stanciu A, Mircescu G. Can the response to iron therapy be predicted in anemic nondialysis patients with chronic kidney disease? Clin J Am Soc Nephrol. 2010;5(3):409–16.
47. Coyne D. Iron indices: what do they really mean? Kidney Int Suppl. 2006;101:S4–8.
48. Eisenga MF, Nolte IM, van der Meer P, Bakker SJL, Gaillard CAJM. Association of different iron deficiency cutoffs with adverse outcomes in chronic kidney disease. BMC Nephrol. 2018;19(1):225.
49. Cho ME, Hansen JL, Peters CB, Cheung AK, Greene T, Sauer BC. An increased mortality risk is associated with abnormal iron status in diabetic and non-diabetic Veterans with predialysis chronic kidney disease. Kidney Int. 2019;96(3):750–60.
50. Koulaouzidis A, Said E, Cottier R, Saeed AA. Soluble transferrin receptors and iron deficiency, a step beyond ferritin. A systematic review. J Gastrointest Liver Dis. 2009;18(3):345–52.
51. Ponikowska B, Suchocki T, Paleczny B, Olesinska M, Powierza S, Borodulin-Nadzieja L, et al. Iron status and survival in diabetic patients with coronary artery disease. Diabetes Care. 2013;36(12):4147–56.

52. Sierpinski R, Josiak K, Suchocki T, Wojtas-Polc K, Mazur G, Butrym A, et al. High soluble transferrin receptor in patients with heart failure: a measure of iron deficiency and a strong predictor of mortality. Eur J Heart Fail. 2021;23(6):919–32.
53. Alcaide-Aldeano A, Garay A, Alcoberro L, Jiménez-Marrero S, Yun S, Tajes M, et al. Iron deficiency: impact on functional capacity and quality of life in heart failure with preserved ejection fraction. J Clin Med. 2020;9(4):1199.
54. Chiang WC, Tsai TJ, Chen YM, Lin SL, Hsieh BS. Serum soluble transferrin receptor reflects erythropoiesis but not iron availability in erythropoietin-treated chronic hemodialysis patients. Clin Nephrol. 2002;58(5):363–9.
55. Tarng DC, Huang TP. Determinants of circulating soluble transferrin receptor level in chronic haemodialysis patients. Nephrol Dial Transplant. 2002;17(6):1063–9.
56. Skikne BS, Punnonen K, Caldron PH, Bennett MT, Rehu M, Gasior GH, et al. Improved differential diagnosis of anemia of chronic disease and iron deficiency anemia: a prospective multicenter evaluation of soluble transferrin receptor and the sTfR/log ferritin index. Am J Hematol. 2011;86(11):923–7.
57. Batchelor EK, Kapitsinou P, Pergola PE, Kovesdy CP, Jalal DI. Iron deficiency in chronic kidney disease: updates on pathophysiology, diagnosis, and treatment. J Am Soc Nephrol. 2020;31(3):456–68.
58. Minamisawa M, Miura T, Motoki H, Ueki Y, Nishimura H, Shoin W, et al. Abstract 14876: prognostic impact of cardio-renal-anemia syndrome in patients at risk for heart failure. Circulation. 2017;136(suppl_1):A14876.
59. Kim CJ, Choi IJ, Park HJ, Kim TH, Kim PJ, Chang K, et al. Impact of Cardiorenal anemia syndrome on short- and long-term clinical outcomes in patients hospitalized with heart failure. Cardiorenal Med. 2016;6(4):269–78.
60. Klip IT, Comin-Colet J, Voors AA, Ponikowski P, Enjuanes C, Banasiak W, et al. Iron deficiency in chronic heart failure: an international pooled analysis. Am Heart J. 2013;165(4):575–582.e3.
61. Alnuwaysir RIS, Grote Beverborg N, Hoes MF, Markousis-Mavrogenis G, Gomez KA, van der Wal HH, et al. Additional burden of iron deficiency in heart failure patients beyond the cardio-renal anaemia syndrome: findings from the BIOSTAT-CHF study. Eur J Heart Fail. 2022;24(1):192–204.
62. House AA, Wanner C, Sarnak MJ, Piña IL, CW MI, Komenda P, et al. Heart failure in chronic kidney disease: conclusions from a Kidney Disease: Improving Global Outcomes (KDIGO) controversies conference. Kidney Int. 2019;95(6):1304–17.
63. Akaishi M, Hiroe M, Hada Y, Suzuki M, Tsubakihara Y, Akizawa T, et al. Effect of anemia correction on left ventricular hypertrophy in patients with modestly high hemoglobin level and chronic kidney disease. J Cardiol. 2013;62(4):249–56.
64. Swedberg K, Young JB, Anand IS, Cheng S, Desai AS, Diaz R, et al. Treatment of anemia with darbepoetin alfa in systolic heart failure. N Engl J Med. 2013;368(13):1210–9.
65. Kang J, Park J, Lee JM, Park JJ, Choi DJ. The effects of erythropoiesis stimulating therapy for anemia in chronic heart failure: a meta-analysis of randomized clinical trials. Int J Cardiol. 2016;218:12–22.
66. Palmer SC, Navaneethan SD, Craig JC, Johnson DW, Tonelli M, Garg AX, et al. Meta-analysis: erythropoiesis-stimulating agents in patients with chronic kidney disease. Ann Intern Med. 2010;153(1):23–33.
67. McCullough PA, Barnhart HX, Inrig JK, Reddan D, Sapp S, Patel UD, et al. Cardiovascular toxicity of epoetin-alfa in patients with chronic kidney disease. Am J Nephrol. 2013;37(6):549–58.
68. Eisenga MF, Emans ME, van der Putten K, Cramer MJ, Diepenbroek A, Velthuis BK, et al. Epoetin Beta and C-terminal fibroblast growth factor 23 in patients with chronic heart failure and chronic kidney Disease. J Am Heart Assoc. 2019;8(16):e011130.
69. Jackevicius CA, Co MJ, Warner AL. Predictors of erythropoietin use in patients with cardiorenal anaemia syndrome. Int J Pharm Pract. 2015;23(3):199–204.

70. Okonko DO, Grzeslo A, Witkowski T, Mandal AKJ, Slater RM, Roughton M, et al. Effect of intravenous iron sucrose on exercise tolerance in anemic and nonanemic patients with symptomatic chronic heart failure and iron deficiency FERRIC-HF: a randomized, controlled, observer-blinded trial. J Am Coll Cardiol. 2008;51(2):103–12.
71. Anker SD, Comin Colet J, Filippatos G, Willenheimer R, Dickstein K, Drexler H, et al. Ferric carboxymaltose in patients with heart failure and iron deficiency. N Engl J Med. 2009;361(25):2436–48.
72. Ponikowski P, van Veldhuisen DJ, Comin-Colet J, Ertl G, Komajda M, Mareev V, et al. Beneficial effects of long-term intravenous iron therapy with ferric carboxymaltose in patients with symptomatic heart failure and iron deficiency†. Eur Heart J. 2015;36(11):657–68.
73. Ponikowski P, Kirwan BA, Anker SD, McDonagh T, Dorobantu M, Drozdz J, et al. Ferric carboxymaltose for iron deficiency at discharge after acute heart failure: a multicentre, double-blind, randomised, controlled trial. Lancet (Lond Engl). 2020;396(10266):1895–904.
74. Kalra PR, Cleland JGF, Petrie MC, Thomson EA, Kalra PA, Squire IB, et al. Intravenous ferric derisomaltose in patients with heart failure and iron deficiency in the UK (IRONMAN): an investigator-initiated, prospective, randomised, open-label, blinded-endpoint trial. Lancet (Lond Engl). 2022;400(10369):2199–209.
75. Mentz RJ, Garg J, Rockhold FW, Butler J, De Pasquale CG, Ezekowitz JA, et al. Ferric Carboxymaltose in heart failure with iron deficiency. N Engl J Med. 2023;389(11):975–86.
76. Graham FJ, Pellicori P, Ford I, Petrie MC, Kalra PR, Cleland JGF. Intravenous iron for heart failure with evidence of iron deficiency: a meta-analysis of randomised trials. Clin Res Cardiol. 2021;110(8):1299–307.
77. Ponikowski P, Mentz RJ, Hernandez AF, Butler J, Khan MS, van Veldhuisen DJ, et al. Efficacy of ferric carboxymaltose in heart failure with iron deficiency: an individual patient data meta-analysis. Eur Heart J. 2023;44(48):5077–91.
78. Salah HM, Savarese G, Rosano GMC, Ambrosy AP, Mentz RJ, Fudim M. Intravenous iron infusion in patients with heart failure: a systematic review and study-level meta-analysis. ESC Heart Fail. 2023;10(2):1473–80.
79. Anker SD, Karakas M, Mentz RJ, Ponikowski P, Butler J, Khan MS, et al. Systematic review and meta-analysis of intravenous iron therapy for patients with heart failure and iron deficiency. Nat Med. 2025;31(8):2640–6.
80. Lewis GD, Malhotra R, Hernandez AF, McNulty SE, Smith A, Felker GM, et al. Effect of Oral iron repletion on exercise capacity in patients with heart failure with reduced ejection fraction and iron deficiency: the IRONOUT HF randomized clinical trial. JAMA. 2017;317(19):1958–66.
81. Macdougall IC, Bock AH, Carrera F, Eckardt KU, Gaillard C, Van Wyck D, et al. FIND-CKD: a randomized trial of intravenous ferric carboxymaltose versus oral iron in patients with chronic kidney disease and iron deficiency anaemia. Nephrol Dial Transplant. 2014;29(11):2075–84.
82. Fishbane S, Block GA, Loram L, Neylan J, Pergola PE, Uhlig K, et al. Effects of ferric citrate in patients with nondialysis-dependent CKD and iron deficiency anemia. J Am Soc Nephrol. 2017;28(6):1851–8.
83. Block GA, Block MS, Smits G, Mehta R, Isakova T, Wolf M, et al. A pilot randomized trial of ferric citrate coordination complex for the treatment of advanced CKD. J Am Soc Nephrol. 2019;30(8):1495–504.
84. Bhandari S, Allgar V, Lamplugh A, Macdougall I, Kalra PA. A multicentre prospective double blinded randomised controlled trial of intravenous iron (ferric Derisomaltose (FDI)) in Iron deficient but not anaemic patients with chronic kidney disease on functional status. BMC Nephrol. 2021;22(1):115.
85. Pergola PE, Kopyt NP. Oral ferric Maltol for the treatment of iron-deficiency anemia in patients with CKD: a randomized trial and open-label extension. Am J Kidney Dis. 2021;78(6):846–856.e1.

86. Shepshelovich D, Rozen-Zvi B, Avni T, Gafter U, Gafter-Gvili A. Intravenous versus Oral iron supplementation for the treatment of anemia in CKD: an updated systematic review and meta-analysis. Am J Kidney Dis. 2016;68(5):677–90.
87. O'Lone EL, Hodson EM, Nistor I, Bolignano D, Webster AC, Craig JC. Parenteral versus oral iron therapy for adults and children with chronic kidney disease. Cochrane Database Syst Rev. 2019;2(2):CD007857.
88. Topic [Internet]. [cited 2025 Oct 7]. Available from: https://kdigo.org/wp-content/uploads/2024/11/KDIGO-2025-Anemia-in-CKD-Guideline_Public-Review-Draft_Nov42024.pdf.
89. Ben-Assa E, Shacham Y, Shashar M, Leshem-Rubinow E, Gal-Oz A, Schwartz IF, et al. Target hemoglobin may be achieved with intravenous iron alone in anemic patients with Cardiorenal syndrome: an observational study. Cardiorenal Med. 2015;5(4):246–53.
90. Macdougall IC, Ponikowski P, Stack AG, Wheeler DC, Anker SD, Butler J, et al. Ferric Carboxymaltose in iron-deficient patients with hospitalized heart failure and reduced kidney function. Clin J Am Soc Nephrol. 2023;18(9):1124–34.
91. Schödel J, Ratcliffe PJ. Mechanisms of hypoxia signalling: new implications for nephrology. Nat Rev Nephrol. 2019;15(10):641–59.
92. Haase VH. Hypoxia-inducible factor-prolyl hydroxylase inhibitors in the treatment of anemia of chronic kidney disease. Kidney Int Suppl. 2021;11(1):8–25.
93. Bruick RK, McKnight SL. A conserved family of prolyl-4-hydroxylases that modify HIF. Science. 2001;294(5545):1337–40.
94. Gupta N, Wish JB. Hypoxia-inducible factor prolyl hydroxylase inhibitors: a potential new treatment for anemia in patients with CKD. Am J Kidney Dis. 2017;69(6):815–26.
95. Martin ER, Smith MT, Maroni BJ, Zuraw QC, deGoma EM. Clinical trial of Vadadustat in patients with anemia secondary to stage 3 or 4 chronic kidney disease. Am J Nephrol. 2017;45(5):380–8.
96. Chen N, Hao C, Peng X, Lin H, Yin A, Hao L, et al. Roxadustat for anemia in patients with kidney Disease not receiving dialysis. N Engl J Med. 2019;381(11):1001–10.
97. Singh AK, Carroll K, McMurray JJV, Solomon S, Jha V, Johansen KL, et al. Daprodustat for the treatment of anemia in patients not undergoing dialysis. N Engl J Med. 2021;385(25):2313–24.
98. Chertow GM, Pergola PE, Farag YMK, Agarwal R, Arnold S, Bako G, et al. Vadadustat in patients with anemia and non-dialysis-dependent CKD. N Engl J Med. 2021;384(17):1589–600.
99. Cunningham JW, Claggett BL, Lopes RD, McMurray JJV, Perkovic V, Carroll K, et al. Daprodustat and heart failure in CKD. J Am Soc Nephrol. 2024;35(5):607–17.
100. Ku E, Del Vecchio L, Eckardt KU, Haase VH, Johansen KL, Nangaku M, et al. Novel anemia therapies in chronic kidney disease: conclusions from a kidney Disease: improving global outcomes (KDIGO) controversies conference. Kidney Int. 2023;104(4):655–80.
101. Liu J, Meng Z, Feng L, Zhuo L, Liang Y, Yang M, et al. Efficacy and safety of roxadustat for treating anaemia in patients with chronic kidney disease and heart failure: a retrospective cohort study. Clin Kidney J. 2025;18(4):sfaf061.
102. Singh YS, Matsue Y, Iso T, Fujimoto Y, Yanagisawa N, Shitara J, et al. Daprodustat for patients with heart failure and renal anemia: a pilot multicenter, open-label, randomized controlled study. J Cardiol. 2025;86(6):592–8. https://doi.org/10.1016/j.jjcc.2025.09.011.
103. Docherty KF, Curtain JP, Anand IS, Bengtsson O, Inzucchi SE, Køber L, et al. Effect of dapagliflozin on anaemia in DAPA-HF. Eur J Heart Fail. 2021;23(4):617–28.
104. Ferreira JP, Anker SD, Butler J, Filippatos G, Iwata T, Salsali A, et al. Impact of anaemia and the effect of empagliflozin in heart failure with reduced ejection fraction: findings from EMPEROR-Reduced. Eur J Heart Fail. 2022;24(4):708–15.
105. Fuchs Andersen C, Omar M, Glenthøj A, El Fassi D, Møller HJ, Lindholm Kurtzhals JA, et al. Effects of empagliflozin on erythropoiesis in heart failure: data from the Empire HF trial. Eur J Heart Fail. 2023;25(2):226–34.

106. Koshino A, Schechter M, Chertow GM, Vart P, Jongs N, Toto RD, et al. Dapagliflozin and anemia in patients with chronic kidney disease. NEJM Evid. 2023;2(6):EVIDoa2300049.
107. Mazer CD, Hare GMT, Connelly PW, Gilbert RE, Shehata N, Quan A, et al. Effect of Empagliflozin on erythropoietin levels, iron stores, and red blood cell morphology in patients with type 2 diabetes mellitus and coronary artery disease. Circulation. 2020;141(8):704–7.
108. Sano M, Goto S. Possible mechanism of hematocrit elevation by sodium glucose cotransporter 2 inhibitors and associated beneficial renal and cardiovascular effects. Circulation. 2019;139(17):1985–7.
109. Packer M. Potential interactions when prescribing SGLT2 inhibitors and intravenous iron in combination in heart failure. JACC Heart Fail. 2023;11(1):106–14.
110. Packer M, Cleland JGF. Combining iron supplements with SGLT2 inhibitor-stimulated erythropoiesis in heart failure: should we be worried about thromboembolic events? J Card Fail. 2023;29(3):403–6.

Chapter 15
Metabolic Implications in Cardio-Renal Syndromes

B. Timar, L. Gaita, V. Avram, and A. Braha

15.1 Introduction to the Metabolic Dysfunctions of Cardio-Renal Syndromes

Cardio-renal syndromes (CRS) represent, as discussed in the previous chapters, a complex pathologic interaction between the heart and the kidney, in which the acute or chronic dysfunction of one organ contributes to the deterioration of the other. Beyond hemodynamic and neurohormonal mechanisms, metabolic dysfunctions play a key role in the progression of these syndromes and contribute to the development of a cardio-renal-metabolic vicious cycle in which metabolite accumulation, chronic inflammation, and dysregulation of mineral homeostasis simplify the deterioration of both organs [1–3].

Recently, another syndrome has been defined, that alongside the cardiovascular (CV) and renal dysfunction, includes the metabolic component represented by obesity and/or diabetes, namely the cardiovascular-kidney-metabolic (CKM) syndrome. This new integrative concept refers to the systemic disorder caused by pathological interactions between metabolic risk factors, chronic kidney disease (CKD), and CV disease (CVD), leading to multiorgan dysfunction, poor health outcomes, and an increased rate of adverse CV and renal outcomes. The CKM syndrome can be classified into 5 stages, from 0 (no CKM risk factors), to 1 (excess or dysfunctional adiposity), 2 (metabolic risk factors and CKD), 3 (subclinical CVD in CKM) and 4 (clinical CVD in CKM) [4].

B. Timar (✉) · L. Gaita · V. Avram · A. Braha
Second Department of Internal Medicine —Diabetes, Nutrition, Metabolic Diseases, and Systemic Rheumatology, "Victor Babes" University of Medicine and Pharmacy, Timisoara, Romania

Clinic of Diabetes, Nutrition and Metabolic Diseases, "Pius Brînzeu" Emergency Clinical County University Hospital, Timisoara, Romania
e-mail: bogdan.timar@umft.ro

A. Covic, A. Burlacu (eds.), *Renal Dysfunction in Cardiovascular Pathologies*,
https://doi.org/10.1007/978-3-032-25434-4_15

Nevertheless, not only aspects related to obesity, insulin resistance, dysglycemia, and dyslipidemia are included among the metabolic dysfunctions encountered in CRS, but also metabolic acidosis, hyperkalemia, and dysregulation of mineral and bone metabolism, all of which represent essential determinants of CV and renal mortality. This complex association begins with crosstalk between the heart and kidney, involving hemodynamic, neurohormonal, and inflammatory markers. The activation of the renin-angiotensin-aldosterone system (RAAS) and the sympathetic nervous system, two of the most important pathogenic mechanisms of this syndrome, which are usually triggered by a decrease in cardiac output, contribute to sodium and water retention, systemic vasoconstriction, and maladaptive cardiac remodeling. Consecutive renal hypoperfusion leads to deterioration of kidney function, decreased estimated glomerular filtration rate (eGFR), and accumulation of uremic toxins, metabolic acidosis, and electrolyte imbalance. All of these disturbances increase systemic inflammation and oxidative stress, which directly affect the myocardium, endothelium, and vascular system. The result is a vicious cardiorenal-metabolic cycle in which each component amplifies the other, creating a self-perpetuating cycle of morbidity [5, 6].

In more detail, the activation of the RAAS, alongside low-grade chronic inflammation and endothelial dysfunction, contributes to profound metabolic changes, from shifts in myocardial energetic metabolism to disruptions in calcium and phosphate homeostasis, which also explain the progressive and treatment-refractory characteristics of the CRS. Moreover, the accumulation of uremic toxins due to their inefficient excretion becomes more evident as eGFR decreases. The increased plasmatic concentration of waste products of catabolism, such as urea, creatinine, guanidine, or phenols, can have a cytotoxic effect and induce endothelial dysfunction, reduce nitric oxide activity, and also contribute to an increased systemic oxidative stress [2, 7].

Additionally, patients with CKD often associate insulin resistance with the previously mentioned systemic inflammation, uremic toxin accumulation, and altered muscle insulin signaling. The accompanying atherogenic dyslipidemia, characterized by increased levels of small, dense low-density lipoprotein (LDL) particles, hypertriglyceridemia, and decreased levels of high-density lipoprotein cholesterol (HDLc), further accelerates the development of atherosclerosis and coronary artery disease (CAD). The link between the kidney and the heart is also evident, as a decrease in eGFR contributes to sodium and water retention, leading to congestion, hypertension, and ventricular remodeling. The alteration of the clearance of various cardioprotective pharmacologic agents further complicates the management of these patients, showing, once again, the cyclicity of the process, with the decreased eGFR being both a consequence of heart failure (HF) and also a major key factor in a cascade of metabolic imbalances with negative effects on the heart [4, 8].

One of the most frequent and, yet, in some cases, life-threatening metabolic complications of the CRS is hyperkalemia, caused by the decrease of renal excretion of potassium associated with increases in this electrolyte in the context of administering guideline-directed medical therapy that usually includes RAAS inhibitors and mineralocorticoid receptor antagonists. The risk of hyperkalemia is further increased by an accentuated muscle catabolism, metabolic acidosis, and, in some patients, an inadequate diet, with severe cardiac effects such as the alteration of the resting potential of cardiomyocytes, conduction disorders, disruptions of the myocardial contractility, ventricular arrhythmias, and, in severe cases, cardiac arrest. To prevent these outcomes, the treatment with RAAS inhibitors and/or mineralocorticoid receptor antagonists is often stopped or limited, which further contributes, indirectly, to the progression of heart and renal failure [2, 9].

Another metabolic consequence of CRS is metabolic acidosis caused by the reduced renal excretion of hydrogen ions and reduced renal ammoniagenesis which further contribute to an accelerated catabolism of proteins, systemic inflammation and insulin resistance, while also stimulating calcium and phosphate release from bones and, thus, becoming not only a marker of kidney dysfunction, but also an active causal factor that impacts CV and renal health outcomes. The CKD-mineral and bone disorder (CKD-MBD) thus becomes another essential component of the metabolic dysfunction in CRS, in which decreased eGFR leads to phosphate retention, reduced renal synthesis of 1,25-dihydroxyvitamin D, and hypocalcemia. These changes stimulate parathyroid hormone (PTH) secretion, leading to secondary hyperparathyroidism, and also increase calcium release from bones, increasing their fragility [1, 2].

Another key factor in the pathogenesis of CKD-MBD is the increased level of fibroblast growth factor-23 (FGF23), a hormone produced by osteocytes that regulates phosphate homeostasis by increasing its excretion and suppressing vitamin D activation. These metabolic disturbances, along with vitamin D deficiency and the hypercalcemia observed in some advanced CKD cases, contribute to vascular calcification, arterial stiffness, left ventricular hypertrophy, and alterations in myocardial perfusion. As a result, CKD-MBD contributes to cardiac remodeling and has a negative impact on CV morbidity and mortality by amplifying the global CV, renal, and metabolic dysfunction [10, 11].

The vicious cycle of CRS is also aggravated by therapeutic limitations induced by metabolism, or, in other words, the context in which metabolic dysfunction restricts the possibility of administering guideline-directed medical therapy. At the same time, the lack of an optimal treatment itself accentuates the metabolic dysfunction and increases the severity of HF or CKD, with multiple consecutive exacerbations. Specifically, the presence of hyperkalemia and metabolic acidosis usually necessitates a reduction in, or even elimination of, pharmacologic agents that have proven pleiotropic beneficial effects in patients with CVD or CKD, such as RAAS inhibitors, angiotensin receptor-neprilysin inhibitors (ARNI), and nonsteroidal/steroidal mineralocorticoid receptor antagonists. Additionally, patients with a serum potassium level >5,5 mmol/L or an eGFR <30 mL/min/1,73m^2 are usually excluded from most clinical trials and, thus, are underrepresented and do not benefit from optimal cardio-renoprotective treatment. It is also known that chronic metabolic acidosis itself contributes to a reduced efficacy of diuretics and increases sodium retention. In order to correct these metabolic disturbances, various drugs are already or currently being introduced into clinical practice or are in development with promising results, such as potassium binders, alkalizing agents, and anti-FGF23 therapies [10, 12, 13].

With regard to the cardio-renal-metabolic vicious cycle, once it is started, the progression of the disease becomes self-sustained. Chronic metabolic dysfunctions such as hyperkalemia, metabolic acidosis, CKD-MBD, and, additionally, malnutrition, increase even more the oxidative stress, chronic systemic inflammation, and mitochondrial dysfunction, with subsequent fibrotic myocardial remodeling, reduction of cardiac contractility, and aggravation of heart and kidney failure, with dramatic effects on the myocardium and renal parenchyma. Furthermore, the reduction in cardiac output contributes to renal hypoperfusion and tubular ischemia, leading to a progressive loss of functional nephrons. In contrast, simultaneously, uremic toxins contribute to endothelial dysfunction and microangiopathy, further accentuating deterioration in kidney perfusion. The anemia, which is often encountered in patients with CKD, also contributes to the tissular hypoxia and to the myocardial oxidative stress, while the malnutrition-inflammation-cachexia syndrome (MICS), another complex consequence of chronic diseases such as CKD or HF, reduces the metabolic regenerative capacity and aggravates the previous metabolic imbalances [2, 14].

Understanding this interdependence between organs, in which the damage of one of them generates systemic metabolic disturbances which, in turn, affect, structurally and functionally, the other organ, and so on, has led to a change of paradigm: the main goal in treating these patients is not just to maintain the renal and cardiac function, but also to correct the metabolic dysfunction to break the vicious cycle.

Current research focuses on developing drugs which will help with the correction of metabolic dysfunction, while pharmacologic agents already in use include the sodium-glucose cotransporter-2 inhibitors (SGLT2i) which have redefined the treatment of CKM syndrome, alongside drugs such as patiromer or sodium zirconium cyclosilicate (for hyperkalemia), sodium bicarbonate (for metabolic acidosis) or FGF23 inhibitors, all of the above in the context of a personalized diet. Through early diagnosis, periodic monitoring of metabolic markers, and a multidisciplinary, individualized therapeutic approach, significant benefits in the prognosis of patients with CRS can be achieved, with reduced progression of CV and renal disease and lower cardiorenal mortality. The following subchapters will present, in detail, these components of the metabolic dysfunction in CRS, specifically, the glycemic control, metabolic acidosis, dyslipidemia, CKD-MBD, and personalized therapeutic approach [2, 4, 15].

15.2 Glycemic Control in Cardio-Renal Syndrome

The assessment of glycemic control in patients with CRS requires a careful and differentiated approach, considering the pathophysiological complexity generated by the simultaneous dysfunction of the CV system and renal function. In this context, glycemic monitoring strategies must be tailored to each patient, taking into account the severity of the condition, associated comorbidities, and individual response to treatment. Therefore, therapeutic interventions must be individualized, taking into account the patient's metabolic profile, the medications used, and the potential pathological interactions between diabetes treatments and those for cardiac or renal pathologies.

In clinical practice, short-term glycemic control is most often assessed with a glucometer, which measures fasting or 2-h postprandial glycemia, enabling immediate adjustment of antidiabetic treatment and detection of hypoglycemia [16]. However, this method does not capture glycemic variability or detect nocturnal or asymptomatic hypoglycemia. The main method for assessing long-term glycemic control is measuring glycated hemoglobin A1c (HbA1c). HbA1c reflects the percentage of glucose that binds irreversibly to hemoglobin, and both median blood glucose levels and the duration of exposure to hyperglycemia influence its level. Therefore, HbA1c estimates the average glycemic level over the past 2–3 months. Although this method represents the gold standard for the long-term assessment of glycemic control in diabetes mellitus, the accuracy of this marker decreases significantly in patients with advanced CKD associated with diabetes, especially in those with secondary anemia, those receiving erythropoietin treatment, or those with reduced red blood cell turnover. In such situations, HbA1c values tend to be overestimated or underestimated compared to the patient's actual average blood glucose level. For this reason, guidelines recommend the use of complementary markers, such as fructosamine or glycated albumin, which can provide additional information on glycemic control. However, it is important to remember that these biomarkers can also be influenced by protein status, and hypoalbuminemia can introduce additional interpretational errors [17].

Albumin glycation is a non-enzymatic, continuous process that is directly dependent on the average blood glucose concentration, and changes in this marker quickly follow any fluctuations in blood glucose levels. Glycated albumin reflects the average blood glucose over a relatively short term (2–3 weeks), since the life span of plasma albumin is about 14–21 days [18]. Unlike HbA1c, glycated albumin values are not influenced by red blood cell lifespan, anemia, erythropoietin treatments, hemolytic states, or hemoglobin variants. Thus, it is extremely useful in patients with advanced chronic renal failure, dialysis patients, pregnant women, or those with anemia, where HbA1c may be inaccurate [18, 19].

The amount of glycated albumin largely determines the fructosamine level. Normal fructosamine values are between 200 and 285 μmol/L when serum albumin is approximately 5 g/dL. A decrease in serum albumin lowers fructosamine levels, and its interpretation becomes uncertain when serum albumin falls below 3.0 g/dL, as seen in conditions such as liver cirrhosis or nephrotic syndrome. For this reason, some guidelines or experts prefer glycated albumin as a marker, as it is considered more specific and of additional utility in monitoring patients with advanced CKD [20]. At the same time, studies have shown that glycated albumin is closely correlated with the risk of microvascular complications (retinopathy, diabetic nephropathy) [18, 19, 21]. Fructosamine dosing is recommended in the presence of anemia, hemoglobinopathies, erythropoietin treatment, or in any situation with altered red blood cell turnover, when glycemic monitoring by HbA1c is not reliable [22, 23].

Continuous glucose monitoring (CGM) technology has gained increasing interest in this population. CGM provides detailed information, such as the percentage of "time in range" (TIR, time spent with blood glucose between 70 and 180 mg/dl), glycemic variability (GV), or the percentage of time spent in hypoglycemia (TBR) or hyperglycemia (TAR), aspects that are difficult to access through classic monitoring [24].

The use of CGM metrics (TIR, TBR, GV) has been validated in patients with CRS to reduce the risk of arrhythmias, hospitalizations, and hypoglycemia [24, 25]. The Glucose Management Indicator (GMI) is a complementary marker derived from the average of blood glucose values recorded by CGM systems, converted into an HbA1c equivalent to facilitate the assessment of glycemic control, especially in patients in whom HbA1c is not relevant (e.g., emia, erythropoietin treatment, advanced renal failure) [24].

GMI provides an estimate of HbA1c and is calculated based on the average CGM blood glucose over the last 14–28 days, using the formula: GMI $(\%) = 3.31 + 0.02392 \times$ average blood glucose (mg/dL) [26]. Unlike HbA1c, which is sensitive to red blood cell turnover and hematological factors, GMI reflects only the most recent blood glucose values measured by CGM. In studies involving CRS, GMI correlated with TIR and successfully detected the risk of hyperglycemia or hypoglycemia. However, GMI cannot replace clinical assessment or other CGM parameters, but it is useful when HbA1c has limitations. The American Diabetes Association (ADA) [16] şi Kidney Disease Improving Global Outcomes (KDIGO) [27] Guidelines support the use of GMI as an alternative/complementary parameter to HbA1c in cardiorenal syndrome, together with other CGM metrics (TIR, GV) [24, 28].

In patients with reduced renal function or on renal replacement therapy, CGM accuracy may be affected in extreme situations (hypoglycemia or hyperglycemia), where the observed deviations may exceed the reference capillary glucose values by 10–20% [29, 30]. It is also important to note the physiological delay of 10–20 min between plasma glucose and interstitial glucose measured by the sensor. This lag may be accentuated in patients with low tissue perfusion, hypotension, or edema, which are common among those undergoing dialysis and those with HF [30]. CGM sensors may overestimate or underestimate blood glucose during and immediately after hemodialysis due to sudden changes in blood glucose concentrations and fluid volume. There have been reports of post-dialysis blood glucose "nadirs" that are not fully captured by CGM [24].

Thus, current guidelines recommend a target TIR of >70% in young adults and > 65% in elderly, frail patients or those at high risk of hypoglycemia. HbA1c targets should also be individualized: in the elderly with frailty or those with HF or dialysis, more permissive values (7.5–8%) are acceptable [24]. The use of CGM in patients with HF or advanced CKD offers a decisive advantage in identifying silent hypoglycemia, reducing GV, and optimally adjusting therapy. Severe hypoglycemia increases the risk of arrhythmias and repeated hospitalizations, and metrics such as TBR, TIR, and day-to-day variability help minimize these risks [30].

As shown in Table 15.1 below, the therapeutic targets for glycemic control in patients with CRS are based exclusively on data from the ADA [16, 25], KDIGO [27], and the Renal Association [31] Guidelines. These therapeutic targets need to be adjusted to each patient's specific characteristics (age, comorbidities, risk of hypoglycemia, dialysis status, and frailty).

These therapeutic targets in patients with diabetes and cardiorenal syndrome are addressed by a modern treatment designed for long-term protection of cardiac and renal function, optimizing benefits and minimizing specific risks. At the same time, early and staged association of renin-angiotensin system inhibitors (angiotensin-converting enzyme inhibitors (ACEIs) or angiotensin II receptor antagonists (ARBs)), angiotensin receptor-prilysin inhibitors (ARNIs), mineralocorticoid receptor antagonists (MRAs), and diuretics is recommended [34]. Careful monitoring of volume status and potassium levels is mandatory to prevent hyperkalemia, acute renal failure, or HF decompensation. Adjustment of diuretics and MRA is based on clinical and biological reassessments to optimize hemodynamic and metabolic balance [2].

Table 15.1 Therapeutic targets for glycemic control in people with diabetes and CRS

Parameter	Timing	General therapeutic target	Therapeutic targets in advanced CRM
Fasting glycemia [16]	Daily	80–130 mg/dl (4.4–7.2 mmol/L)	90–150 mg/dl (5.0–8.3 mmol/L)
2-h postprandial glycemia [16]	Daily	<180 mg/dl (<10.0 mmol/L)	<200 mg/dl (≤11.1 mmol/L)
HbA1c [16]	Glycemic control over the last 2–3 months	<7.0% (53 mmol/mol)	<7.5–8.0% (58–64 mmol/mol) (29)
Fructosamine [22]	Glycemic control over the last 2–3 weeks	200–285 µmol/L (equivalent with HbA1c <7%)	<350 µmol/L
Glycated albumin [19, 32, 33]	Glycemic control over the last 2–3 weeks	<13–16%	<20%
TIR [16]	Daily	>70% between 70–180 mg/dl;	>65% between 70–180 mg/dl
TBR [16]	Daily	<4% below 70 mg/dl; <1% below 54 mg/dl	<5% below 70 mg/dl
TAR [16]	Daily	<25% above 180 mg/dl <5% above 250 mg/dl	<30%
GV [16]	Daily	<36%	Individualized
GMI [16]	Daily	<7.0% (53 mmol/mol)	<7.5–8%

Abbreviations: *HbA1c* glycated hemoglobin, *TIR* time in range. *TBR* time below range, *TAR* time above range, *GV* glycemic variability, *GMI* glucose management indicator, *CRM* cardio-reno-metabolic syndrome

SGLT2 inhibitors (e.g., dapagliflozin, empagliflozin, canagliflozin) represent the mainstay of therapy for cardiac and renal protection, with indications including patients with and without diabetes, across the entire spectrum of estimated glomerular filtration rate (eGFR), starting at 20 mL/min/1.73 m^2 [35]. Clinical trials (EMPA-REG-OUTCOME [36], CREDENCE [24], DAPA-CKD [25], EMPA-KIDNEY [24]) and recent real-world data confirm reductions in the risks of progression of renal disease, HF, and major CV events, independent of glycemic control. It acts by inhibiting SGLT2 in the renal proximal tubule, thereby reducing glucose and sodium reabsorption. This induces glycosuria and natriuresis, with an osmotic diuretic effect, resulting in decreased intravascular volume, reduced intraglomerular pressure, and albuminuria. It also improves cardiac remodeling and reduces oxidative stress, inflammation, and fibrosis. The result is a slowdown in the progression of renal disease, a reduction in hospitalizations for HF, and a decrease in CV mortality, independent of glycemic control [37]. However, SGLT2i should be temporarily stopped in cases of dehydration, severe infections, perioperatively, or reduced fluid intake, to reduce the risk of euglycemic ketoacidosis or volume decompensation [38].

GLP-1 receptor agonists (GLP-1 RAs), such as semaglutide, dulaglutide, and liraglutide, and dual agents, such as tirzepatide, are associated with weight loss, improved glycemic control, reduced risk of atherosclerotic CV events (ASCVD), and, according to recent meta-analyses, significantly reduce progression to end-stage renal disease and major renal events [39]. GLP-1 RAs and duals can be used in patients with advanced CKD, with some molecules approved up to dialysis. Because gastrointestinal adverse effects (nausea, vomiting) are common, slow titration is preferred. This may be problematic in patients with fragile nutritional status; discontinuation of treatment due to these is more common than with a placebo in major trials [40]. GLP-1 RAs act by mimicking incretins, causing increased glucose-dependent insulin secretion, decreased glucagon secretion, delayed gastric emptying, and reduced appetite. These effects lead to decreased body mass, reduced inflammation, improved metabolic parameters, decreased incidence of ASCVD events, and slowed progression of nephropathy (by reducing proteinuria, inflammation, and oxidative stress at the renal level) [41].

Insulin is the mainstay option in patients with diabetes and severe CKD, especially those on dialysis and with advanced HF [34]. It promotes effective glycemic control in patients with absolute or relative insulin deficiency, prevents protein catabolism and the development of ketoacidosis, but has no direct CV or renal organ protective effects. Careful monitoring prevents hypoglycemia, which may increase the risk of arrhythmia and adverse CV events in this population. As renal clearance decreases, insulin requirements decrease due to the risk of hypoglycemia, especially on dialysis days. Reducing or suspending the rapid/bolus insulin dose during dialysis is recommended [42]. In frail patients, the "basal plus" regimen (adding a single bolus to the basal insulin dose) is preferred over the classic basal-bolus regimen.

Dipeptidyl peptidase-4 (DPP-4) inhibitors (sitagliptin, vildagliptin, linagliptin) have a neutral CV profile and a low risk of hypoglycemia, making them safe to use in patients with CKD. They act by inhibiting the degradation of incretins, thereby increasing glucose-dependent insulin secretion and reducing glucagon secretion. The dose should be adjusted according to GFR, except for linagliptin, which does not require adjustment [34].

Metformin remains a basic therapeutic option in type 2 diabetes, but its use is strictly dependent on renal function. Administration is allowed only in patients with GFR $\geq$30 mL/min/1.73 m^2. In the range of 30–45 mL/min/1.73 m^2, dose reduction and periodic renal function assessment are recommended. Below the GFR threshold of 30 mL/min/1.73 m^2, the treatment must be discontinued due to the significant risk of lactic acidosis [42].

Sulfonylureas stimulate insulin secretion, but in patients with advanced CKD, they cause a major risk of hypoglycemia, which is why their use is generally discouraged. In addition, these drugs do not offer proven organ-protective benefits and are not recommended in the setting of cardiorenal syndrome [38]. Thiazolidinediones (TZDs), such as pioglitazone, are insulin-sensitizing agents that reduce hepatic glucose production and increase peripheral glucose utilization. Although they may improve insulin resistance and have favorable metabolic effects, their use is limited by the risk of fluid retention and worsening of HF; therefore, they are contraindicated or used with great caution in these patients. In the context of CKD, TZDs have not demonstrated organ-protective benefits [34].

15.3 Metabolic Acidosis in Cardiorenal Syndrome

15.3.1 Mechanisms [43, 44]

Metabolic acidosis in CKD occurs when the kidney is unable to excrete the daily acid load (endogenous and exogenous). Various factors contribute to this:

- Reduction in the excretion of NH_4^+
- Reduction in the excretion of H^+
- Accumulation of uremic toxins
- Reduction in the production of HCO_3^-

Furthermore, accumulation of lactate due to cardiogenic shock or through the accumulation of metformin in diabetic patients can exacerbate metabolic acidosis [45, 46].

In the case of patients with diabetes mellitus, another cause of metabolic acidosis could be an acute metabolic complication, such as diabetic ketoacidosis. This can occur in patients with type 1 diabetes who are either untreated or have taken their insulin treatment improperly. Another situation is the case of patients with diabetes (either type 1 or type 2) who are suffering from an acute condition that generates severe insulin resistance, such as acute pancreatitis, myocardial infarction, stroke, etc. The absolute or relative lack of insulin promotes the use of fatty acids for energy when glucose is unavailable, thereby leading to ketone production. In most cases, metabolic acidosis is associated with hyperpotassemia, as H+ and K+ ions are exchanged to maintain acid-base balance. Diabetic ketoacidosis provides a unique medical challenge as it can present high, normal, or low levels of serum potassium. After the exchange of H+ and K+ ions, the unique situation created by high blood glucose and consequent glycosuria promotes volume depletion, leading to a reduction in total body potassium [47].

Due to severe dehydration, patients with diabetic ketoacidosis may also experience acute kidney injury that further aggravates the metabolic acidosis by reducing renal excretion of ketones and impairing HCO_3^- regeneration, significantly impacting recovery [47, 48].

Emphasis should be placed on patients with type 2 diabetes utilizing SGLT2i. By eliminating glucose through the urine, SGLT2i alter the insulin-to-glucagon ratio, promoting lipolysis and secondary ketone production. This not only increases the likelihood of diabetic ketoacidosis but also makes diagnosis more difficult, as it generates a particular form of euglycemic diabetic ketoacidosis, as excess glucose is eliminated through the urine [49].

15.3.2 Consequences of Metabolic Acidosis [50–57]

Muscle metabolism suffers under acidotic conditions. The higher intracellular H+ concentration competes with Ca2+, which is needed for muscle fiber contraction· reducing physical output in both skeletal and cardiac muscles. Acidotic conditions also interfere with mitochondrial bioenergetics, reducing muscle ATP and phosphocreatine resynthesis, generating fatigue, and inhibiting protein synthesis.

Acidotic conditions alter hemoglobin's structure, reducing its oxygen affinity and promoting hypoxia, thereby generating or aggravating lactic acidosis.

Moreover, muscle turnover is increased as catabolism is favored over synthesis, leading to muscle wasting, reducing muscle contraction force, and further increasing fatigue.

Metabolic acidosis also contributes to mineral-bone disease associated with CKD. Excess H^+ also penetrates the bone matrix, altering its structure, releasing Ca^{2+}, and buffering H^+ at the expense of bone demineralization, increasing the risk of renal lithiasis and fractures.

There is a complex interplay between inflammation and acidosis. While it is known that inflammation can cause acidosis by generating tissue hypoxia through local damage to small blood vessels, with secondary lactic acid accumulation, and by producing other acidic byproducts from immune cells and bacteria. Acidotic conditions can increase inflammation by activating the inflammasome via monocytes and macrophages, increasing IL-1β production. This proinflammatory state impairs insulin signaling.

Changes in insulin receptor structure under acidic conditions limit insulin binding, thereby promoting insulin resistance. Insulin production and release from pancreatic β cells are highly dependent on ATP production. Furthermore, the insulin receptor is a tyrosine kinase receptor that requires ATP to function. Mitochondrial dysfunction, present in both CKD and HF, is further aggravated by metabolic acidosis, which increases insulin resistance by limiting ATP production.

Increased insulin resistance will worsen metabolic control of diabetes mellitus and affect both the kidney and the heart in the long term.

This plethora of modifications leads to the worsening of CKD and aggravating HF, creating a vicious cycle of disease progression for both pathologies.

15.3.3 Workup [58–62]

Blood gas analysis is mandatory in evaluating acid-base disorders. A practical approach to this would be as follows:

- Establishing the type of acid-base disorder:
  - pH < 7,35—acidosis
  - pH > 7,45—alkalosis
- Differentiating between the main causes of acid-base disorders. If the pH and $[HCO_3^-]$ change in the same direction, the main cause is metabolic. If the pH and $[HCO_3^-]$ change in the opposite direction, the main cause is respiratory
- Establishing if the disorder is compensated for or not:
  - Primary decrease of $[HCO_3^-]$ < 22 mmol/L and pH < 7,35: metabolic acidosis
    - Normal $PaCO_2$—uncompensated
    - Decreased $PaCO_2$, with decreased pH—partial compensation
    - Decreased $PaCO_2$, with normal pH—total compensation
  - Primary increase of $[HCO_3^-]$ > 26 mmol/L and pH > 7,45: metabolic alkalosis
    - Normal $PaCO_2$—uncompensated
    - Increased $PaCO_2$, with increased pH—partial compensation
    - Increased $PaCO_2$, with normal pH—total compensation
  - Primary increase of $PaCO_2$ > 45 mmHg and pH < 7,35: respiratory acidosis
    - Normal $[HCO_3^-]$—uncompensated
    - Increased $[HCO_3^-]$, with decreased pH—partial compensation
    - Increased $[HCO_3^-]$, with normal pH—total compensation
  - Primary decrease of $PaCO_2$ < 35 mmHg and pH > 7,45: respiratory alkalosis
    - Normal $[HCO_3^-]$—uncompensated
    - Decreased $[HCO_3^-]$, with increased pH—partial compensation
    - Decreased $[HCO_3^-]$, with normal pH—total compensation
- In cases in which $PaCO_2$ and $[HCO_3^-]$ change in opposite directions and the pH presents extreme deviations, the patient presents a mixed disorder

  - Mixed acidosis—an association of metabolic and respiratory acidosis with an extremely low pH
  - Mixed alkalosis—an association of metabolic and respiratory alkalosis with an extremely high pH

- In the case of metabolic acidosis, evaluating the anionic gap is mandatory
  $AG = [Na^+ + K^+] - [Cl^- + HCO_3^-]$ (normal values = 12–16 mmol/L)
- While common in CKD due to the accumulation of phosphates and sulphates, high anionic gap metabolic acidosis can also be caused by:
  - Increases in ketones
    - Diabetic ketoacidosis
    - Alcoholic ketosis
    - Starvation ketosis
  - Increases in glycol
  - Increases in methanol
  - Increases in lactate
  - Increases in salicylates

- Normal anionic gap metabolic acidosis occurs when the decrease in $[HCO_3^-]$ is compensated by an increase in $[Cl^-]$ and requires calculating the urine anion gap as an indirect measure of renal ammonia excretion
  when urine pH is <6.5 – UAG = Urine Na^++ Urine K^+ – Urine Cl^-
  when urine pH is >6.5 – UAG = Urine Na^+ + Urine K^+ - (Urine Cl^- + Urine HCO_3^-)
  - Negative UAG—indicates increased renal ammonia excretion, suggesting a normal kidney response to the acidosis
  - Positive UAG—indicates impaired renal ammonia excretion, suggesting renal tubular acidosis
  - Type 1
    - Occurs due to the decrease in H^+ in the distal renal tubules
    - Frequently associated with hypokalemia
    - Urinary pH > 5,3
    - Associates high urine calcium output with a risk of nephrocalcinosis
  - Type 2
    - Occurs due to the decrease in $HCO3^-$ reabsorption in the proximal renal tubules
    - Frequently associated with hypokalemia
    - Urinary pH < 5,3
    - Frequently found with Fanconi syndrome
  - Type 3 is a rare form of disease that associates both defects described in Type 1 and Type 2
  - Type 4
    - Occurs due to hypoaldosteronism or aldosterone resistance

  - Frequently associated with hyperkalemia
  - Urinary pH < 5,3
  - Typically found in elderly persons with diabetes mellitus with mild to moderate renal impairment

- Possible confounders of the blood workup
  - Arterial and venous blood samples should both be used to measure $HCO3^-$ values, and if the two values vary by more than 2 mmol/l, the use of heparin is required in arterial blood sample analysis in the blood gas measurement, which may dilute the sample
  - Hypoalbuminemia can influence the anionic gap, as albumin has a negative charge. In cases of lower albumin levels, the anionic gap may appear less severe. The corrected Anion Gap can be calculated with the following formula:

$$\text{measured AG} + \left[0.25\,\text{X}\left(\text{normal albumin} - \text{measured albumin}\right)\right]$$

15.3.4 Treatment [47, 53, 61, 63–68]

The main objectives are correcting the fluid and electrolyte imbalances and removing the cause of the acidosis.

- Using crystalloid isotonic solutions such as NaCl 0,9% is preferred.
- Care should be taken when restoring the fluid balance so as not to aggravate HF in the patient. Fluid intake and output should be closely monitored.
- Oxygen therapy should be considered in cases of lactic acidosis, acute HF, or respiratory failure:
- Hyperkalemia can be addressed with insulin (activates Na^+/K^+ ATPase) and glucose solutions (to allow the use of insulin without the risk of hypoglycemia).
- $NaHCO_3$ can be administered using the following dosage: $(24\text{-}[HCO_3^-]_{current}) \times$ weight (in kg) $\times$ 0,5 (for $NaHCO_3$ 8,4% solution—1 ml = 1 mmol).
- The use or cessation of diuretics should be decided depending on the state of hydration, serum K^+ values, and the cause of the acidosis.
- Insulin should be administered in case of diabetic ketoacidosis.
- Fomepizole (alcohol dehydrogenase inhibitor) should be used in cases of methanol or ethylene glycol poisoning. As an alternative, if fomepizole is not available, the use of alcohol could be considered, as it has a higher affinity for alcohol dehydrogenase.
- Hemodialysis should be considered if appropriate to eliminate the main toxic factor causing metabolic acidosis.
- Ultrafiltration could be used to prevent hypoperfusion when removing excess volume, thereby avoiding increasing lactate concentrations and aggravating acidosis.

- Dietary considerations:
  - Restrict Na^+ intake to 1500–2000 mg/day.
  - Avoid consuming more than 1,3 g/kg/day of protein.
  - Choose complete, lean protein sources. Red meat should be avoided.
  - Choose a healthy source of mono- and polyunsaturated fats.
  - Avoid simple carbohydrates (especially if the patient has diabetes mellitus).
  - Avoid phosphorus additives and limit phosphorus intake.
- Currently under development, Veverimer is a polymer that removes HCl from the digestive system, providing a treatment for acidosis that raises serum bicarbonate without a sodium load.

15.4 Dyslipidemia in Cardio-Reno-Metabolic Syndrome

Dyslipidemia in patients with CKD is characterized by increased triglycerides (TG) and very low density lipoproteins (VLDL and remnant), decreased HDLc, with the appearance of HDL dysfunction (loss of CV protective effect), and the appearance of small and dense LDLc particles, proatherogenic, and increased lipoprotein (a) (Lp(a)), another proatherogenic marker, which progressively accumulates with the decline of renal function [69–71].

The relationship between CKD and hypertriglyceridemia is bidirectional, generating a pathophysiological "vicious circle" in which each condition worsens the other [70]. In CKD, significant alterations in lipid metabolism occur: the activity of lipoprotein lipase and hepatic lipase decreases, which reduces the degradation of chylomicrons and VLDL [72], increased hepatic production of VLDL, stimulated by CKD-specific insulin resistance [73], as well as inhibition of VLDL remnant clearance by increasing cholesteryl ester transfer protein (CETP) and reducing apolipoprotein C-II (apoC-II) activity, worsening hypertriglyceridemia, and favoring the appearance of small, dense LDL particles. Chronic inflammation, oxidative stress, and accumulation of uremic toxins alter lipoprotein composition and function [70].

On the other hand, hypertriglyceridemia also worsens CKD. Lipid accumulation in the kidney triggers inflammation, oxidative stress, and fibrogenesis, which progresses to glomerulosclerosis, microalbuminuria, and accelerated decline in GFR. TG and VLDL remnants increase the risk of atherosclerosis in the renal microcirculation, worsening ischemia and renal function. Changes in HDL and LDL composition reduce renal antioxidant and anti-inflammatory potential. Most of the time, CKD initiates lipid metabolism dysregulation; however, pre-existing hypertriglyceridemia (e.g., obesity, diabetes, metabolic syndrome) accelerates the progression of kidney disease, resulting in a self-perpetuating relationship between the two pathologies. In advanced stages, this vicious circle becomes difficult to break, requiring active therapeutic intervention on both mechanisms [70].

The risk of CV events in patients with CKD increases exponentially with decreasing eGFR. Even after achieving LDLc targets with intensive therapies (statins ± Ezetimibe), a significant "residual risk" remains, explained by the persistence of hypertriglyceridemia, HDL dysfunction, and the accumulation of small and dense LDLc particles, as well as CKD-specific proinflammatory and procoagulant factors [71, 74]. CV risk stratification in patients with CKD [75, 76] should be performed using dedicated calculators that include eGFR and albuminuria (SCORE2 CKD Add-on [77], u-prevent [78], PREVENT [79]) for relevant predictions and optimal adaptation of interventions. Recent meta-analyses, confirmed by professional guidelines such as the ESC [80]/ADA [25], have shown that CKD stage ≥3b or severe albuminuria increases the relative risk by 2–3 times compared to the general population, justifying the preventive intensification and aggressive use of CV therapies.

Each therapeutic class used for dyslipidemia in patients with cardiorenometabolic syndrome (CKD, HF) has specific indications, benefits, and limitations, according to the most recent guidelines and large clinical trials. In Table 15.2, we detail the main therapeutic classes used in dyslipidemia associated with cardiorenometabolic syndrome, including their mechanism of action, dose adjustments based on eGFR, target lipids, notable studies, and relevant adverse effects in this context.

Statins are the therapy of choice for reducing LDLc and CV risk in all stages of pre-dialysis CKD, with strong evidence for reducing mortality, the risk of infarction, and stroke. They act by inhibiting the enzyme HMG-CoA reductase, thereby reducing hepatic cholesterol synthesis, increasing the number of LDL receptors in the liver, enhancing LDL clearance from plasma, lowering LDLc levels, and exhibiting anti-inflammatory and atherosclerotic plaque-stabilizing effects. Studies show efficacy and safety in CKD up to advanced stages, even in hemodialysis patients. However, the clinical benefit decreases in dialysis [98]. Statins are also effective in HF with reduced ejection fraction, especially in patients with atherosclerotic risk [99]. Atorvastatin can be used at usual doses (10–80 mg) regardless of GFR, including in dialysis patients, without requiring major dose adjustments; however, adverse reactions are closely monitored.

In contrast, Rosuvastatin requires a dose reduction to 5–10 mg/day when GFR <30 ml/min/1.73 m^2, avoiding high doses in advanced renal failure to prevent accumulation and the risk of myopathy. Possible adverse effects include rhabdomyolysis, myositis, hepatotoxicity, and, very rarely, worsening renal function in advanced CKD. Data from the SHARP study [83] showed that statin use in dialysis patients is not consistently beneficial, and initiation is not routinely recommended; however, continuation is possible if they were already part of the therapeutic regimen.

By blocking intestinal cholesterol absorption, Ezetimibe lowers LDLc in combination with statins. The SHARP study [83] has shown that Ezetimibe reduces the risk of CV events in advanced CKD, including dialysis, with a very good safety profile. It does not require adjustment based on GFR and is well tolerated, except for the rare risk of liver dysfunction.

PCSK9 inhibitors (alirocumab, evolocumab) reduce the degradation of the hepatic LDL receptor, increasing the number of active receptors on the surface of

Table 15.2 Particularities of therapeutic interventions in dyslipidemia associated with cardiorenal syndrome

Therapeutic class	Mechanism of action	Dose adjustments (eGFR/ml/min)	Targeted lipids	Clinical trials	Adverse effects
Statins (atorvastatin, rosuvastatin)	Inhibits HMG-CoA reductase, ↑ LDLc clearance	Atorvastatin: 10–80 mg/day at any stage of CKD; Rosuvastatin: max 10 mg/day at GFR < 30 ml/min, start with 5 mg	↓ LDLc, ↓ TG, ↑ HDLc	4D [81], TNT [82], SHARP [83], JUPITER [84]	Rhabdomyolysis, myopathy, hepatotoxicity, very rarely renal injury or de novo diabetes
Ezetimibe	Inhibits intestinal absorption of cholesterol	No adjustment until dialysis	↓ LDLc	SHARP [83], IMPROVE-IT [85]	Rare liver dysfunctions
PCSK9i	Inhibits hepatic LDL receptor degradation	No restrictions based on GFR, but not administered during dialysis	↓ LDLc, ↓ Lp(a)	FOURIER [86], ODYSSEY [87], SHARP [83]	Injection site reactions, flu-like symptoms
Inclisiran	Interfering RNA, ↓ synthesis of PCSK9	No dose adjustment is necessary for renal disease, but caution is recommended in severe renal impairment or dialysis due to limited experience	↓ LDLc, ↓ Lp(a)	ORION [88]	Mild local reactions
Bempedoic acid	Inhibits ACL, ↓ hepatic cholesterol synthesis	No adjustment for moderate CKD	↓ LDLc	CLEAR Outcomes [89], Harmony [90]	Hyperuricemia/gout, increased transaminases, muscle pain
Fibrate (fenofibrate)	PPARα agonist, ↑ fatty acid oxidation	GFR between 30–59 ml/min/1.73 m^2: maximum 100 mg fenofibrate; GFR < 30 ml/min/1.73 m^2: discontinue	↓ TG, ↑ HDLc, ↓ LDLc	FIELD [91], ACCORD Lipid [92]	Rhabdomyolysis (especially in combination with statins), renal failure, hyperkalemia
Omega-3 (icosapent ethyl)	↓ hepatic TG synthesis, anti-inflammatory role	No restrictions for moderate CKD, caution in dialysis	↓ TG, ↓ LDLc	REDUCE-IT [93], EVOLVE [94]	Bleeding (increased risk in combination with anticoagulants), rare arrhythmias, edema

Bile acid sequestrants	Binds intestinal bile acids	Do not administer if TG > 300 mg/dL, or on dialysis	↓ LDLc, ↑ HDLc, ↑/→ TG	Lipid Research Clinics [95]	Increased TG, constipation, impaired absorption of fat-soluble vitamins
Niacin	↓ hepatic synthesis of VLDL and LDL	Avoided in advanced CKD	↓ LDLc, ↓ TG, ↑ HDLc	AIM-HIGH [96], HPS2-THRIVE [97]	Flushing, hepatotoxicity, increased blood sugar, and uric acid levels

Abbreviations: *4D Study* Die Deutsche Diabetes Dialyse Studie, *TNT Study* Treating to New Targets, *SHARP Study* Study of Heart and Renal Protection, *JUPITER Trial* Justification for the Use of Statins in Prevention: an Intervention Trial Evaluating Rosuvastatin, *IMPROVE-IT* IMproved Reduction of Outcomes: Vytorin Efficacy International Trial, *FOURIER Trial* Further Cardiovascular Outcomes Research with PCSK9 Inhibition in Subjects with Elevated Risk, *ODYSSEY OUTCOMES Trial* Evaluation of Cardiovascular Outcomes after an Acute Coronary Syndrome during Treatment with Alirocumab, *CLEAR* Cholesterol Lowering via Bempedoic Acid, an ACL-Inhibiting Regimen, *FIELD* Fenofibrate Intervention and Event Lowering in Diabetes, *ACCORD Lipid* Action to Control Cardiovascular Risk in Diabetes Lipid arm, *REDUCE-IT* Reduction of Cardiovascular Events With Icosapent Ethyl–Intervention Trial, *EVOLVE* EpanoVa fOr Lowering Very high triglycerideEs, *AIM-HIGH* Atherothrombosis Intervention in Metabolic Syndrome with Low HDL/High Triglycerides: Impact on Global Health Outcomes, *HPS2-THRIVE* Heart Protection Study 2–Treatment of HDL to Reduce the Incidence of Vascular Events, *RNA* Ribonucleic Acid, *CKD* Chronic Kidney Disease, *eGFR* estimated glomerular filtration rate, HMG-CoA: 3-hydroxy-3-methylglutaryl coenzyme A, *VLDL* very low-density lipoprotein, *HDLc* high-density lipoprotein cholesterol, *TG* triglycerides, *Lp(a)* lipoprotein (a), *LDLc* low density lipoprotein cholesterol, *PCSK9i* Subtilisin/kexin type 9 proprotein convertase inhibitors, *ACL* adenosine triphosphate-citrate lyase, *PPARα* Peroxisome Proliferator-Activated Receptor alpha hepatocytes; thus, LDL clearance from plasma is accelerated, and LDLc decreases by 50–60%, also reducing Lp(a). Inclisiran is an interfering RNA that inhibits hepatic PCSK9 synthesis, with effects on LDL receptors and LDLc reduction similar to those of PCSK9 inhibitors. They are useful in very high-risk patients or those who do not reach the target with statins and Ezetimibe. FOURIER [86], ODYSSEY [49], and ORION [88] studies have shown efficacy and reductions in CV events, including in moderate-severe CKD. This therapeutic class does not require dose adjustment until GFR < 30 ml/min; however, data in patients on dialysis are limited, so initiation in patients newly enrolled in renal replacement programs is not recommended. Adverse effects are rare and clinically insignificant, such as local injection reactions, flu-like symptoms, and do not present an increased risk of rhabdomyolysis or renal toxicity.

Bempedoic acid reduces LDLc by inhibiting the enzyme ATP-citrate lyase (ACL) in the hepatic cholesterol synthesis pathway. It is indicated especially in patients with intolerance to statins or in combination with them, and in those with very high CV risk. CLEAR Outcomes [89] and Harmony [90] studies have demonstrated efficacy, including in moderate CKD, without exacerbation of proteinuria or further loss of renal function. They do not require adjustment in moderate CKD, but are administered with caution in advanced CKD. They may cause relevant adverse reactions, including hyperuricemia and gout, as well as increased transaminases.

Fibrates (fenofibrates) are peroxisome proliferator-activated receptor alpha (PPARα) agonists that stimulate fatty acid oxidation and VLDL/TG clearance, increasing HDL and substantially lowering TG. Fibrates are indicated in patients with persistent hypertriglyceridemia or residual CV risk. The benefit of CKD progression is controversial, but the occurrence of rhabdomyolysis when combined with statins is worth considering. The dose must be reduced in patients with an eGFR <60 ml/min. It is contraindicated in those with eGFR <30 ml/min due to the risk of renal accumulation/toxicity, rhabdomyolysis, increased creatinine, and hyperkalemia [100].

Omega-3 polyunsaturated fatty acids (icosapent ethyl, EPA) lower TG and reduce the risk of major CV events in mixed dyslipidemia, according to REDUCE-IT [93] and EVOLVE [94] studies. They are well tolerated in patients with moderate CKD and have anti-inflammatory benefits. They do not require adjustment in moderate CKD, but are administered with caution in those on dialysis. When combined with anticoagulants/antiplatelet agents, they slightly increase the risk of bleeding. Peripheral edema or gastrointestinal disorders have also been described as rare adverse effects.

Bile acid sequestrants lower LDLc and raise HDLc and are useful when other options are contraindicated. They can be used in the early stages of CKD in patients with pure hypercholesterolemia, but are not recommended when TG exceeds 300 mg/dL or in those on dialysis, as they may increase even more the TG and the risk of severe constipation, vitamin malabsorption, or may worsen metabolic balance [95]. Niacin lowers LDLc and TG, and increases HDLc. Usefulness in CKD is minimal, and recent studies show no benefit on CV risk in patients with CKD or HF [97].

15.5 Alterations of the Mineral Metabolism. Metabolic Bone Disease in CKD

15.5.1 Mechanisms

One of the key components of the CRS is the CKD—mineral and bone disorder (CKD-MBD), characterized by phosphate retention, a reduction in the renal synthesis of 1,25-dihydroxyvitamin D and hypocalcemia, which stimulates the PTH secretion, with secondary hyperparathyroidism, and also contributes to the release of calcium from bones, increasing their fragility. CKD leads to early disturbances in phosphate and calcium homeostasis, which progress alongside a decrease in the estimated glomerular filtration rate (eGFR) and contribute significantly to both pathological bone remodeling and associated CV mortality. Although multiple aspects of CRS have been known for a long time, a large part of the pathogenesis of CKD-MBD remains unexplained [2, 3, 15, 101].

The maybe surprising association between bone and heart—the bone-heart axis—relies, as key mediators, on the PTH, fibroblast growth factor-23 (FGF23) and 1,25-dihydroxyvitamin D (calcitriol), the active form of vitamin D, all 3 of them being the main factors that regulate phosphate and calcium homeostasis through their effects on the kidneys, bone and intestine. Often, in the initial stages of CKD, FGF23 secreted by osteocytes undergoes a compensatory increase, which reduces tubular phosphate reabsorption but decreases renal calcitriol synthesis. However, in the long term, phosphate retention increases to a level that cannot be compensated for, leading to secondary hyperparathyroidism, increased bone turnover (in some phenotypes), and contributing to vascular calcification through osteogenic mechanisms [2, 10, 15, 102].

This pro-osteogenic role of phosphate in the vascular wall develops through the induction of the smooth muscle cell transition to an "osteoblast-like" phenotype, promoting the formation of hydroxyapatite deposits. As already mentioned, the initial increase in FGF23 secretion has adaptive effects; later, it can cause adverse CV effects, such as left ventricular hypertrophy and an increased risk of HF. Concomitantly with the decrease of the eGFR and with this hormonal imbalance, calcium levels fluctuate; the reduction of the circulating calcium contributes to the stimulation of the parathyroid glands, contributing even more to the bone-kidney vicious cycle, with an increased risk of fractures in the fragile bones [103].

Although the metabolic profile of patients with CKD includes hypocalcemia alongside elevated FGF23, PTH, and phosphate, and a lower level of calcitriol, paradoxically, in patients with prolonged secondary hyperparathyroidism, calcium levels can be elevated, especially when patients are treated with calcium-containing pharmacologic agents. Both hypo- and hypercalcemia can have a negative impact on patients with CKD-MBD; hypocalcemia can contribute to the release of calcium from bones, potentially leading to fractures, whereas hypercalcemia can lead to extraskeletal calcifications and an increased CV risk. The risk of fractures in patients with CKD is much higher than that in the general population, with a 2-times higher risk in stage G3 and a 4-times higher risk in stage G5D [103–105]. Nevertheless, not all bone abnormalities in CKD-BMD—also called renal osteodystrophy—are the same, but, considering their high or low turnover and their main cause, can be categorized in hyperparathyroidism-related bone disease (osteitis fibrosa cystica), mixed uremic osteodystrophy, osteomalacia, or adynamic bone disease [106].

Klotho is a co-receptor of FGF23 and contributes to the regulation of calcitriol and phosphate metabolism, as well as to the prevention of aging and neurodegeneration. In patients with CKD, alongside the reduction in eGFR, Klotho levels also decline, with consequences including vascular aging, predisposition to vascular calcification, arterial stiffness, and loss of the protective effect of the FGF23-Klotho axis on mineral metabolism. It is, therefore, evident that the CKD-MBD contributes to vascular and, later, to left ventricular dysfunction that can lead to an increased CV morbidity and mortality [107].

Vascular calcification in patients with CKD is not merely a passive mineral deposition but an active, regulated process that mirrors multiple aspects of osteogenesis, including the phenotypic conversion of vascular smooth muscle cells to osteoblast-like cells. Additionally, persistently elevated serum phosphate and calcium concentrations, alongside oxidative stress and chronic systemic inflammation, trigger vascular calcification, leading to a subsequent increase in arterial stiffness, as evidenced by increased pulse wave velocity [108]. Not only are the vessels the ones that undergo calcification in patients with CKD-MBD, but also the valves—especially the aortic and the mitral valves—even more so in patients undergoing dialysis or those with hypercalcemia and prolonged exposure to calcium-based pharmacologic agents [109]. Both the arterial stiffness and the valvular calcification contribute to an increased CV and even all-cause mortality risk, according to recent studies, through the development of left ventricular hypertrophy and diastolic dysfunction. Additionally, these pathological changes, together with the mineral imbalances, hyperphosphatemia, hypocalcemia, occasionally hypercalcemia, and, in some cases, hypomagnesemia, and the increased levels of FGF23, can alter the electric properties of the myocardium, change its structure, and increase its vulnerability and, consequently, contribute to the development of arrhythmias [110, 111].

15.5.2 Assessment

The routine assessment of patients with CKD starting at stage G3a should include at least the following parameters: serum calcium, phosphate, and PTH levels, which should be monitored regularly based on the presence and magnitude of abnormalities and the rate of progression of CKD. Additionally, in these patients, 25-hydroxyvitamin D (calcidiol) levels might be measured and monitored. Another marker that can be used to assess, indirectly, the bone turnover, in patients starting stage G3a CKD, except serum PTH, is the bone-specific alkaline phosphatase, while bone-derived turnover markers of collagen synthesis, such as the procollagen type I C-terminal propeptide (P1CP) or collagen breakdown, such as type I collagen cross-linked telopeptide, are not routinely measured. Similarly, although FGF23 levels can provide prognostic information, they are not yet part of the routine monitoring algorithm used in clinical practice. Nevertheless, the interpretation of these results should be done in the context of the CKD stage, concomitant medications (vitamin D, calcimimetics), and clinical and nutritional status, since misinterpretation can occur in the setting of inflammation, malnutrition, or dialysis [2, 15].

Imaging techniques such as standard radiography, bone densitometry (DXA—dual-energy X-ray absorptiometry), or CT scans are recommended only when their results would influence patient management, such as in assessing global CV risk or to avoid excessive use of calcium-based pharmacologic agents. Standard radiography is sometimes used to highlight advanced calcification. In contrast, CT with Agatston scoring is used to assess coronary calcification and identify the risk of CV events. These results can influence the choice between calcium-based and non-calcium-based phosphate binders. DXA is recommended to evaluate bone mineral density and fracture risk, while bone biopsy is very rarely used in cases where the diagnosis is unclear and is required to choose the appropriate therapy [2, 112].

15.5.3 Management

One key aspect of managing CKD-MBD is reducing phosphate intake, for which nutritional education is essential. Phosphate is naturally found in animal products such as dairy, liver, and other organs, and can be added to various processed foods, such as processed meat or sodas. When dietary measures are insufficient, phosphate binders can be used. This category of pharmacologic agents can be calcium- or non-calcium-based, and the choice for each patient is based on the patient's serum calcium levels, the presence of vascular calcifications, and CV risk. On the one hand, calcium-based phosphate binders are efficient and readily available. Yet they expose the patient to a higher calcium level, which could lead to chronic hypercalcemia and vascular calcifications. On the other hand, non-calcium-based phosphate binders such as sevelamer carbonate or lanthanum carbonate are preferable alternatives, especially since some studies have shown the beneficial effects of sevelamer carbonate on lipids and inflammation, although the results on mortality reduction remain unclear. Given the adverse effects, phosphate binders can cause gastrointestinal disturbances such as constipation, nausea, or abdominal discomfort, and their pharmacological interactions with certain antibiotics, iron supplements, digoxin, and other drugs should be managed on a case-by-case basis [15, 113, 114].

Another important pathway in the management of CKD-MBD is the control of the secondary hyperparathyroidism for which active vitamin D analogues or calcimimetics are used. Vitamin D analogues such as calcitriol, paricalcitol, or alfacalcidol reduce PTH levels through negative feedback and also improve bone turnover, but they also increase intestinal absorption of calcium and phosphate, potentially leading to hypercalcemia and hyperphosphatemia if their use is not adjusted according to these parameters [115]. Calcimimetics such as cinacalcet or etelcalcetide also reduce PTH levels, but, unlike the vitamin D analogues, they activate the parathyroid calcium-sensing receptor and do not increase calcium uptake, a key advantage for patients with hypercalcemia or vascular calcifications. However, since calcimimetics can cause hypocalcemia, frequent monitoring of this parameter is necessary after initiation or dosage adjustment. In practice, the combination of these classes of pharmacologic agents at low doses can control PTH levels without causing calcium disturbances [115, 116].

This avoidance of chronic hypercalcemia is a key objective in the management of CKD-MBD when calcium-based phosphate binders, calcium supplements, or vitamin D analogues are used without monitoring serum calcium levels, as it can contribute to the progression of vascular and valvular calcifications and to the development of diastolic dysfunction. In this context, recent guidelines recommend limiting calcium intake and adjusting the therapeutic strategy based on plasma calcium levels. Recent studies have shown that magnesium has a protective effect against vascular calcification and arterial stiffness—possibly by inhibiting phosphate-calcium crystallization and directly impacting vascular cells—while results regarding the long-term benefits on CV events and mortality, and on bone health, are still relatively unknown. Nevertheless, the use of potassium binders containing magnesium as well as magnesium-based supplements represents a promising new therapeutic strategy that should still be applied with caution, taking into account renal function and the risk of hypermagnesemia [117].

When choosing the optimal therapeutic strategy for patients with CKD-MBD, personalized care must be at the center of attention, considering both CV and bone-related risks. Although additional long-term clinical trials are still needed to assess the impact of these pharmacologic agents on CV morbidity and mortality, for the moment, maintaining the balance between the PTH control and the avoidance of calcium/phosphate disturbances, while assessing the kidney function and CV risk, is considered to be the best approach for these patients [2, 15].

15.6 Special Considerations

15.6.1 Managing the RAAS Blockade [118–120]

- Angiotensin-converting enzyme inhibitors and angiotensin II receptor blockers reduce the progression of CKD through various mechanisms, and current guidelines recommend titration to the maximum dose.
- Serum K^+ values must be monitored as RAAS inhibition promotes hyperkalemia, which increases the risk of arrhythmia and sudden cardiac death.
- To maintain the use of angiotensin-converting enzyme inhibitors, angiotensin II receptor blockers, and mineralocorticoid receptor antagonists, potassium binders such as patiromer and sodium zirconium cyclosilicate can be used to limit the risk of hyperkalemia.

- Mineralocorticoid receptor antagonists are among the main pillars of HF management, contributing to the reduction of inflammation, fibrosis, and volume retention.
- Steroidal mineralocorticoid receptor antagonists such as spironolactone and eplerenone exhibit greater kidney binding than in the heart and more off-target binding, thereby causing more side effects than nonsteroidal mineralocorticoid receptor antagonists such as finerenone, balcinrenone, apararenone, and esaxerenone.
- Steroidal mineralocorticoid receptor can cause certain side-effects, such as gynecomastia, sexual or menstrual dysfunction and metabolic issues (hyperglycemia).
- Recent trials using nonsteroidal mineralocorticoid receptor antagonists in patients with diabetes, HF, and CKD have shown promise in reducing CV risk while also being well tolerated.
- Nonsteroidal mineralocorticoid receptor antagonists are more selective and safer in CKD patients as their use is associated with a lower risk of hyperkalemia compared to steroidal mineralocorticoid receptor agonists due to a more balanced distribution between the heart and the kidneys, also generating greater heart and kidney protection.

15.6.2 Diuretics [121–127]

- Both hypo- and hyperkalemia can be present in CKD, depending on the type of diuretics used and their dosage.
- Hypokalemia promotes ammonia excretion and is often accompanied by refractory metabolic alkalosis until serum K+ levels are restored, a process made more difficult by the fact that alkalosis promotes urinary K^+ loss.
- Both hypo- and hyperkalemia contribute to worsening of mortality and an increased number of CV events; however, only hypokalemia has been associated with increased progression of CKD.
- Loop diuretics are more commonly used in CKD as they increase fractional sodium excretion to a greater extent compared to thiazide diuretics (20% versus 5–10%).
- Loop diuretics are effective regardless of eGFR, whereas thiazide diuretics have limited effects below an eGFR of 30 ml/min/1,73 m^2.
- It should be noted that patients who associate both loop and thiazide diuretics present with higher mortality and have a greater risk of hypokalemia.
- The use of SGLT2i offers benefits for both CKD and HF, as they reduce progression and improve clinical outcomes in both diseases.
- SGLT2i have synergistic effects with other diuretics by limiting proteinuria, reducing blood pressure and volume overload, and contributing to the limitation of inflammation and fibrosis.

- Use of SGLT2i can also contribute to limiting the side effects of mineralocorticoid receptor antagonists in HF and CKD.
- Further metabolic benefits of SGLT2i use come from controlling glycaemia and uric acid levels.
- Both CKD and HF are associated with mitochondrial dysfunction. SGLT2i increases the number of mitochondria per cell, increases ATP production, limits disease progression, and improves clinical outcomes and patient quality of life.

15.6.3 Nutrition: [118, 128–130]

- High protein intake (>1.3 g/kg body weight) damages the kidneys, causing glomerular injury and increasing albumin excretion; as such, lower protein intake should be considered to avoid muscle catabolism due to increased acid load, which can further lead to muscle wasting and renal hypertrophy.
- As lower protein intake is important, equal importance should be given to maintaining quality protein intake.
- Lower protein intake also improves metabolic acidosis.
- Consuming plant-based proteins in favor of animal-based proteins consumes excess H^+ due to the higher concentration of glutamate and potassium salts and the lower concentration of sulfur-containing amino acids.
- 0.8 g/kg of protein should be considered for patients with CKD not on hemodialysis.
- 1–1,2 g/kg of protein should be considered in patients with CKD undergoing hemodialysis.
- Sodium intake should be limited to <2300 mg/day.
- Avoid ingestion of NaCl substitutes that contain K^+.
- Avoid K^+ rich foods, especially those that contain K^+ additives.
- Consuming foods with a low phosphorus-to-protein ratio should be encouraged.
- Intake of food with high inorganic absorbable phosphorus additives should be avoided.
- High calcium intake via food or supplements should be avoided.
- Phosphorus binders can help overcome high dietary intake of absorbable phosphorus.
- The diet should be adapted to the individual's specific needs. The DASH and Mediterranean diets are best suited to the particular needs of patients with cardiorenal syndrome. They should be considered as viable treatment options to improve both CV and kidney outcomes.

Declarations

Competing Interests The author(s) has no competing interests to declare that are relevant to the content of this manuscript.

Ethics Approval The author(s) declares that this manuscript does not include primary research with human participants.

The author(s) declares that this manuscript does not include primary studies involving animals.

References

1. Beghini A, Sammartino AM, Papp Z, von Haehling S, Biegus J, Ponikowski P, et al. 2024 update in heart failure. ESC Heart Fail. 2025;12(1):8–42. [cited 2025 Oct 30] Available from: https://pubmed.ncbi.nlm.nih.gov/38806171/.
2. Stevens PE, Ahmed SB, Carrero JJ, Foster B, Francis A, Hall RK, et al. KDIGO 2024 Clinical Practice Guideline for the evaluation and Management of Chronic Kidney Disease. Kidney Int. 2024;105(4):S117–314. [cited 2025 Oct 30] Available from: https://pubmed.ncbi.nlm.nih.gov/38490803/.
3. Rangaswami J, Bhalla V, Blair JEA, Chang TI, Costa S, Lentine KL, et al. Cardiorenal syndrome: classification, pathophysiology, diagnosis, and treatment strategies: a scientific statement from the American Heart Association. Circulation. 2019;139(16):E840–78. [cited 2025 Oct 30] Available from: https://www.ahajournals.org/doi/pdf/10.1161/CIR.0000000000000664?download=true.
4. Ndumele CE, Rangaswami J, Chow SL, Neeland IJ, Tuttle KR, Khan SS, et al. Cardiovascular-kidney-metabolic health: a presidential advisory from the American Heart Association. Circulation. 2023;148(20):1606–35. [cited 2025 Oct 30] Available from: https://pubmed.ncbi.nlm.nih.gov/37807924/.
5. Marx-Schütt K, Cherney DZI, Jankowski J, Matsushita K, Nardone M, Marx N. Cardiovascular disease in chronic kidney disease. Eur Heart J. 2025;46(23):2148–60. [cited 2025 Oct 30] Available from: https://pubmed.ncbi.nlm.nih.gov/40196891/.
6. Noels H, van der EPC V, Rubin S, Emmett A, Marx N, Tomaszewski M, et al. Renal-cardiac crosstalk in the pathogenesis and progression of heart failure. Circ Res. 2025;136(11):1306–34. [cited 2025 Oct 30] Available from: https://cris.maastrichtuniversity.nl/en/publications/renal-cardiac-crosstalk-in-the-pathogenesis-and-progression-of-he/.
7. Charytan DM, Fishbane S, Malyszko J, McCullough PA, Goldsmith D. Cardiorenal syndrome and the role of the bone-mineral Axis and anemia. Am J Kidney Dis. 2015;66(2):196–205. [cited 2025 Oct 30] Available from: https://pubmed.ncbi.nlm.nih.gov/25727384/.
8. Guaricci AI, Sturdà F, Russo R, Basile P, Baggiano A, Mushtaq S, et al. Assessment and management of heart failure in patients with chronic kidney disease. Heart Fail Rev. 2024;29(2):379–94. [cited 2025 Oct 30] Available from: https://pubmed.ncbi.nlm.nih.gov/37728751/.
9. Wang AYM. Optimally managing hyperkalemia in patients with cardiorenal syndrome. Nephrol Dial Transplant. 2019;34(Suppl 3):III36–44. [cited 2025 Oct 30] Available from: https://pubmed.ncbi.nlm.nih.gov/31800079/.
10. Binnenmars SH, Hoogslag GE, Yeung SMH, Brouwers FP, Bakker SJL, van Gilst WH, et al. Fibroblast growth factor 23 and risk of new onset heart failure with preserved or reduced ejection fraction: the PREVEND Study. J Am Heart Assoc. 2022;11(15) [cited 2025 Oct 30] Available from: https://pubmed.ncbi.nlm.nih.gov/35876420/.
11. Wang Y, Zhang D, Zhou R, Yang X, Wang X, Jiang Y, et al. Baseline fibroblast growth factor 23 predicts incident heart failure and cardiovascular mortality in patients with chronic kidney disease: a 3-year follow-up study. IJC Heart Vasc. 2025:56. [cited 2025 Oct 30] Available from: https://pubmed.ncbi.nlm.nih.gov/39807363/.
12. Leon SJ, Tangri N. Balancing hyperkalemia risks with clinical benefits of renin-angiotensin-aldosterone inhibitors/mineralocorticoid receptor antagonists blockade: it's apples and

oranges. Kidney360. 2022;3(8):1442–4. [cited 2025 Oct 30] Available from: https://pubmed.ncbi.nlm.nih.gov/36176652/.
13. Natale P, Palmer SC, Ruospo M, Saglimbene VM, Strippoli GFM. Potassium binders for chronic hyperkalaemia in people with chronic kidney disease. Cochrane Database Syst Rev. 2020;6(6) [cited 2025 Oct 30] Available from: https://pubmed.ncbi.nlm.nih.gov/32588430/.
14. Sarnaik KS, Mirzai S. When the heart, kidneys, and body waste away: a review of Cachexia in cardiorenal syndrome. Curr Heart Fail Rep. 2025;22(1):1–14. [cited 2025 Oct 30] Available from: https://link.springer.com/article/10.1007/s11897-025-00711-2.
15. Valson A, Sahay M, Prasad N, Agarwal S, Varughese S, Gang S. KDIGO 2017 Clinical Practice Guideline update for the diagnosis, evaluation, prevention and prevention of Chronic Kidney Disease-Mineral and Bone Disorder (CKDMBD): Indian Commentary. Indian J Nephrol. 2020;30(4):221–33. [cited 2025 Oct 30] Available from: https://pubmed.ncbi.nlm.nih.gov/33273784/.
16. Committee ADAPP, ElSayed NA, McCoy RG, Aleppo G, Balapattabi K, Beverly EA, et al. 6. Glycemic goals and hypoglycemia: standards of care in diabetes—2025. Diabetes Care. 2025;48(Supplement_1):S128–45. [cited 2025 Sep 27] Available from: https://doi.org/10.2337/dc25-S006.
17. Kaminski CY, Galindo RJ, Navarrete JE, Zabala Z, Moazzami B, Gerges A, et al. Assessment of glycemic control by continuous glucose monitoring, hemoglobin A1c, fructosamine, and glycated albumin in patients with end-stage kidney disease and burnt-out diabetes. Diabetes Care. 2024;47(2):267–71. [cited 2025 Sep 27] Available from: https://doi.org/10.2337/dc23-1276.
18. Vos FE, Schollum JB, Walker RJ. Glycated albumin is the preferred marker for assessing glycaemic control in advanced chronic kidney disease. NDT Plus. 2011;4(6):368. [cited 2025 Sep 27] Available from: https://pmc.ncbi.nlm.nih.gov/articles/PMC4421676/.
19. Freitas PAC, Ehlert LR, Camargo JL. Glycated albumin: a potential biomarker in diabetes. Arch Endocrinol Metab. 2022;61(3):296. [cited 2025 Sep 27] Available from: https://pmc.ncbi.nlm.nih.gov/articles/PMC10118799/.
20. What is the difference between fructosamine and glycated albumin?. | myadlm.org. [cited 2025 Sep 27]. Available from: https://myadlm.org/science-and-research/scientific-shorts/2023/what-is-the-difference-between-fructosamine-and-glycated-albumin.
21. Kim H, Tang O, Rebholz CM, Grams ME, Coresh J, Christenson RH, et al. Associations of glycated albumin and HbA1c with chronic kidney disease in US adults. J Appl Lab Med. 2022;7(4):842. [cited 2025 Sep 27] Available from: https://pmc.ncbi.nlm.nih.gov/articles/PMC9246894/.
22. Fructosamine: Reference Range, Interpretation, Collection and Panels. [cited 2025 Sep 27]. Available from: https://emedicine.medscape.com/article/2089070-overview.
23. Gounden V, Anastasopoulou C, Zubair M, Jialal I. Clinical utility of fructosamine and glycated albumin. StatPearls; 2025. [cited 2025 Sep 27] Available from: https://www.ncbi.nlm.nih.gov/books/NBK470185/.
24. Rhee CM, Gianchandani RY, Kerr D, Philis-Tsimikas A, Kovesdy CP, Stanton RC, et al. Consensus report on the use of continuous glucose monitoring in chronic kidney disease and diabetes. J Diabetes Sci Technol. 2024;19(1):19322968241292040. [cited 2025 Sep 27] Available from: https://pmc.ncbi.nlm.nih.gov/articles/PMC11607725/.
25. Committee ADAPP, ElSayed NA, McCoy RG, Aleppo G, Balapattabi K, Beverly EA, et al. 11. Chronic kidney disease and risk management: standards of care in diabetes—2025. Diabetes Care. 2025;48(Supplement_1):S239–51. [cited 2025 Sep 27] Available from: https://doi.org/10.2337/dc25-S011.
26. Bergenstal RM, Beck RW, Close KL, Grunberger G, Sacks DB, Kowalski A, et al. Glucose management indicator (GMI): a new term for estimating A1C from continuous glucose monitoring. Diabetes Care. 2018;41(11):2275–80. [cited 2025 Sep 27] Available from: https://doi.org/10.2337/dc18-1581.

27. Navaneethan SD, Zoungas S, Caramori ML, Chan JCN, Heerspink HJL, Hurst C, et al. Diabetes management in chronic kidney disease: synopsis of the KDIGO 2022 clinical practice guideline update. Ann Intern Med. 2023;176(3):381–7.
28. Ling J, Ng JKCC, Lau ESH, Ma RCW, Kong APS, Luk AOY, et al. Continuous glucose monitoring metrics in the assessment of glycemia in moderate-to-advanced CKD in diabetes. Kidney Int Rep. 2022;7(6):1354. [cited 2025 Sep 27] Available from: https://pmc.ncbi.nlm.nih.gov/articles/PMC9171696/.
29. Narasaki Y, Kalantar-Zadeh K, Daza AC, You AS, Novoa A, Peralta RA, et al. Accuracy of continuous glucose monitoring in hemodialysis patients with diabetes. Diabetes Care. 2024;47(11):1922–9. [cited 2025 Sep 27] Available from: https://doi.org/10.2337/dc24-0635.
30. Huang P, He J, Ren L, Yang R, Feng D, Li L, et al. Research progress on the application of CGM in patients with diabetes and hemodialysis. Int J Med Sci. 2024;21(15):3083–90. [cited 2025 Sep 27] Available from: https://www.medsci.org://creativecommons.org/licenses/by/4.0/.
31. ABCD and Renal Association Clinical practice guidelines for management of hyperglycaemia in adults with diabetic kidney disease (DKD) | The Association of British Clinical Diabetologists. [cited 2025 Sep 27] Available from: https://abcd.care/resource/archived/abcd-and-renal-association-clinical-practice-guidelines-management-hyperglycaemia.
32. Hwang YC, Jung CH, Ahn HY, Jeon WS, Jin SM, Woo J-T, et al. Optimal glycated albumin cutoff value to diagnose diabetes in Korean adults: a retrospective study based on the oral glucose tolerance test. Clin Chim Acta. 2014;437:1–5. [cited 2025 Sep 27] Available from: https://www.sciencedirect.com/science/article/pii/S000989811400285X.
33. Gan T, Liu X, Xu G. Glycated albumin versus HbA1c in the evaluation of glycemic control in patients with diabetes and CKD. Kidney Int Rep. 2017;3(3):542. [cited 2025 Sep 27] Available from: https://pmc.ncbi.nlm.nih.gov/articles/PMC5976809/.
34. Bonifant G, Davis SN, Weir MR. Treatment of diabetes in patients with advanced chronic kidney disease or kidney failure. Nephrol Dial Transplant. 2025; [cited 2025 Sep 27] Available from: https://doi.org/10.1093/ndt/gfaf083.
35. Padda IS, Mahtani AU, Parmar M. Sodium-Glucose Transport 2 (SGLT2) inhibitors. StatPearls; 2025. [cited 2025 Sep 27] Available from: https://www.ncbi.nlm.nih.gov/books/NBK576405/.
36. Zinman B, Wanner C, Lachin JM, Fitchett D, Bluhmki E, Hantel S, et al. Empagliflozin, cardiovascular outcomes, and mortality in type 2 diabetes. N Engl J Med. 2015;373(22):2117–28. [cited 2025 Sep 7] Available from: http://www.nejm.org/doi/10.1056/NEJMoa1504720.
37. Hou YC, Zheng CM, Yen TH, Lu KC. Molecular mechanisms of SGLT2 inhibitor on cardiorenal protection. Int J Mol Sci. 2020;21(21):1–25. [cited 2025 Sep 27] Available from: https://pubmed.ncbi.nlm.nih.gov/33105763/.
38. KDIGO. Clinical practice guideline for diabetes management in chronic kidney disease. Kidney Int. 2022;102(5):S1–127. [cited 2025 Jul 6]; Available from: https://pubmed.ncbi.nlm.nih.gov/36272764/.
39. Nardi E, Prastaro M, Santoro C, Gallo L, Simeoli L, Fontanarosa S, et al. Therapeutic tailored approach in patients with diabetes, cardiovascular and renal comorbidities: a cardiologist's view. Nutr Metab Cardiovasc Dis. 2025;35(9):104033. [cited 2025 Sep 27] Available from: https://www.sciencedirect.com/science/article/pii/S0939475325001875.
40. Badve SV, Bilal A, Lee MMY, Sattar N, Gerstein HC, Ruff CT, et al. Effects of GLP-1 receptor agonists on kidney and cardiovascular disease outcomes: a meta-analysis of randomised controlled trials. Lancet Diabetes Endocrinol. 2025;13(1):15–28. [cited 2025 Sep 27] Available from: https://pubmed.ncbi.nlm.nih.gov/39608381/.
41. Halimi JM, Fauchier L, Karras A, Amouyal C, Eladari D, Rossignol P, et al. Expert perspectives on incorporating glucagon-like peptide-1 receptor agonist in diabetes and chronic kidney disease: challenges and opportunities. Eur J Prev Cardiol. 2025; [cited 2025 Sep 27] Available from: https://doi.org/10.1093/eurjpc/zwaf426.

42. Karalliedde J, McCafferty K, Winocour P, Chowdhury TA, Kanumilli N, De P, et al. Association of British Clinical Diabetologists and UK Kidney Association Joint Clinical Practice Guidelines for the pharmacological management of Hyperglycemia in Adults With Type 2 Diabetes Mellitus and CKD. Kidney Int Rep. 2025;10:3318. [cited 2025 Sep 27] Available from: https://www.sciencedirect.com/science/article/pii/S2468024925004723.
43. Verma S, Graham MM, Lecamwasam A, Romanovsky A, Duggan S, Bagshaw S, et al. Cardiorenal interactions: a review. CJC Open. 2022;4(10):873–85. [cited 2025 Oct 6]; Available from: https://www.sciencedirect.com/science/article/pii/S2589790X22001354.
44. Raphael KL. Metabolic acidosis in CKD: Core curriculum 2019. Am J Kidney Dis. 2019;74(2):263–75. Available from: https://doi.org/10.1053/j.ajkd.2019.01.036.
45. Klemm G, Markart S, Hermann A, Staudinger T, Hengstenberg C, Heinz G, et al. Lactate as a predictor of 30-day mortality in cardiogenic shock. J Clin Med. 2024;13(7):1932.
46. Greenberg KI, Lecker SH. Metabolic acidosis. In: W.B. Saunders, editor. Advances in kidney disease and health, vol. 32; 2025. p. 61–8.
47. Umpierrez GE, Davis GM, ElSayed NA, Fadini GP, Galindo RJ, Hirsch IB, et al. Hyperglycemic crises in adults with diabetes: a consensus report. Diabetes Care. 2024;47(8):1257–75. Available from: https://doi.org/10.2337/dci24-0032.
48. Huang SK, Huang CY, Lin CH, Cheng BW, Chiang YT, Lee YC, et al. Acute kidney injury is a common complication in children and adolescents hospitalized for diabetic ketoacidosis. PLoS One. 2020;15(10):e0239160.
49. Baek HS, Jeong C, Yang Y, Lee J, Lee J, Lee SH, et al. Diabetic ketoacidosis as an effect of sodium-glucose cotransporter 2 inhibitor: real world insights. Diabetes Metab J. 2024;48(6):1169–75.
50. Shamseddin MK, Parfrey PS. Mechanisms of the cardiorenal syndromes. Nat Rev Nephrol. 2009;5:641–9.
51. Kraut JA, Madias NE. Metabolic acidosis: pathophysiology, diagnosis and management. Nat Rev Nephrol. 2010;6:274–85.
52. Collister D, Ferguson TW, Funk SE, Reaven NL, Mathur V, Tangri N. Metabolic acidosis and cardiovascular disease in CKD. Kidney Med. 2021;3(5):753–761.e1.
53. Kim HJ. Metabolic acidosis in chronic kidney disease: pathogenesis, clinical consequences, and treatment. Electrolyte Blood Press. 2021;19:29–37. Korean Society of Electrolyte and Blood Pressure Research.
54. Ho JQ, Abramowitz MK. Clinical consequences of metabolic acidosis—muscle. Adv Chronic Kidney Dis. 2022;29(4):395–405. [cited 2025 Oct 17]; Available from: https://www.sciencedirect.com/science/article/abs/pii/S1548559522000787.
55. Swenson ER. The many acid–base manifestations and consequences of hypoxia. Curr Opin Physiol. 2019;7:72–81. [cited 2025 Oct 18]; Available from: https://www.sciencedirect.com/science/article/abs/pii/S2468867319300033.
56. Avram VF, Merce AP, Hâncu IM, Bătrân AD, Kennedy G, Rosca MG, et al. Impairment of mitochondrial respiration in metabolic diseases: an overview. Int J Mol Sci. 2022;23(16) Available from: https://www.mdpi.com/1422-0067/23/16/8852.
57. Erra Díaz F, Dantas E, Geffner J. Unravelling the interplay between extracellular acidosis and immune cells. Mediat Inflamm (Hindawi Limited). 2018;2018:1218297.
58. Bajwa GS, Hussain A, Javaid MM. How to work up an adult patient with metabolic acidosis. Br J Hosp Med. 2022;83(8):1–11. https://doi.org/10.12968/hmed.2021.0582.
59. Gezer M, Bulucu F, Ozturk K, Kilic S, Kaldirim U, Eyi YE. Effectiveness of the Stewart method in the evaluation of blood gas parameters. Turk J Emerg Med. 2015;15(1):3–7.
60. Batlle D, Chin-Theodorou J, Tucker BM. Metabolic acidosis or respiratory alkalosis? Evaluation of a low plasma bicarbonate using the urine anion gap. Am J Kidney Dis. 2017;70(3):440–4.
61. Rice M, Ismail B, Pillow MT. Approach to metabolic acidosis in the emergency department. Emerg Med Clin North Am. 2014;32(2):403–20. [cited 2025 Jul 27];Available from: https://www.sciencedirect.com/science/article/abs/pii/S0733862714000030.

62. Palmer BF, Kelepouris E, Clegg DJ. Renal tubular acidosis and management strategies: a narrative review. Adv Ther. 2021;38(2):949–68. https://doi.org/10.1007/s12325-020-01587-5.
63. McGuire LC, Cruickshank AM, Munro PT. Alcoholic ketoacidosis. Emerg Med J. 2006;23:417–20.
64. Kraut JA, Madias NE. Lactic acidosis. N Engl J Med. 2014;371(24):2309–19. Available from: http://www.nejm.org/doi/10.1056/NEJMra1309483.
65. Drugs.com. Drugs.com. 2024 Sodium Bicarbonate Dosage. [cited 2025 Jul 27] Available from: https://www.drugs.com/dosage/sodium-bicarbonate.html.
66. Editorial Board. Kidney Int. 2024;105(4):A1.
67. McDonagh TA, Metra M, Adamo M, Baumbach A, Böhm M, Burri H, et al. ESC Guidelines for the diagnosis and treatment of acute and chronic heart failure. Eur Heart J. 2021;42:3599–726. Oxford University Press.
68. Bart BA, Goldsmith SR, Lee KL, Givertz MM, O'Connor CM, Bull DA, et al. Ultrafiltration in decompensated heart failure with cardiorenal syndrome. N Engl J Med. 2012;367(24):2296–304.
69. Suh SH, Kim SW. Dyslipidemia in patients with chronic kidney disease: an updated overview. Diabetes Metab J. 2023;47(5):612. [cited 2025 Sep 27] Available from: https://pmc.ncbi.nlm.nih.gov/articles/PMC10555535/.
70. Tramontano D, D'Erasmo L, Larouche M, Brisson D, Lauzière A, Di Costanzo A, et al. The vicious circle of chronic kidney disease and hypertriglyceridemia: what is first, the hen or the egg? Atherosclerosis. 2025;403:119146. [cited 2025 Sep 27] Available from: https://www.sciencedirect.com/science/article/pii/S0021915025000437.
71. Kon V, Yang H, Fazio S. Residual cardiovascular risk in chronic kidney disease: role of high-density lipoprotein. Arch Med Res. 2015;46(5):379. [cited 2025 Sep 27] Available from: https://pmc.ncbi.nlm.nih.gov/articles/PMC4805367/.
72. Tsimihodimos V, Mitrogianni Z, Elisaf M. Dyslipidemia associated with chronic kidney disease. Open Cardiovasc Med J. 2011;5(1):41. [cited 2025 Sep 27] Available from: https://pmc.ncbi.nlm.nih.gov/articles/PMC3106357/.
73. Bermúdez-López M, Betriu À, Valdivielso JM, Bretones del Pino T, Arroyo D, Fernández E. Beyond the traditional lipid parameters in chronic kidney disease. Nefrología (Engl Ed). 2018;38(2):109–13. [cited 2025 Sep 27] Available from: https://www.revistanefrologia.com/en-beyond-traditional-lipid-parameters-in-articulo-S2013251417302006.
74. Reijnders E, van der Laarse A, Jukema JW, Cobbaert CM. High residual cardiovascular risk after lipid-lowering: prime time for predictive, preventive, personalized, participatory, and psycho-cognitive medicine. Front Cardiovasc Med. 2023;10:1264319. [cited 2025 Sep 27] Available from: https://pmc.ncbi.nlm.nih.gov/articles/PMC10613690/.
75. Ortiz A, Wanner C, Gansevoort RT, Cozzolino M, Fliser D, Gambaro G, et al. Chronic kidney disease as cardiovascular risk factor in routine clinical practice: a position statement by the Council of the European Renal Association. Clin Kidney J. 2023;16(3):403–7. [cited 2025 Sep 28] Available from: https://doi.org/10.1093/ckj/sfac199.
76. Khan SS, Coresh J, Pencina MJ, Ndumele CE, Rangaswami J, Chow SL, et al. Novel prediction equations for absolute risk assessment of total cardiovascular disease incorporating cardiovascular-kidney-metabolic health: a scientific statement from the American Heart Association. Circulation. 2023;148(24):1982–2004.
77. Matsushita K, Kaptoge S, Hageman SHJ, Sang Y, Ballew SH, Grams ME, et al. Including measures of chronic kidney disease to improve cardiovascular risk prediction by SCORE2 and SCORE2-OP. Eur J Prev Cardiol. 2023;30(1):8. [cited 2025 Sep 28] Available from: https://pmc.ncbi.nlm.nih.gov/articles/PMC9839538/.
78. U-Prevent. [cited 2025 Sep 28] Available from: https://u-prevent.com/manual/information?returnUrl=%2Fcalculators.
79. Khan SS, Matsushita K, Sang Y, Ballew SH, Grams ME, Surapaneni A, et al. Development and validation of the American Heart Association's PREVENT equations. Circulation. 2024;149(6):430–49.

80. Visseren F, Mach F, Smulders YM, Carballo D, Koskinas KC, Bäck M, et al. 2021 ESC Guidelines on cardiovascular disease prevention in clinical practice. Eur Heart J. 2021;42(34):3227–337.
81. Wanner C, Krane V, März W, Olschewski M, Mann JFE, Ruf G, et al. Atorvastatin in patients with type 2 diabetes mellitus undergoing hemodialysis. N Engl J Med. 2005;353(3):238–48. [cited 2025 Sep 28] Available from: https://pubmed.ncbi.nlm.nih.gov/16034009/.
82. LaRosa JC, Grundy SM, Waters DD, Shear C, Barter P, Fruchart JC, et al. Intensive lipid lowering with atorvastatin in patients with stable coronary disease. N Engl J Med. 2005;352(14):97–9. [cited 2025 Sep 28] Available from: https://pubmed.ncbi.nlm.nih.gov/15755765/.
83. Baigent C, Landray MJ, Reith C, Emberson J, Wheeler DC, Tomson C, et al. The effects of lowering LDL cholesterol with simvastatin plus ezetimibe in patients with chronic kidney disease (Study of Heart and Renal Protection): a randomised placebo-controlled trial. Lancet. 2011;377(9784):2181–92. [cited 2025 Sep 28] Available from: https://pubmed.ncbi.nlm.nih.gov/21663949/.
84. Ridker PM, Danielson E, Fonseca FAH, Genest J, Gotto AM, Kastelein JJP, et al. Rosuvastatin to prevent vascular events in men and women with elevated C-reactive protein. N Engl J Med. 2008;359(21):2195–207. [cited 2025 Sep 28] Available from: https://pubmed.ncbi.nlm.nih.gov/18997196/.
85. Cannon CP, Blazing MA, Giugliano RP, McCagg A, White JA, Theroux P, et al. Ezetimibe added to statin therapy after acute coronary syndromes. N Engl J Med. 2015;372(25):2387–97. [cited 2025 Sep 28] Available from: https://pubmed.ncbi.nlm.nih.gov/26039521/.
86. Sabatine MS, Giugliano RP, Keech AC, Honarpour N, Wiviott SD, Murphy SA, et al. Evolocumab and clinical outcomes in patients with cardiovascular disease. N Engl J Med. 2017;376(18):1713–22. [cited 2025 Sep 28] Available from: https://pubmed.ncbi.nlm.nih.gov/28304224/.
87. Schwartz GG, Steg PG, Szarek M, Bhatt DL, Bittner VA, Diaz R, et al. Alirocumab and cardiovascular outcomes after acute coronary syndrome. N Engl J Med. 2018;379(22):2097–107. [cited 2025 Sep 28] Available from: https://pubmed.ncbi.nlm.nih.gov/30403574/.
88. Ray KK, Wright RS, Kallend D, Koenig W, Leiter LA, Raal FJ, et al. Two phase 3 trials of Inclisiran in patients with elevated LDL cholesterol. N Engl J Med. 2020;382(16):1507–19. [cited 2025 Sep 28] Available from: https://pubmed.ncbi.nlm.nih.gov/32187462/.
89. Nissen SE, Lincoff AM, Brennan D, Ray KK, Mason D, Kastelein JJP, et al. Bempedoic acid and cardiovascular outcomes in statin-intolerant patients. N Engl J Med. 2023;388(15):1353–64. [cited 2025 Sep 28] Available from: https://www.nejm.org/doi/pdf/10.1056/NEJMoa2215024.
90. Ray KK, Bays HE, Catapano AL, Lalwani ND, Bloedon LT, Sterling LR, et al. Safety and efficacy of bempedoic acid to reduce LDL cholesterol. N Engl J Med. 2019;380(11):1022–32. [cited 2025 Sep 28] Available from: https://pubmed.ncbi.nlm.nih.gov/30865796/.
91. Keech A, Simes RJ, Barter P, Best J, Scott R, Taskinen MR, et al. Effects of long-term fenofibrate therapy on cardiovascular events in 9795 people with type 2 diabetes mellitus (the FIELD study): randomised controlled trial. Lancet. 2005;366(9500):1849–61. [cited 2025 Sep 28] Available from: https://research.bond.edu.au/en/publications/effects-of-long-term-fenofibrate-therapy-on-cardiovascular-events.
92. Ginsberg HN, Elam MB, Lovato LC, Crouse JR 3rd, Leiter LA, Linz P, et al. Effects of combination lipid therapy in type 2 diabetes mellitus. N Engl J Med. 2010;362(17):1563–74. [cited 2025 Sep 28] Available from: https://pubmed.ncbi.nlm.nih.gov/20228404/.
93. Bhatt DL, Steg PG, Miller M, Brinton EA, Jacobson TA, Ketchum SB, et al. Cardiovascular risk reduction with Icosapent ethyl for hypertriglyceridemia. N Engl J Med. 2019;380(1):11–22. [cited 2025 Sep 28] Available from: https://www.nejm.org/doi/pdf/10.1056/NEJMoa1812792.
94. Kastelein JJP, Maki KC, Susekov A, Ezhov M, Nordestgaard BG, Machielse BN, et al. Omega-3 free fatty acids for the treatment of severe hypertriglyceridemia: the EpanoVa for

Lowering Very high triglyceridEs (EVOLVE) trial. J Clin Lipidol. 2014;8(1):94–106. [cited 2025 Sep 28] Available from: https://pubmed.ncbi.nlm.nih.gov/24528690/.
95. Rifkind B, Levy R, Fisher G. Plasma lipid distributions in selected North American populations: the Lipid Research Clinics Program Prevalence Study. The Lipid Research Clinics Program Epidemiology Committee. Circulation. 1979;60(2):427–39. [cited 2025 Sep 28] Available from: https://pubmed.ncbi.nlm.nih.gov/312704/.
96. Boden WE, Probstfield JL, Anderson T, Chaitman BR, Desvignes-Nickens P, Koprowicz K, et al. Niacin in patients with low HDL cholesterol levels receiving intensive statin therapy. N Engl J Med. 2011;365(24):2255–67. [cited 2025 Sep 28] Available from: https://pubmed.ncbi.nlm.nih.gov/22085343/.
97. Landray MJ, Haynes R, Hopewell JC, Parish S, Aung T, Tomson J, et al. Effects of extended-release niacin with laropiprant in high-risk patients. N Engl J Med. 2014;371(3):203–12. [cited 2025 Sep 28] Available from: https://pubmed.ncbi.nlm.nih.gov/25014686/.
98. Lin YC, Lai TS, Wu HY, Chou YH, Chiang WC, Lin SL, et al. Effects and safety of statin and ezetimibe combination therapy in patients with chronic kidney disease: a systematic review and meta-analysis. Clin Pharmacol Ther. 2020;108(4):833–43. [cited 2025 Sep 28] Available from: https://pubmed.ncbi.nlm.nih.gov/32320058/.
99. Anderson JL, May HT, Le VT, Muhlestein JB, Horne BD, Bair TL, et al. Impact of statin therapy in heart failure patients: results of a large real-world experience. JACC: Adv. 2023;2(4). [cited 2025 Sep 28] Available from: https://doi.org/10.1016/j.jacadv.2023.100385.
100. Davidson MH, Armani A, McKenney JM, Jacobson TA. Safety considerations with fibrate therapy. Am J Cardiol. 2007;99(6 SUPPL. 1) [cited 2025 Jul 15] Available from: https://pubmed.ncbi.nlm.nih.gov/17368275/.
101. Salera D, Merkel N, Bellasi A, de Borst MH. Pathophysiology of chronic kidney disease–mineral bone disorder (CKD-MBD): from adaptive to maladaptive mineral homeostasis. Clin Kidney J. 2025;18(Supplement_1):13–4. [cited 2025 Sep 7] Available from: https://doi.org/10.1093/ckj/sfae431.
102. Murray SL, Wolf M. Calcium and phosphate disorders: core curriculum 2024. Am J Kidney Dis. 2024;83(2):241–56. [cited 2025 Oct 30] Available from: https://pubmed.ncbi.nlm.nih.gov/38099870/.
103. Hill Gallant KM, Spiegel DM. Calcium balance in chronic kidney disease. Curr Osteoporos Rep. 2017;15(3):214–21. [cited 2025 Oct 30] Available from: https://pubmed.ncbi.nlm.nih.gov/28474258/.
104. Nakano T, Kishimoto H, Tokumoto M. Direct and indirect effects of fibroblast growth factor 23 on the heart. Front Endocrinol (Lausanne). 2023;14. [cited 2025 Oct 30] Available from: https://pubmed.ncbi.nlm.nih.gov/36909314/.
105. Vilaca T, Salam S, Schini M, Harnan S, Sutton A, Poku E, et al. Risks of hip and nonvertebral fractures in patients with CKD G3a-G5D: a systematic review and meta-analysis. Am J Kidney Dis. 2020;76(4):521–32. [cited 2025 Oct 30] Available from: https://pubmed.ncbi.nlm.nih.gov/32654892/.
106. Srisuwarn P, Eastell R, Salam S. Clinical utility of bone turnover markers in chronic kidney disease. J Bone Metab. 2024;31(4):264–78. [cited 2025 Oct 30] Available from: https://pubmed.ncbi.nlm.nih.gov/39701107/.
107. Kanbay M, Copur S, Ozbek L, Mutlu A, Cejka D, Ciceri P, et al. Klotho: a potential therapeutic target in aging and neurodegeneration beyond chronic kidney disease-a comprehensive review from the ERA CKD-MBD working group. Clin Kidney J. 2023;17(1) [cited 2025 Oct 30] Available from: https://pubmed.ncbi.nlm.nih.gov/38213484/.
108. Temmar M, Liabeuf S, Renard C, Czernichow S, Esper NE, Shahapuni I, et al. Pulse wave velocity and vascular calcification at different stages of chronic kidney disease. J Hypertens. 2010;28(1):163–9. [cited 2025 Oct 30] Available from: https://pubmed.ncbi.nlm.nih.gov/19927012/.
109. Hénaut L, Candellier A, Huish S, Issa N, Sinha S, Massy ZA. Valvular calcification in chronic kidney disease: new insights from recent clinical and preclinical studies. Clin Kidney

J. 2025;18(Suppl 1):i27–45. [cited 2025 Oct 30] Available from: https://pubmed.ncbi.nlm.nih.gov/40083956/.
110. Kaur R, Singh R. Mechanistic insights into CKD-MBD-related vascular calcification and its clinical implications. Life Sci. 2022;311(Pt B) [cited 2025 Oct 30] Available from: https://pubmed.ncbi.nlm.nih.gov/36336124/.
111. Jankowski J, Floege J, Fliser D, Böhm M, Marx N. Cardiovascular disease in chronic kidney disease pathophysiological insights and therapeutic options. Circulation. 2021;143(11):1157–72.
112. Ketteler M, Evenepoel P, Holden RM, Isakova T, Jørgensen HS, Komaba H, et al. Chronic kidney disease-mineral and bone disorder: conclusions from a Kidney Disease: Improving Global Outcomes (KDIGO) Controversies Conference. Kidney Int. 2025;107(3):405–23. [cited 2025 Oct 30] Available from: https://pubmed.ncbi.nlm.nih.gov/39864017/.
113. Suki WN, Zabaneh R, Cangiano JL, Reed J, Fischer D, Garrett L, et al. Effects of sevelamer and calcium-based phosphate binders on mortality in hemodialysis patients. Kidney Int. 2007;72(9):1130–7. [cited 2025 Oct 30] Available from: https://pubmed.ncbi.nlm.nih.gov/17728707/.
114. Patel L, Bernard LM, Elder GJ. Sevelamer versus calcium-based binders for treatment of hyperphosphatemia in CKD: a meta-analysis of randomized controlled trials. Clin J Am Soc Nephrol. 2016;11(2):232–44. [cited 2025 Oct 30] Available from: https://pubmed.ncbi.nlm.nih.gov/26668024/.
115. Wetmore JB, Quarles LD. Calcimimetics or vitamin D analogs for suppressing parathyroid hormone in end-stage renal disease: time for a paradigm shift? Nat Clin Pract Nephrol. 2009;5(1):24–33. [cited 2025 Oct 30] Available from: https://pubmed.ncbi.nlm.nih.gov/18957950/.
116. Goto S, Hamano T, Fujii H, Taniguchi M, Abe M, Nitta K, et al. Hypocalcemia and cardiovascular mortality in cinacalcet users. Nephrol Dial Transplant. 2024;39(4):637–47. [cited 2025 Oct 30] Available from: https://pubmed.ncbi.nlm.nih.gov/37777840/.
117. Zaslow SJ, Oliveira-Paula GH, Chen W. Magnesium and vascular calcification in chronic kidney disease: current insights. Int J Mol Sci. 2024;25(2) [cited 2025 Oct 30] Available from: https://pubmed.ncbi.nlm.nih.gov/38256228/.
118. Triozzi JL, Parker Gregg L, Virani SS, Navaneethan SD. Management of type 2 diabetes in chronic kidney disease. BMJ Open Diabetes Res Care (BMJ Publishing Group). 2021;9 https://doi.org/10.1136/bmjdrc-2021-002300.
119. Fonseca C, Garagarza C, Silva G, Caires G, Marques I, Lopes JA, et al. Hyperkalemia management: a multidisciplinary expert panel's perspective on the role of new potassium binders. Heart Fail Rev (Springer). 2024;30:271.
120. Harrington JL, Canonico ME, El Rafei A, Solomon SD, Teerlink JR, Vaduganathan M, et al. Nonsteroidal and steroidal mineralocorticoid antagonists: rationale, evidence, and unanswered questions. JACC: Heart Fail. 2025;13:102637. Elsevier Inc.
121. Dussol B, Moussi-Frances J, Morange S, Somma-Delpero C, Mundler O, Berland Y. A pilot study comparing furosemide and hydrochlorothiazide in patients with hypertension and stage 4 or 5 chronic kidney disease. J Clin Hypertens. 2012;14(1):32–7.
122. Sung LC, Chiu HW, Yu SMW, Tsou LLA, Hsu YH, Wu MS, et al. Thiazide diuretics versus loop diuretics in stage 3-5 CKD: impact on cardiorenal outcomes. Postgrad Med. 2024;136(7):738–48. Available from: https://doi.org/10.1080/00325481.2024.2396796.
123. Iordan L, Gaita L, Timar R, Avram V, Sturza A, Timar B. The Renoprotective Mechanisms of Sodium-Glucose Cotransporter-2 Inhibitors (SGLT2i)—a narrative review. Int J Mol Sci. 2024;25:7057. Multidisciplinary Digital Publishing Institute (MDPI)
124. Zhang B, Deng L. Application of SGLT-2 inhibitors in non-diabetic CKD: mechanisms, efficacy, and safety. Front Med. 2025;12:1574693. Frontiers Media SA.
125. Dhondup T, Qian Q. Acid-Base and electrolyte disorders in patients with and without chronic kidney disease: an update. Kidney Dis. 2017;3(4):136–48.

126. Gilligan S, Raphael KL. Hyperkalemia and hypokalemia in CKD: prevalence, risk factors, and clinical outcomes. Adv Chronic Kidney Dis. 2017;24(5):315–8. [cited 2025 Oct 26] Available from: https://www.sciencedirect.com/science/article/abs/pii/S1548559517300927.
127. Murakami Y, Kiuchi S, Hisatake S, Ikeda T. Combination of SGLT2 inhibitors and loop diuretics in the treatment of heart failure. J Pers Med. 2025;15(3):99.
128. Kalantar-Zadeh K, Moore LW, Tortorici AR, Chou JA, St-Jules DE, Aoun A, et al. North American experience with low protein diet for non-dialysis-dependent chronic kidney disease. BMC Nephrol. 2016;17(1):90.
129. Adeva MM, Souto G. Diet-induced metabolic acidosis. Clin Nutr. 2011;30(4):416–21. [cited 2025 Oct 19] Available from: https://www.sciencedirect.com/science/article/abs/pii/S0261561411000604.
130. Kalantar-Zadeh K. Patient education for phosphorus management in chronic kidney disease. Patient Prefer Adherence. 2013;7:379–90.

Chapter 16
Therapeutic Adjustments in Cardiorenal Syndrome: An Integrated Approach to Heart and Kidney Care

Shreeyukta Bhattarai, Binoy Shah, Edgar Lerma, and Ankur Shah

16.1 Introduction

Cardiorenal syndrome (CRS) represents one of the most challenging clinical scenarios in contemporary medicine, reflecting the intricate bidirectional relationship between cardiac and renal dysfunction. First formally defined by the National Heart, Lung, and Blood Institute in 2004 [1, 2], CRS encompasses a complex group of disorders wherein acute or chronic dysfunction in one organ induces acute or chronic dysfunction in the other. The Acute Dialysis Quality Initiative refined this definition in 2008, establishing a classification system that recognizes both cardiorenal and renal-cardiac syndromes across five distinct subtypes (Table 16.1) [3, 4].

The goal of this definition facilitated clinicians in overcoming some of the initial ambiguity in defining CRS for diagnostic and therapeutic purposes, streamlining epidemiological studies, and identifying treatment populations, among other benefits [3]. It also recognized the fact that clinically it will be challenging to identify the initial insult and there will be overlap between different classes.

The management of CRS requires a sophisticated understanding of the pathophysiological interplay between the heart and kidneys, coupled with therapeutic adjustments that address both organs simultaneously. This chapter explores the evidence-based therapeutic strategies for CRS, emphasizing the critical pharmacokinetic and pharmacodynamic modifications necessary in the setting of concurrent cardiac and renal dysfunction.

S. Bhattarai · B. Shah · A. Shah (✉)
Warren Alpert Medical School of Brown University, Providence, RI, USA

Division of Kidney Disease and Hypertension, Rhode Island Hospital, Providence, RI, USA
e-mail: ankur.shah@brownphysicians.org

E. Lerma
Division of Nephrology, University of Illinois at Chicago, Chicago, IL, USA

A. Covic, A. Burlacu (eds.), *Renal Dysfunction in Cardiovascular Pathologies*,
https://doi.org/10.1007/978-3-032-25434-4_16

Table 16.1 Classification of CRS based upon the acute dialysis quality initiative [3, 4]

Phenotype	Official nomenclature	Pathophysiologic description	Typical clinical scenarios
Type 1	Acute cardiorenal	Primary acute cardiac dysfunction leading to acute kidney injury (AKI)	Cardiogenic shock; acute coronary syndrome (ACS); acute decompensated heart failure
Type 2	Chronic cardiorenal	Persistent chronic heart failure causing progressive chronic kidney disease (CKD)	Long-term congestive heart failure (CHF) with chronic renal congestion
Type 3	Acute renocardiac	Primary acute kidney injury (AKI) triggering acute cardiac dysfunction	Fluid overload or uremic toxins from sudden renal failure causing heart failure
Type 4	Chronic renocardiac	Primary chronic kidney disease (CKD) leading to cardiac failure or hypertrophy	CKD-associated cardiomyopathy; left ventricular hypertrophy (LVH) due to renal disease
Type 5	Secondary CRS	Systemic conditions causing simultaneous heart and kidney dysfunction	Sepsis; amyloidosis; cirrhosis; multi-organ failure

16.2 Pathophysiology

While the physiology of cardiorenal syndrome is likely incompletely understood, there are multifactorial mechanisms underlying CRS that are essential to understand rational therapeutic intervention. The traditional paradigm of simple hemodynamic pump dysfunction leading to arterial underfilling and subsequent neurohumoral activation has evolved considerably [5]. Contemporary understanding recognizes that venous congestion plays a pivotal role, as demonstrated by the ADHERE registry findings that serum creatinine elevation occurs in both reduced and preserved ejection fraction heart failure, suggesting congestion as a key mediator rather than cardiac output alone [6].

The pathophysiology of CRS revolves around several interconnected mechanisms. Venous congestion decreases renal blood flow while simultaneously increasing tubular sodium avidity and activating fibrotic and inflammatory pathways. This leads to endothelial activation and cytokine release, creating a self-perpetuating cycle. The neurohumoral systems including the renin-angiotensin-aldosterone system (RAAS), sympathetic nervous system (SNS), and arginine vasopressin (AVP) become hyperactivated in response to perceived volume depletion despite actual fluid overload. Inflammatory mediators such as tumor necrosis factor-alpha, interleukin-1, and interleukin-6 contribute to myocardial depression and endothelial dysfunction. In chronic CRS, fibroblast growth factor-23 (FGF-23) promotes left ventricular hypertrophy and microvascular ischemia, further complicating the clinical picture [2, 7].

16.2.1 Principles of Therapeutic Adjustment

Management of cardiorenal syndrome requires simultaneously addressing short-term hemodynamic instability and long-term disease progression. In the acute setting, the primary therapeutic goal is to relieve congestion and restore adequate perfusion to both organs, because venous hypertension and low forward flow are major drivers of worsening kidney and heart function. As stabilization is achieved, the goals broaden to preventing recurrence of decompensation and interrupting the neurohormonal and inflammatory pathways that perpetuate organ injury. Across both phases, clinical judgment must prioritize integrated physiologic improvement rather than isolated laboratory changes, ensuring that treatment for one organ does not undermine the function of the other.

In the acute setting, the dominant goal is restoration of effective perfusion and relief of venous hypertension, because persistent congestion is a major driver of both renal injury and hemodynamic deterioration. Clinicians should target clear physiologic improvements, reduced filling pressures, improved dyspnea, and adequate urine output, rather than focusing narrowly on short-term changes in serum creatinine. Decisions should follow a hemodynamic rationale: achieve and maintain euvolemia, support forward flow when needed, and avoid interventions that correct laboratory values at the expense of worsening organ congestion.

Chronic management focuses on suppressing maladaptive neurohormonal activation to slow structural deterioration in both the heart and kidneys and preventing recurrence of decompensation. The principal aims are to sustain hemodynamic stability, suppress maladaptive neurohormonal activation, reduce inflammation and fibrosis, and preserve functional reserve in both organs.

16.2.2 Decongestive Therapy: The Foundation of Acute Management

Decongestion represents the cornerstone of acute CRS management, with achievement of euvolemia associated with improved clinical outcomes. The pharmacological approach to decongestion requires careful consideration of drug selection, dosing strategies, and monitoring parameters, all modified by the presence of kidney dysfunction.

Diuretics are classified according to the site of action in the nephron and the mechanism by which they inhibit the Nephron. The loop diuretics furosemide, bumetanide, and torsemide act from the lumen to inhibit the Na-K-2Cl cotransporter (NKCC2) along the thick ascending limb and macula densa. As organic anions, they bind within the translocation pocket on the transport protein by interacting with the chloride-binding site. Because they are larger than chloride, they are not transported through the pocket and thereby inhibit the transporter. Distal convoluted tubule diuretics (thiazides and thiazide-like drugs) are also organic anions that act in much the same manner but bind to the thiazide-sensitive NaCl cotransporter (NCC) along the distal convoluted tubule. These drugs both exert their effect from the luminal side of the tubule. Potassium-sparing diuretics include drugs that block apical sodium channels (amiloride and triamterene) and those that antagonize mineralocorticoid receptors (spironolactone, eplerenone and finerenone). The mineralocorticoid receptor antagonists act intracellularly and do not require tubular secretion. By contrast, loop diuretics must be secreted into the tubular lumen via organic anion transporters to inhibit NKCC2 from the luminal side [8].

16.2.3 Loop Diuretics: Pharmacokinetic Considerations in CKD

Loop diuretics inhibit the Na-K-2Cl cotransporter (NKCC2) along the thick ascending limb of Henle. As organic anions, these agents must be secreted into the tubular lumen to exert their effects, a process that becomes impaired in chronic kidney disease (CKD) as endogenous toxins and metabolic acidosis compete for organic anion transporters.

The pharmacokinetic profiles of these agents differ significantly, with important implications for CKD management. Furosemide exhibits absorption-limited kinetics with variable bioavailability, particularly in edematous states where gastrointestinal absorption may be further compromised. Its half-life is prolonged in kidney failure, necessitating dose adjustments. In contrast, bumetanide and torsemide demonstrate more predictable pharmacokinetics with preserved half-lives in CKD, though their relative potency compared to furosemide changes in the setting of kidney dysfunction. The traditionally cited equipotent dose ratio of 40:1 between furosemide and bumetanide declines in CKD [8, 9]. The DOSE-AHF trial randomized 308 patients to bolus versus continuous infusion and low-dose (equivalent to home dose) versus high-dose (2.5× home dose) strategies. No significant differences emerged between bolus and continuous infusion regarding symptom relief ($P = 0.47$) or renal function changes ($P = 0.45$). However, high-dose therapy showed a trend toward greater symptom improvement ($P = 0.06$) without significantly worsening renal function ($P = 0.21$) [9].

CKD substantially predisposes to a state of diuretic resistance, characterized by three key phenomena. First, the natriuretic dose-response curve shifts rightward due to impaired tubular secretion, requiring higher doses to achieve threshold concentrations in the tubular lumen [8]. Second, the ceiling natriuresis shifts downward; while fractional sodium excretion may be maintained, absolute sodium excretion is markedly reduced due to lower glomerular filtration rate [8]. Third, the braking phenomenon wherein natriuresis wanes despite persistent volume overload occurs through sympathetic nervous system stimulation, RAAS activation, and distal nephron remodeling that increases sodium reabsorption capacity in segments beyond the loop of Henle [10].

Practical management requires confirming that doses exceed the natriuretic threshold, typically assessed by observing increased urine output within 6 h of administration. If no effect occurs, doubling the dose based on the dose-response curve is appropriate. Increasing beyond the ceiling dose can still enhance net natriuresis by prolonging the duration above threshold concentration [8].

16.2.4 Sequential Nephron Blockade: Evidence-Based Adjuncts

When loop diuretics alone are insufficient, the logical next step is sequential nephron blockade. The traditional approach has been to add a thiazide or thiazide-like diuretic, which works by inhibiting the NaCl cotransporter (NCC) in the distal convoluted tubule (DCT), targeting the adaptive increased sodium reabsorption capacity that develops distally [11].

This strategy of sequential nephron blockade still holds true in CKD; although the conventional teaching was to avoid thiazide-like diuretics when the GFR falls below 30 because of concerns of lack of effectiveness. There is no head-to-head comparison trial between thiazides and thiazide-like drugs in cardiorenal syndrome. But the data from the HTN outcome trial suggests that chlorthalidone and metolazone are effective even at lower GFR and favors them over hydrochlorothiazide. Many clinicians prefer chlorthalidone to HCTZ because of its use in large clinical trials, greater potency, and longer half-life [12–15].

The CLOROTIC trial examined the addition of oral hydrochlorothiazide to standard loop diuretic therapy in acute decompensated heart failure. While combination treatment produced greater diuresis and weight loss at 72 h compared to placebo, this came at the expense of more frequent renal dysfunction. Sequential distal blockade thus offers enhanced natriuresis in resistant cases but requires careful renal monitoring and thoughtful agent selection based on baseline kidney function [16].

Another promising strategy for sequential blockade has emerged from recent trials targeting the proximal tubule, where approximately 65% of sodium reabsorption occurs. This physiologically rational approach blocks upstream sodium reabsorption to enhance the effectiveness of loop diuretics acting downstream. Two classes of agents, carbonic anhydrase inhibitors and SGLT-2 inhibitors, act at this proximal nephron segment and have demonstrated compelling benefits in acute decompensated heart failure with superior safety profiles compared to traditional distal tubular blockade [17, 18].

Acetazolamide was found to be a highly effective adjunctive agent in the ADVOR (Acetazolamide in Acute Decompensated Heart Failure with Volume Overload) trial, which randomized 519 patients to receive intravenous acetazolamide (500 mg daily) or placebo added to standard loop diuretics. Acetazolamide significantly improved successful decongestion within 3 days (42.2% vs 30.5%; RR 1.46) without worsening renal function or increasing adverse events, providing robust evidence as a safe, effective strategy for diuretic resistance [17]. The EMPULSE trial demonstrated that early initiation of empagliflozin during hospitalization improved the composite of mortality, heart failure events, and quality of life (win ratio 1.36; P = 0.0054), with benefits extending even to patients with eGFR as low as 20 mL/min/1.73 m [18].

16.2.5 Salvage Therapies

When conventional pharmacologic strategies, including optimized loop diuretics with sequential nephron blockade with distal and/or proximal tubular agents, fail to achieve adequate decongestion, salvage therapies may be considered for patients with refractory volume overload.

Hypertonic Saline Solution represents a counterintuitive but mechanistically sound salvage strategy for patients with severe diuretic resistance. The SMAC-HF study of 1771 patients with NYHA class III heart failure compared the combination of high-dose furosemide, hypertonic saline solution (HSS), and moderate sodium restriction (120 mmol/day) versus high-dose diuretics with stricter sodium restriction (80 mmol/day). Patients receiving HSS achieved significantly faster decongestion, shorter hospitalization (3.5 vs 5.5 days; $P < 0.0001$), and improved renal function [19]. The proposed mechanisms include expansion of intravascular volume leading to improved renal perfusion, enhanced delivery of loop diuretics to the nephron, mobilization of water from interstitial spaces into circulation, and attenuation of neurohormonal activation. This approach may benefit select patients with severe diuretic resistance and preserved renal reserve, though careful monitoring for hypernatremia and volume overload remains essential.

Ultrafiltration, in contrast, has failed to demonstrate superiority over optimized pharmacologic therapy and carries significant safety concerns. The CARRESS-HF trial randomized patients with acute heart failure and worsening renal function to stepped pharmacologic diuresis versus ultrafiltration. Despite theoretical advantages of controlled mechanical fluid removal, ultrafiltration resulted in greater increases in serum creatinine (mean change +0.23 mg/dL vs −0.04 mg/dL, $P = 0.003$) without additional weight loss (12.6 lbs. vs 12.1 lbs., $P = 0.58$) and was associated with a higher rate of serious adverse events (72% vs 57%; $P = 0.03$). These findings establish stepped pharmacologic therapy as the preferred approach, with ultrafiltration best reserved as a last resort for truly refractory cases unresponsive to all optimized pharmacologic strategies [20].

16.2.6 Integrating the Evidence—A Pragmatic Approach

The effective management of cardiorenal syndrome blends pharmacologic knowledge, physiologic assessment, and evidence-based trial data. Relieving congestion improves outcomes, but treatment must be individualized—guided by drug pharmacokinetics, renal function, and the adaptive responses of the kidney.

Loop diuretics remain first-line therapy for decongestion; choose the agent and route (IV versus oral) based on absorption considerations and renal function and escalate to achieve clear urine response (Table 16.2). If natriuresis is inadequate, consider sequential nephron blockade: (1) add a distal thiazide-like agent (metolazone or chlorthalidone) and monitor electrolytes closely—and recognize HCTZ may be ineffective at low GFR; (2) consider short course of proximal blockade with acetazolamide (supported by ADVOR) for augmenting early decongestion, particularly when loop diuretic response is suboptimal [17]; (3) SGLT-2 inhibitors should be used early in suitable patients given consistent cardiorenal benefit and modest decongestive effects [18, 21–23] and (4) MRAs should be continued or instituted for long-term neurohormonal benefit while watching for hyperkalemia—acute use for decongestion has not demonstrated short-term benefit (ATHENA-HF) [24]. Reserve ultrafiltration for refractory volume overload after optimized pharmacologic escalation given safety concerns (CARRESS-HF) [20]. Consider hypertonic saline strategies in select patients with diuretic resistance and preserved renal reserve (SMAC-HF), understanding patient selection and center experience influence outcomes [19].

Table 16.2 Pharmacologic characteristics and kidney function considerations for common diuretic classes

Class & examples	Mechanism	Key pharmacokinetics	GFR considerations & dosing	Clinical implications
Loop diuretics (furosemide, bumetanide, torsemide) [8] [15]	Inhibit NKCC2 in the thick ascending limb leading to increased sodium, potassium, and chloride excretion; increase magnesium and calcium excretion	Oral bioavailability: furosemide ~50% (variable); bumetanide and torsemide >80%. Furosemide has absorption-limited kinetics. Highly protein-bound; secreted via OAT1/3. Elimination: furosemide primarily renal (~50% unchanged; remainder glucuronidated); bumetanide renal and hepatic; torsemide predominantly hepatic. Half-lives: Furosemide 1.3–2 h; bumetanide 1–1.5 h; torsemide 3–6 h	CKD reduces loop diuretic responsiveness (higher threshold, lower ceiling) and often requires higher doses. Furosemide half-life increases in kidney failure; bumetanide and torsemide half-lives remain stable. Equipotent dose ratios (e.g., furosemide: bumetanide 40:1) narrow in CKD	Furosemide absorption can be impaired in edema. Torsemide and bumetanide have more predictable pharmacokinetics
Thiazide and thiazide-like diuretics (hydrochlorothiazide, chlorthalidone, metolazone) [8]	Inhibit the sodium–chloride cotransporter in the distal convoluted tubule. Metolazone also modestly inhibits proximal tubular sodium reabsorption	Oral bioavailability: Hydrochlorothiazide and chlorthalidone ~60–70%; metolazone ~70–90%. Half-lives: Hydrochlorothiazide ~6–15 h; chlorthalidone 40–60 h; metolazone 8–14 h. primarily excreted unchanged in urine	Chlorthalidone and metolazone retain antihypertensive and diuretic effects at GFR <30 mL/min. Metolazone often remains effective at GFR <20 mL/min. Hydrochlorothiazide is generally ineffective at GFR <30 mL/min. Half-lives may be prolonged in CKD	Use only after optimizing loop diuretics. Combination therapy increases the risk of hyponatremia, hypokalemia, and volume depletion

Mineralocorticoid receptor antagonists (spironolactone, eplerenone, finerenone) [25]	Block aldosterone at mineralocorticoid receptors. Spironolactone is steroidal and non-selective; eplerenone is steroidal and more selective; finerenone is non-steroidal and highly selective with added anti-inflammatory and antifibrotic activity	Metabolized primarily in the liver. Spironolactone metabolites have long half-lives (10–35 h) and accumulate in CKD. Eplerenone half-life 4–6 h. Finerenone half-life 2–3 h	High hyperkalemia risk in CKD often requires dose reduction, potassium binders, and close monitoring. Finerenone dosing is based on GFR and serum potassium and is not recommended at GFR <25 mL/min	Spironolactone causes more endocrine adverse effects
Carbonic anhydrase inhibitor (acetazolamide) [26]	Inhibits proximal tubular bicarbonate reabsorption leads to bicarbonate loss with modest natriuresis	Rapid absorption; half-life 4–8 h. Effect limited by downstream compensation	Limited diuretic benefit in CKD and may worsen metabolic acidosis. No dose adjustment needed for a single 500 mg IV dose but use cautiously in severe CKD	Can be used as an adjunct for decongestion when metabolic status allows; monitor for acidosis, hypokalemia, and hypotension
SGLT-2 inhibitors (empagliflozin, dapagliflozin) [27]	Block SGLT-2 in the proximal tubule leads to osmotic diuresis, mild natriuresis via reduced NHE3 activity, preferential interstitial fluid removal, and attenuation of RAAS and sympathetic activation	Half-life ~12 h. Metabolized by glucuronidation. Highly protein-bound; not removed by dialysis	Clearance decreases with impaired kidney function. Empagliflozin has been studied down to GFR 20 mL/min (avoid below this). Dapagliflozin should not be initiated at GFR <25 mL/min	Produces modest diuresis with relative preservation of intravascular volume and favorable neurohormonal effects

16.3 Neurohumoral Modulation and Novel Metabolic Agents

In chronic cardiorenal syndrome (CRS), maladaptive activation of neurohormonal pathways drives progressive heart and kidney dysfunction. Over time, key systems become hyperactivated—the renin–angiotensin–aldosterone system (RAAS), sympathetic nervous system (SNS), vasopressin axis, and inflammatory mediators—while counter-regulatory natriuretic peptides are downregulated. Interrupting this vicious cycle is critical to slowing disease progression. RAAS inhibitors (ACE inhibitors, ARBs) have long been cornerstones of therapy, providing mortality benefit in heart failure with reduced ejection fraction (HFrEF) and decreasing proteinuria chronic kidney disease (CKD) progression [28].

Similarly, angiotensin receptor–neprilysin inhibition (ARNI) enhances endogenous natriuretic peptides, augmenting cardiorenal protection [29]. Mineralocorticoid receptor antagonists (MRAs) counteract aldosterone-driven fibrosis in both organs. More recently, novel metabolic therapies (SGLT-2 inhibitors and GLP-1 receptor agonists) have shown powerful dual kidney–heart benefits beyond glycemic control. In each case, careful dose titration and monitoring (especially of renal function and potassium) is essential in CKD [30, 31]. Below we summarize the current evidence and practical considerations for each drug class, focusing on CKD patients.

16.3.1 Blockade of the RAAS System

Angiotensin-converting enzyme inhibitors and angiotensin receptor blockers interrupt the fundamental RAAS-mediated pathways driving sodium retention, vasoconstriction, and myocardial and renal fibrosis. These agents provide mortality benefit in heart failure with reduced ejection fraction (HFrEF) and slow progression of proteinuric CKD. In HFrEF, ACEi/ARBs are class I-recommended to reduce mortality [28]. 2020 Cochrane review of 31 CKD-stratified HF trials concluded that effects of ACEi/ARB on mortality and HF hospitalization in CKD remain uncertain because confidence intervals spanned benefit and harm (e.g., RR for all-cause mortality 0.85, 95% CI 0.70–1.02; 4 trials, 5003 CKD participants) [32].

Initiating and maintaining RAAS blockade in CRS requires monitoring and produces predictable changes in renal indices. Serum creatinine, eGFR, and potassium should be checked 3–7 days after initiation. An acceptable creatinine rise, typically up to 30% from baseline, often represents hemodynamic adjustment rather than true renal injury. Hyperkalemia is also a risk and can be managed with diet, medically, or require dialysis. Typical interventions include reducing the RAAS blocker dose, discontinue other potassium-raising medications, implement dietary potassium restriction, consider augmenting loop diuretic therapy if volume status permits, or add gastrointestinal potassium binders [31].

Sacubitril–valsartan combines neprilysin inhibition with AT1 receptor blockade. Neprilysin inhibition increases the level of endogenous natriuretic peptides, promoting vasodilation, natriuresis and improved hemodynamics. A 2020 meta-analysis specifically examining patients with heart failure and chronic kidney disease (3460 individuals) found that sacubitril/valsartan significantly increased eGFR (MD = 1.90 ml/min/1.73 m^2) and decreased blood pressure and NT-proBNP compared to RAS inhibitors [33].

Sacubitril is a prodrug that is converted by hepatic esterases into its active metabolite, LBQ657, which is predominantly eliminated through the urine. In CKD, reduced renal clearance leads to higher drug exposure, requiring careful dose adjustment at lower GFR levels. Safety and efficacy data are limited when GFR falls below 20 mL/min/1.73 m^2. Because LBQ657 is 94–97% protein-bound and not removed by either hemodialysis or peritoneal dialysis, dosing for dialysis patients is typically approached as if the GFR were <30 mL/min/1.73 m^2. The medication should also be avoided in cases of significant hepatic impairment. Initiation of sacubitril/valsartan can cause transient GFR drop and hyperkalemia, similar to ACEi/ARBs. Trials report slightly more hypotension but less cough or renal impairment than ACEi [29].

Aldosterone promotes sodium retention, myocardial and vascular fibrosis, endothelial dysfunction, and pro-inflammatory signaling, worsening both cardiac remodeling and renal fibrosis [34]. A Cochrane meta-analysis on heart failure medications in CKD found that aldosterone antagonists had uncertain effects on death (2 studies, 34 participants: RR 0.61, 95% CI 0.06 to 6.59; very low certainty evidence), but may increase the risk of hyperkalemia (3 studies, 826 participants: RR 2.91, 95% CI 2.03 to 4.17; $I^2 = 0\%$; low certainty evidence) [32]. A separate Cochrane review (44 studies, 5745 participants) examining aldosterone antagonists added to ACEi or ARBs for CKD progression found uncertain effects on kidney failure, death, and cardiovascular events, though they may reduce proteinuria. This analysis was limited by the inclusion of smaller, heterogeneous studies without adequate power for patient-level outcomes [35].

The non-steroidal MRA finerenone has shown substantial benefits in diabetic CKD. The FIDELITY pooled analysis combined data from FIDELIO-DKD and FIGARO-DKD trials in patients with CKD and type 2 diabetes, demonstrating a 14% reduction in composite cardiovascular outcomes (HR 0.86, 95% CI 0.78–0.95) and a 23% reduction in composite kidney outcomes (HR 0.77, 95% CI 0.67–0.88) with finerenone versus placebo. Importantly, this analysis confirmed benefits across the spectrum of CKD, irrespective of baseline atherosclerotic cardiovascular disease history (excluding those with HFrEF) [36].

When initiating or continuing MRAs in CKD, proactive potassium management is essential. Check serum potassium within 1 week of initiation, particularly in patients with eGFR <45 mL/min/1.73 m^2. Strategies to maintain MRA therapy include dietary potassium restriction, reducing or discontinuing other potassium-raising medications, optimizing loop diuretic dosing, and using gastrointestinal potassium binders (patiromer, sodium zirconium cyclosilicate).

16.3.2 SGLT-2 Inhibitors: Metabolic and Hemodynamic Benefits

SGLT-2 inhibitors have emerged as transformative agents in CRS, providing benefits through multiple mechanisms. They produce osmotic diuresis and natriuresis, preferentially reducing congestive volume, restore tubuloglomerular feedback, thereby reducing glomerular hyperfiltration and intraglomerular pressure, lower blood pressure and body weight, improve glycemic control in diabetes, and exhibit anti-inflammatory and antifibrotic effects [28].

The most comprehensive recent evidence comes from the SGLT-2 Inhibitor Meta-Analysis Cardio-Renal Trialists' Consortium (SMART-C), which pooled data from 11 trials with 78,607 patients across three major populations: diabetes at high atherosclerotic cardiovascular disease risk, heart failure, and chronic kidney disease [37]. This collaborative meta-analysis demonstrated that SGLT-2 inhibitors reduced major adverse cardiovascular events by 9% (HR 0.91, 95% CI 0.87–0.96) with consistent effects across all populations and subgroups. The benefit for cardiovascular death was driven primarily by reductions in HF death (HR 0.68) and sudden cardiac death (HR 0.86). For kidney outcomes specifically, the SMART-C analyses showed SGLT-2 inhibitors reduced CKD progression by 38% (HR 0.62, 95% CI 0.57–0.68) regardless of baseline eGFR or albuminuria, with benefits extending to patients with eGFR <30 mL/min/1.73 m^2 (HR 0.71, 95% CI 0.60–0.83) [36, 37].

SGLT-2i cause an initial eGFR dip that stabilizes, followed by a flatter decline over time. This reflects reduced hyperfiltration rather than injury and should not prompt discontinuation. Volume depletion and hypotension are possible, especially in patients on high diuretic doses, so blood pressure should be monitored. Genitourinary infections are slightly more common.

16.3.3 Beta-Blockers: Modulating Sympathetic Overactivity

Beta-blockers blunt the maladaptive sympathetic overactivity that increases heart rate, myocardial oxygen demand, and arrhythmic risk while promoting adverse remodeling. These agents reduce cardiovascular mortality, heart failure hospitalizations, and sudden cardiac death in HFrEF [38].

A Cochrane meta-analysis found that treatment with beta-blockers may reduce the risk of all-cause death in CKD patients with heart failure (4 studies including CIBIS-II, MERIT-HF, and SENIORS subgroups, 3136 participants: RR 0.69, 95% CI 0.60 to 0.79; I^2 = 0%; moderate certainty evidence). Beta-blockers may also decrease hospitalization for heart failure (3 studies, 2287 participants: RR 0.67, 95% CI 0.43 to 1.05; I^2 = 87%; low certainty evidence) [32].

16.3.4 GLP-1 Receptor Agonists: Emerging Cardiorenal Protection

Glucagon-like peptide-1 receptor agonists provide cardiorenal benefits through multiple mechanisms. Large, sustained weight reductions, improved glycemic control, and lower systolic blood pressure reduce cardiac workload, insulin resistance, and hyperfiltration. Proposed direct renal mechanisms include albuminuria reduction, improved endothelial function, decreased inflammation and oxidative stress, and favorable intrarenal hemodynamic effects. Cardiovascular benefits include proven reduction in major adverse cardiovascular events. The FLOW study randomly assigned patients with type 2 diabetes and an eGFR of 50 to 75 ml/min and uACR of >300 and <5000 mg/G or an eGFR of 25 to <50 ml/min and uACR of >100 and <5000 mg/G to receive subcutaneous semaglutide at a dose of 1.0 mg weekly or placebo and found a 20% lower hazard of all-cause mortality, 29% lower hazard of cardiovascular mortality, and improved annual eGFR slope of 1.16 ml/min. Subgroup analysis demonstrated a more pronounced benefit in patients with chronic heart failure (HR of composite outcome of 0.67 vs 0.79 [39].

Because most GLP-1 RAs are not renally cleared (except exenatide, which is contraindicated if eGFR <30 mL/min/1.73 m^2), agents such as liraglutide, semaglutide, and dulaglutide can be used in moderate CKD without dose adjustment. They are especially valuable in diabetic CKD with obesity or uncontrolled glucose, as they address multiple cardiometabolic risk factors simultaneously. The FLOW trial excluded patients with eGFR <25 mL/min/1.73 m^2, so data in advanced CKD remain limited. When initiating GLP-1 receptor agonists in patients with cardiorenal syndrome, clinicians must anticipate gastrointestinal side effects (nausea, vomiting), which can lead to volume depletion and acute kidney injury, particularly in patients already on aggressive diuretic regimens. A proactive reduction in loop diuretic dose may be necessary upon initiation to prevent hypotension and prerenal azotemia. Additionally, because these agents delay gastric emptying, they may alter the absorption kinetics of oral medications [8].

16.3.5 Integrating the Evidence: A Practical Framework

The contemporary approach to CRS management has evolved toward a "quadruple therapy" framework in eligible patients, layering multiple complementary mechanisms: RAAS blockade (ACEi/ARB or ARNI), mineralocorticoid receptor antagonism (preferably finerenone in diabetic CKD), SGLT-2 inhibition, and GLP-1 receptor agonism when indicated. This combination addresses sodium retention, neurohormonal activation, fibrosis, inflammation, and metabolic dysfunction simultaneously (Table 16.3).

Table 16.3 Neurohumoral and metabolic agents in chronic cardiorenal syndrome: mechanisms, pharmacology, and kidney function considerations

Class & examples	Mechanism	Key pharmaco-kinetics	Kidney function considerations & dosing	Clinical implications
RAAS inhibitors (ACE inhibitors, ARBs) [28]	Block RAAS-mediated vasoconstriction, sodium retention, and fibrosis. Reduce afterload and proteinuria	Primarily hepatic metabolism; renally excreted metabolites vary by agent	Check creatinine, estimated GFR, and potassium 3–7 days after initiation or dose change. A creatinine rise up to ~30% is expected due to hemodynamic effects. Hyperkalemia risk increases as GFR declines	Foundational therapy in heart failure with reduced ejection fraction and proteinuric CKD. Dose titration often limited by potassium or blood pressure
ARNI (sacubitril–valsartan) [29]	Neprilysin inhibition increases endogenous natriuretic peptides; valsartan blocks AT1 receptor. Improves hemodynamics and reduces fibrosis	Sacubitril metabolized to LBQ657 via esterases; LBQ657 predominantly renally cleared. Valsartan minimally metabolized. Both are highly protein bound	Reduced renal clearance of LBQ657 increases exposure in CKD; use lower starting doses when estimated GFR <30 mL/min per 1.73 m^2. Not removed by hemodialysis or peritoneal dialysis. Safety data limited for estimated GFR <20	May improve kidney function markers and reduce neurohormonal activation. Risk of hypotension and hyperkalemia similar to other RAAS blockers
Mineralocorticoid receptor antagonists (spironolactone, eplerenone, finerenone) [34, 36]	Block aldosterone-mediated sodium retention, inflammation, and fibrosis in heart and kidney	Spironolactone has long-lived active metabolites; eplerenone and finerenone have shorter half-lives and fewer off-target actions. All are hepatically metabolized	Hyperkalemia risk increases as GFR declines. Frequent monitoring is required, especially at estimated GFR <45 mL/min per 1.73 m^2. Finerenone not recommended below estimated GFR 25	Provide cardiac and renal protection but require active potassium management. Finerenone has lower endocrine side effects and lower hyperkalemia risk

(continued)

Table 16.3 (continued)

Class & examples	Mechanism	Key pharmaco-kinetics	Kidney function considerations & dosing	Clinical implications
SGLT-2 inhibitors (empagliflozin, dapagliflozin, canagliflozin) [21–23]	Reduce proximal tubular glucose and sodium reabsorption → natriuresis, osmotic diuresis, restoration of tubuloglomerular feedback, and lower intraglomerular pressure. Also reduce inflammation and fibrosis	Metabolized by glucuronidation. High protein binding. Not dialyzable	Initial estimated GFR dip is expected and usually benign. Empagliflozin supported down to estimated GFR 20; dapagliflozin not initiated below estimated GFR 25. Canagliflozin utilized in GFR 30–90. Volume depletion may occur at low GFR or with high diuretic use	Provide kidney and cardiovascular protection across CKD severity, including advanced CKD, with slower long-term estimated GFR decline
Beta-blockers (carvedilol, metoprolol succinate, bisoprolol) [38]	Reduce sympathetic drive, lower heart rate and arrhythmia risk, and improve myocardial oxygen balance	Hepatic metabolism predominates; renal clearance varies by agent	Generally safe across CKD stages with minimal dose adjustment. Hypotension and bradycardia risk higher in advanced CKD or volume overload	Essential therapy for heart failure with reduced ejection fraction; reduce mortality and sudden cardiac death
GLP-1 receptor agonists (liraglutide, semaglutide, dulaglutide) [40]	Improve glycemic control, reduce body weight and blood pressure, and exert anti-inflammatory and vascular effects. May reduce albuminuria and improve endothelial function	Most agents not renally cleared; exenatide is the exception and should not be used at estimated GFR <30	Liraglutide, semaglutide, and dulaglutide can be used in moderate CKD without dose adjustment. Limited evidence exists when estimated GFR <25	Provide cardiovascular protection and may slow CKD progression, especially in diabetic CKD with obesity or poor glycemic control

Individual treatment must be tailored to renal function with appropriate dose adjustments and vigilant safety monitoring, particularly for hyperkalemia when combining RAAS blockers with MRAs. The evidence supports aggressive use of these agents in CKD to fundamentally alter the natural history of cardiorenal disease, but successful implementation requires systematic monitoring and proactive management of predictable adverse effects.

Declarations

Competing Interests The author(s) has no competing interests to declare that are relevant to the content of this manuscript.

Ethics Approval The author(s) declares that this manuscript does not include primary research with human participants.

The author(s) declares that this manuscript does not include primary studies involving animals.

References

1. Kumar U, Wettersten N, Garimella PS. Cardiorenal syndrome: pathophysiology. Cardiol Clin. 2019;37(3):251–65.
2. Rangaswami J, et al. Cardiorenal syndrome: classification, pathophysiology, diagnosis, and treatment strategies: a scientific statement from the American Heart Association. Circulation. 2019;139(16):e840–78.
3. Ronco C, et al. Cardio-renal syndromes: report from the consensus conference of the acute dialysis quality initiative. Eur Heart J. 2010;31(6):703–11.
4. Ronco C, et al. Cardiorenal syndrome. J Am Coll Cardiol. 2008;52(19):1527–39.
5. Francis GS. Neurohumoral activation and progression of heart failure: hypothetical and clinical considerations. J Cardiovasc Pharmacol. 1998;32(Suppl 1):S16–21.
6. Sweitzer NK, et al. Comparison of clinical features and outcomes of patients hospitalized with heart failure and normal ejection fraction (> or =55%) versus those with mildly reduced (40% to 55%) and moderately to severely reduced (<40%) fractions. Am J Cardiol. 2008;101(8):1151–6.
7. McCallum W, Sarnak MJ. Cardiorenal syndrome in the hospital. Clin J Am Soc Nephrol. 2023;18(7):933–45.
8. Ellison DH. Clinical pharmacology in diuretic use. Clin J Am Soc Nephrol. 2019;14(8):1248–57.
9. Felker GM, et al. Diuretic strategies in patients with acute decompensated heart failure. N Engl J Med. 2011;364(9):797–805.
10. Wilcox CS, et al. Response of the kidney to furosemide. I. Effects of salt intake and renal compensation. J Lab Clin Med. 1983;102(3):450–8.
11. Rao VS, et al. Compensatory distal reabsorption drives diuretic resistance in human heart failure. J Am Soc Nephrol. 2017;28(11):3414–24.
12. Kidney Disease: Improving Global Outcomes (KDIGO) Blood Pressure Work Group. KDIGO 2021 Clinical practice guideline for the management of blood pressure in chronic kidney disease. Kidney Int. 2021;99(3s):S1–S87.
13. Agarwal R, et al. Chlorthalidone for hypertension in advanced chronic kidney disease. N Engl J Med. 2021;385(27):2507–19.
14. Whelton PK, et al. 2017 ACC/AHA/AAPA/ABC/ACPM/AGS/APhA/ASH/ASPC/NMA/PCNA guideline for the prevention, detection, evaluation, and Management of High Blood

Pressure in adults: a report of the American College of Cardiology/American Heart Association Task Force on Clinical Practice Guidelines. J Am Coll Cardiol. 2018;71(19):e127–248.
15. Ali S, et al. Revisiting diuretic choice in chronic kidney disease. Curr Opin Nephrol Hypertens. 2022;31(5):406–13.
16. Trullàs JC, et al. Combining loop with thiazide diuretics for decompensated heart failure: the CLOROTIC trial. Eur Heart J. 2023;44(5):411–21.
17. Mullens W, et al. Acetazolamide in acute decompensated heart failure with volume overload. N Engl J Med. 2022;387(13):1185–95.
18. Voors AA, et al. The SGLT2 inhibitor empagliflozin in patients hospitalized for acute heart failure: a multinational randomized trial. Nat Med. 2022;28(3):568–74.
19. Smith CE, et al. Multidisciplinary group clinic appointments: the self-management and Care of Heart Failure (SMAC-HF) trial. Circ Heart Fail. 2014;7(6):888–94.
20. Bart BA, et al. Ultrafiltration in decompensated heart failure with cardiorenal syndrome. N Engl J Med. 2012;367(24):2296–304.
21. Heerspink HJL, et al. Dapagliflozin in patients with chronic kidney disease. N Engl J Med. 2020;383(15):1436–46.
22. Perkovic V, et al. Canagliflozin and renal outcomes in type 2 diabetes and nephropathy. N Engl J Med. 2019;380(24):2295–306.
23. The EMPA-KIDNEY Collaborative Group. Empagliflozin in Patients with Chronic Kidney Disease. N Engl J Med. 2023;388(2):117–27.
24. Butler J, et al. Efficacy and safety of spironolactone in acute heart failure: the ATHENA-HF randomized clinical trial. JAMA Cardiol. 2017;2(9):950–8.
25. Harrington JL, et al. Nonsteroidal and steroidal mineralocorticoid antagonists: rationale, evidence, and unanswered questions. JACC Heart Fail. 2025;13(10):102637.
26. Van Berkel MA, Elefritz JL. Evaluating off-label uses of acetazolamide. Am J Health Syst Pharm. 2018;75(8):524–31.
27. Lee YH, Lim S, Davies MJ. Cardiometabolic and renal benefits of sodium-glucose cotransporter 2 inhibitors. Nat Rev Endocrinol. 2025;21(12):783–98.
28. Pantelis S, A.U.o.T.H.H.T.G. st Department of Nephrology. Use of ACEi/ARBs, SGLT2 inhibitors and MRAs can help us reach the therapeutic ceiling in CKD. Clin Kidney J. 2025;17(2):sfae014.
29. Reed DN, Preeti P, Mirembe R. Sacubitril-Valsartan. In: StatPearls [Internet]. Treasure Island (FL): StatPearls Publishing; 2024.
30. Spasovski G, et al. A new Hope on the horizon for kidney and cardiovascular protection with SGLT2 inhibitors, GLP-1 receptor agonists, and mineralocorticoid receptor antagonists in type 2 diabetic and chronic kidney disease patients. Metab Syndr Relat Disord. 2024;22(3):170–8.
31. Hundemer GL, Sood MM. Hyperkalemia with RAAS inhibition: mechanism, clinical significance, and management. Pharmacol Res. 2021;172:105835.
32. Lunney M, et al. Pharmacological interventions for heart failure in people with chronic kidney disease. Cochrane Database Syst Rev. 2020;2(2):Cd012466.
33. Kang H, et al. Effects of sacubitril/valsartan in patients with heart failure and chronic kidney disease: a meta-analysis. Eur J Pharmacol. 2020;884:173444.
34. Ferreira João P, et al. Steroidal MRA across the Spectrum of renal function. JACC: Heart Failure. 2022;10(11):842–50.
35. Chung EY, et al. Aldosterone antagonists in addition to renin angiotensin system antagonists for preventing the progression of chronic kidney disease. Cochrane Database Syst Rev. 2020;10(10):Cd007004.
36. Rajiv A, et al. Cardiovascular and kidney outcomes with finerenone in patients with type 2 diabetes and chronic kidney disease: the FIDELITY pooled analysis. Eur Heart J. 2025;43(6):474.
37. Apperloo EM, et al. Efficacy and safety of SGLT2 inhibitors with and without glucagon-like peptide 1 receptor agonists: a SMART-C collaborative meta-analysis of randomised controlled trials. Lancet Diabetes Endocrinol. 2024;12(8):545–57.

38. Badve SV, et al. Effects of beta-adrenergic antagonists in patients with chronic kidney disease: a systematic review and meta-analysis. J Am Coll Cardiol. 2011;58(11):1152–61.
39. Rossing P, et al. The rationale, design and baseline data of FLOW, a kidney outcomes trial with once-weekly semaglutide in people with type 2 diabetes and chronic kidney disease. Nephrol Dial Transplant. 2023;38(9):2041–51.
40. Badve SV, et al. Effects of GLP-1 receptor agonists on kidney and cardiovascular disease outcomes: a meta-analysis of randomised controlled trials. Lancet Diabetes Endocrinol. 2025;13(1):15–28.

Chapter 17
Chronic Kidney Disease and Cardiovascular Surgery: Bridging the Gap

Grigore Tinica, Valeriu Ardei, and Alexandru Burlacu

17.1 Introduction

Chronic kidney disease (CKD) represents one of the most powerful amplifiers of risk in patients undergoing cardiovascular (CV) surgery. As the global burden of CKD continues to rise—largely driven by population aging, diabetes, hypertension, and metabolic syndrome—an increasing proportion of patients referred for coronary artery bypass grafting (CABG), valvular surgery, or thoracic aortic interventions present with impaired renal function. This epidemiologic overlap creates a clinical scenario in which the pathophysiological consequences of CKD intersect with the hemodynamic, inflammatory and metabolic disturbances inherent to cardiac surgery, resulting in a disproportionately high incidence of perioperative morbidity and mortality.

CKD imposes a series of systemic derangements: chronic inflammation, oxidative stress, uremic toxin accumulation, anemia, endothelial dysfunction, vascular calcification, deranged mineral metabolism and impaired volume regulation. These abnormalities collectively shape a biological environment that increases susceptibility to ischemia-reperfusion injury, hemodynamic instability, postoperative acute kidney injury (AKI), prolonged mechanical ventilation, infection, bleeding, arrhythmias and long-term mortality. Importantly, even mild to moderate reductions in estimated glomerular filtration rate (eGFR), traditionally considered low risk, have been consistently shown to predict unfavorable postoperative outcomes.

G. Tinica · A. Burlacu
Institute of Cardiovascular Diseases "Prof. Dr. George I.M. Georgescu", Iasi, Romania

University of Medicine and Pharmacy "Grigore T. Popa", Iasi, Romania

V. Ardei (✉)
Institute of Cardiovascular Diseases "Prof. Dr. George I.M. Georgescu", Iasi, Romania

A. Covic, A. Burlacu (eds.), *Renal Dysfunction in Cardiovascular Pathologies*,
https://doi.org/10.1007/978-3-032-25434-4_17

Despite substantial progress in perioperative medicine, a significant "gap" persists between evidence-based strategies for CKD management and their application in the context of complex cardiac surgical pathways. Existing cardiac surgery risk models, such as EuroSCORE II and the Society of Thoracic Surgeons (STS) score, acknowledge renal dysfunction as a critical variable, yet they often underestimate risk in advanced CKD stages or dialysis-dependent patients. The KDIGO guidelines provide standardized definitions for CKD and AKI, but their integration into perioperative decision-making remains inconsistent across institutions and clinical specialties. Consequently, many high-risk CKD patients enter surgery without optimal preoperative correction of anemia, electrolyte disturbances, metabolic acidosis, mineral bone disease, or volume overload—factors that directly influence postoperative outcomes.

Cardiopulmonary bypass (CPB) introduces another layer of complexity. Nonpulsatile flow, hemodilution, systemic inflammatory activation, oxidative stress, and microembolic phenomena increase the vulnerability of an already compromised kidney. While off-pump CABG has been proposed as a renal-sparing alternative, randomized studies provide mixed results, and benefits appear most pronounced in highly selected advanced-CKD populations. Additionally, emerging data suggest that renal medullary hypoxia, impaired autoregulation and the loss of nephron reserve contribute significantly to postoperative AKI, independent of CPB exposure.

Bridging this gap requires a multidisciplinary, protocol-driven approach that integrates nephrology, cardiology, anesthesiology, and intensive care. Key components include accurate preoperative staging of CKD, optimization of comorbidities, individualized hemodynamic goals, careful fluid and perfusion management, avoidance of nephrotoxic exposures, and early detection of renal stress. Novel strategies—such as machine-learning risk calculators, precision hemodynamics, goal-directed perfusion during CPB, pharmacologic renoprotective agents, and standardized postoperative AKI bundles—are redefining the modern landscape of renal protection in cardiac surgery.

The aim of this chapter is to provide a comprehensive and updated analysis of the interaction between CKD and cardiovascular surgery, integrating the latest evidence, guideline recommendations, mechanistic insights and practical perioperative management strategies. Each section will explore a critical dimension of this complex relationship—epidemiology, pathophysiology, preoperative optimization, intraoperative considerations, postoperative outcomes and emerging directions—ultimately delineating a framework for improving care and reducing risk in this increasingly prevalent patient population.

17.2 Epidemiology and Pathophysiology

17.2.1 Epidemiology of CKD in Patients Undergoing Cardiovascular Surgery

Chronic kidney disease is increasingly prevalent worldwide, affecting an estimated 9–13% of the global population. The burden is even more pronounced among patients requiring cardiovascular surgery, where CKD prevalence ranges from 25% to 40% depending on the cohort and definition used. Several factors contribute to this overlap: the aging population, the rising incidence of diabetes and hypertension, and improved long-term survival of patients with coronary and valvular disease.

Large registry analyses indicate that even early-stage CKD (eGFR 60–89 ml/min/1.73 m^2) independently increases postoperative mortality and major adverse cardiovascular events (MACE) after CABG or valve surgery. Moderate CKD (eGFR 30–59) doubles operative mortality, while severe CKD and dialysis dependence increase risk four-to eight-fold. These risks persist even after adjusting for age, diabetes, left ventricular dysfunction, and procedural complexity.

Patients with CKD also exhibit higher rates of postoperative acute kidney injury, between 30% and 40% in most contemporary series. The KDIGO consortium emphasizes that preexisting CKD is the single most important risk factor for developing cardiac surgery–associated AKI. This creates a compounding effect: CKD predisposes to AKI, and AKI accelerates long-term CKD progression, a phenomenon known as the "cardio-renal continuum."

The epidemiologic burden is further amplified by the increasing use of complex surgical interventions such as redo sternotomies, combined CABG–valve procedures, and extensive aortic repairs—procedures that inherently increase exposure to ischemia, CPB, contrast agents, and hemodynamic instability.

17.2.2 Pathophysiology Linking CKD and Cardiovascular Surgical Risk

The pathophysiological interplay between CKD and cardiovascular surgery is multifactorial, involving structural, inflammatory, metabolic, and hemodynamic mechanisms that synergistically increase perioperative vulnerability.

17.2.2.1 Endothelial Dysfunction and Vascular Calcification

CKD is characterized by pervasive endothelial dysfunction driven by oxidative stress, chronic inflammation, asymmetric dimethylarginine excess, and impaired nitric oxide bioavailability. These abnormalities impair vasoreactivity, promote microcirculatory dysfunction, and exacerbate renal susceptibility to ischemia during CPB.

Simultaneously, CKD accelerates medial and intimal vascular calcification due to hyperphosphatemia, secondary hyperparathyroidism, and dysregulated fibroblast growth factor 23 (FGF-23) signaling. This leads to increased arterial stiffness, impaired autoregulation, and higher myocardial oxygen demand intraoperatively.

17.2.2.2 Chronic Inflammation and Immune Dysregulation

CKD is a pro-inflammatory state characterized by elevated IL-6, TNF-α, CRP, and oxidative stress markers. Cardiopulmonary bypass adds an additional inflammatory insult through complement activation, leukocyte activation, and the release of reactive oxygen species. The synergistic inflammatory response contributes to increased risks of postoperative AKI, vasoplegia, sepsis, delirium, and prolonged mechanical ventilation.

17.2.2.3 Uremic Toxins and Metabolic Derangements

Retention of uremic toxins, such as indoxyl sulfate and p-cresol sulfate, induces mitochondrial dysfunction, endothelial injury and myocardial fibrosis. These toxins impair renal perfusion autoregulation and aggravate susceptibility to ischemia–reperfusion injury. CKD-associated metabolic derangements, including metabolic acidosis and electrolyte imbalances, further impair hemodynamic stability during surgery.

17.2.2.4 Anemia and Impaired Oxygen Delivery

Anemia is prevalent even in early CKD and is frequently under-recognized preoperatively. Reduced hemoglobin diminishes oxygen delivery to the myocardium and kidneys, contributing to perioperative ischemia and higher transfusion requirements—a known predictor of mortality and AKI after cardiac surgery.

17.2.2.5 Volume Overload, RAAS Activation and Hemodynamic Instability

CKD patients have reduced ability to regulate sodium and water balance, predisposing them to volume overload, hypertension, and left ventricular hypertrophy. Activation of the renin–angiotensin–aldosterone system (RAAS) and sympathetic overactivity further amplify perioperative hemodynamic instability. These factors complicate fluid management during and after CPB, where both hypovolemia and excessive hemodilution can worsen renal perfusion.

17.2.2.6 Loss of Nephron Reserve and Impaired Autoregulation

Reduced nephron mass limits the kidney's ability to respond to stress. In CKD, renal autoregulation curves are flattened, meaning that even brief episodes of hypotension during anesthesia or CPB can precipitate ischemic tubular injury. This explains why CKD patients can develop severe AKI even with apparently stable intraoperative hemodynamics.

17.2.3 Summary of Mechanistic Interactions

The convergence of endothelial dysfunction, vascular calcification, inflammation, metabolic derangements, anemia, impaired autoregulation, and uremic toxin burden creates a profoundly vulnerable physiologic substrate. When exposed to the stresses of cardiovascular surgery—ischemia reperfusion, CPB, hemodilution, systemic inflammation—the CKD kidney is uniquely predisposed to injury. This biological vulnerability forms the mechanistic basis for the elevated rates of AKI, prolonged ICU stay, cardiovascular events, and mortality observed in this population.

17.3 Risk Stratification and Preoperative Assessment

17.3.1 Limitations of Traditional Surgical Risk Models in CKD

Traditional perioperative risk models—EuroSCORE II and the Society of Thoracic Surgeons (STS) calculator—incorporate renal dysfunction but often underestimate risk in patients with moderate to severe CKD. Several contemporary studies demonstrate calibration drift of these models in the modern cardiac surgical population, particularly in the context of rising comorbidity burden.

Recent observations from multicenter cohorts indicate that albuminuria, independently of eGFR, is strongly associated with postoperative mortality and AKI but is not included in current cardiac risk models. The KDIGO 2022 update reinforces this, recommending that both eGFR and albuminuria be used to stratify perioperative renal risk.

Thus, the contemporary view is that traditional tools, while useful, must be supplemented with CKD-specific biomarkers, functional assessments, and individualized hemodynamic parameters.

17.3.2 Contemporary Approaches to Renal Risk Stratification

17.3.2.1 KDIGO-Based CKD Staging and Albuminuria

KDIGO's update underscores the prognostic value of albuminuria for both cardiovascular and renal outcomes. Large-scale data from the Chronic Kidney Disease Prognosis Consortium confirm that albuminuria >30 mg/g substantially increases the risk of perioperative AKI, independent of eGFR.

17.3.2.2 Biomarker-Based Risk Prediction

Recent advances highlight the role of novel functional and damage biomarkers in predicting CSA-AKI: TIMP-2 IGFBP7 (cell-cycle arrest markers), validated in high-risk cardiac surgery patients to predict AKI before creatinine rises. NGAL (neutrophil gelatinase-associated lipocalin)—reliable in predicting early AKI in CPB patients. Soluble urokinase-type plasminogen activator receptor (suPAR)—a strong predictor of AKI, cardiac events, and mortality in CKD patients undergoing cardiac surgery. Cystatin C is superior to creatinine in early AKI detection and long-term renal prognostication. In 2023, a consortium of perioperative nephrology experts recommended routine incorporation of at least one early stress biomarker in high-risk CKD surgical patients.

17.3.2.3 Machine-Learning and Predictive Analytics

AI-driven models outperform conventional scoring systems in CKD populations. Examples include: XGBoost algorithms trained on >50,000 CPB procedures predicting AKI with AUC 0.87, outperforming STS and EuroSCORE II; Deep learning–based hemodynamic instability forecasts using intraoperative arterial waveform data; Random forest models integrating creatinine trajectory, albuminuria, and comorbidities showing a 25–30% improvement in AKI prediction accuracy.

17.3.3 Preoperative Optimization of the CKD Patient

17.3.3.1 Hemodynamic Evaluation and Volume Management

Updated perioperative guidelines emphasize: objective volume status assessment using lung ultrasound, IVC ultrasound, or bioimpedance spectroscopy and individualized hemodynamic targets to avoid both hypovolemia and congestion.

Overhydration correlates with increased risk of CPB-associated AKI, while preoperative dehydration increases susceptibility to ischemic tubular injury.

17.3.3.2 Correction of Anemia and Iron Deficiency

CKD-related anemia carries major implications for postoperative outcomes. Evidence-based strategies include: IV iron therapy when TSAT <20% and judicious use of erythropoiesis-stimulating agents (ESAs) in severe anemia. Preoperative anemia doubles the risk of AKI and increases transfusion requirements; each unit of transfused RBCs increases AKI risk by 15–20%.

17.3.3.3 Medication Management

Recent recommendations include:

- Withholding SGLT2 inhibitors 3 days pre-op to avoid euglycemic ketoacidosis.
- Careful consideration of ACEi/ARB continuation vs. temporary withholding.
- Avoiding NSAIDs and nephrotoxic antibiotics before surgery.

17.3.3.4 Evaluation of Mineral Bone Disease and Electrolytes

CKD mineral bone disease contributes to arrhythmogenic risk, vascular stiffness and bleeding.

For preoperative correction of phosphate, calcium, and magnesium, vitamin D deficiency is recommended by recent nephrology reviews.

17.3.3.5 Integrating Multidisciplinary Evaluation

Modern perioperative care requires a coordinated approach. In 2023, the International Cardio-Renal Collaboration Group proposed a structured Cardio-Renal Preoperative Pathway, including:

- Early nephrology involvement (≥2 weeks pre-op).
- KDIGO-based renal staging + albuminuria.
- Biomarker-guided risk assessment.
- Preoperative correction of anemia, electrolytes and volume.
- Decision-making regarding CPB strategies and off-pump feasibility.
- Postoperative AKI surveillance bundle.

17.4 Intraoperative Considerations

17.4.1 Impact of Cardiopulmonary Bypass on the CKD Kidney

CPB imposes significant physiological stress on renal function, which is magnified in CKD due to impaired autoregulatory capacity, endothelial dysfunction and diminished nephron reserve. The kidney's susceptibility arises from nonpulsatile flow, hemodilution, systemic inflammatory activation, oxidative stress and microembolization—mechanisms extensively documented in contemporary mechanistic studies.

17.4.1.1 Nonpulsatile Flow and Autoregulatory Failure

Nonpulsatile perfusion reduces cortical oxygen delivery and disrupts renal microcirculation, especially in CKD patients who already exhibit blunted autoregulatory curves. Because CKD kidneys require higher perfusion pressures to maintain filtration, intraoperative hypotension during CPB—particularly MAP <65 mmHg—is strongly associated with postoperative AKI.

17.4.1.2 Hemodilution and Reduced Oxygen-Carrying Capacity

Excessive hemodilution (hematocrit <24%) reduces oxygen delivery to the renal medulla, leading to ischemic tubular injury. A 2020 multicenter analysis demonstrated that maintaining hematocrit ≥28% during CPB reduced AKI rates by 20%, particularly in CKD stages 3–5. This finding has influenced newer perfusion targets in many high-volume centers.

17.4.1.3 Inflammatory and Oxidative Stress Response

CPB triggers complement activation (C3a, C5a), cytokine release (IL-6, IL-8), and neutrophil-endothelial interactions, amplifying the already heightened inflammatory milieu of CKD. In CKD, accumulation of uremic toxins increases mitochondrial vulnerability to oxidative stress, contributing to a disproportionately high incidence of ischemia–reperfusion injury.

17.4.2 Off-Pump Coronary Artery Bypass Surgery (OPCAB) in CKD

The role of off-pump CABG as a renoprotective strategy remains debated.

17.4.2.1 Evidence Supporting Renal Benefit

Several recent meta-analyses suggest that OPCAB may reduce AKI in high-risk patients:

- A 2021 meta-analysis of >35,000 patients found a 15–20% reduction in AKI with OPCAB, most pronounced in CKD stages 4–5.
- A nationwide registry analysis showed OPCAB reduces the need for postoperative RRT in CKD patients by ~30%.

17.4.2.2 Evidence Against Universal Benefit

Other contemporary trials show mixed results:

The EXCEL-OPCAB follow-up (2023) found no significant difference in kidney injury biomarkers or mortality compared with CPB in moderate CKD.

OPCAB may compromise graft patency, particularly for the right coronary system, which can indirectly worsen long-term outcomes.

17.4.2.3 Consensus Interpretation

OPCAB appears beneficial primarily in advanced CKD or dialysis-dependent patients, and when performed by experienced surgeons; otherwise, benefits are less consistent.

17.4.3 Individualized Perfusion Strategies and Goal-Directed CPB

In the last 5 years, a major paradigm shift has emerged: goal-directed perfusion (GDP). GDP integrates oxygen delivery (DO_2), indexed pump flow, hematocrit targets, and real-time metabolic monitoring.

17.4.3.1 Oxygen Delivery Thresholds

Recent studies indicate that DO_2 <270 mL/min/m^2 during CPB is an independent predictor of postoperative AKI. CKD patients demonstrate even higher vulnerability, with some centers using DO_2 targets of 300–330 mL/min/m^2.

17.4.3.2 Flow Targets and Temperature Management

GDP strategies typically include:

- Maintaining indexed flow ≥2.4 L/min/m^2.
- Limiting hemodilution.
- Avoiding deep hypothermia when possible.

17.4.3.3 Pulsatile vs. Nonpulsatile Perfusion

Modern perfusion technology has enabled both intermittent and continuous pulsatile flow during cardiopulmonary bypass, prompting renewed interest in its potential benefits for renal protection. Although Doppler-based studies consistently show that pulsatile perfusion enhances cortical renal blood flow, large randomized trials have not demonstrated a definitive reduction in acute kidney injury or overall mortality. Despite this incomplete evidence, many specialists recommend considering pulsatile perfusion in patients with advanced CKD or those with marked vascular calcification, since even modest improvements in microcirculatory dynamics may confer clinically meaningful advantages in this particularly fragile population.

17.4.4 Intraoperative Hemodynamic Management

17.4.4.1 Blood Pressure Targets

Maintaining optimal blood pressure during CPB is crucial for preserving renal perfusion in CKD patients. Recent investigations emphasize that mean arterial pressure should be maintained at or above 70–75 mmHg throughout CPB, as short periods of hypotension—particularly MAP values below 60 mmHg lasting more than 10 min—significantly increase the risk of postoperative AKI. These findings underscore the need for vigilant monitoring and rapid intervention to prevent injurious drops in renal perfusion pressure.

17.4.4.2 Vasopressor Selection

The choice of vasopressor plays an equally important role in protecting kidney function during cardiac surgery. Current practice generally favors norepinephrine as the first-line agent due to its balanced hemodynamic effects and limited adverse impact on renal blood flow. When catecholamines prove insufficient, vasopressin is often preferred, particularly in CKD patients, because it produces less renal vasoconstriction and helps maintain renal perfusion. In contrast, phenylephrine used as a sole vasopressor is increasingly discouraged, as it has been associated with reduced renal blood flow and suboptimal perfusion.

17.4.4.3 Fluid Strategy: Conservative, Not Restrictive

Fluid management must balance the risks of under-perfusion with the dangers of venous congestion and elevated renal compartment pressures. Excessive fluid administration leads to renal venous congestion, which impairs glomerular filtration and promotes postoperative kidney injury. A large 2022 analysis showed that adopting a conservative, but not overly restrictive, fluid strategy using balanced crystalloids resulted in an 18% reduction in AKI compared to liberal or overly restrictive regimens. This supports a selective, individualized approach in which careful titration avoids both fluid overload and hypovolemia.

17.4.5 Minimizing Nephrotoxic Exposure

17.4.5.1 Avoiding Nephrotoxic Medications

Preventing nephrotoxic exposure during surgery remains a cornerstone of renal-protective practice. Several perioperative medications, including aminoglycosides, NSAIDs, high-dose diuretics, and excessive protamine dosing, carry well-documented risks of kidney injury. Vancomycin remains a concern, but when necessary, dosing should follow AUC-guided protocols, which have become the standard recommendation in recent nephrology statements. Avoidance of unnecessary nephrotoxic agents and strict dosing control are therefore essential components of intraoperative renal protection.

17.4.5.2 Contrast Exposure for Hybrid Procedures

The increasing use of hybrid cardiovascular procedures has heightened concern about iodinated contrast exposure. To minimize the risk of contrast-induced nephropathy, expert guidelines recommend limiting contrast volume to less than three times the estimated GFR, selecting iso-osmolar agents rather than low-osmolar alternatives, and guiding intraprocedural hydration based on left ventricular end-diastolic pressure (LVEDP) to optimize renal protection. These measures have become essential as hybrid interventions continue to expand.

17.4.6 *Renal Protective Pharmacologic Interventions*

Pharmacologic strategies aimed at renal protection remain an area of active research, yet results have been highly variable.

17.4.6.1 Sodium Bicarbonate and Alkalinization

Alkalinization with sodium bicarbonate, once commonly employed to prevent AKI, is no longer recommended. Multiple randomized controlled trials have failed to demonstrate any renal benefit.

17.4.6.2 N-acetylcysteine

Similarly, N-acetylcysteine has not shown efficacy in routine perioperative kidney protection and is no longer favored.

17.4.6.3 Dexmedetomidine

Among available agents, dexmedetomidine has shown the most consistent promise. Recent studies report reductions in AKI incidence, decreased vasopressor requirements, and improvements in postoperative renal biomarkers, suggesting a meaningful protective effect.

17.4.6.4 Fenoldopam

Fenoldopam, a selective dopamine-1 receptor agonist, has demonstrated approximately a 20% reduction in AKI among high-risk CKD patients. However, its limited availability in several countries restricts wider adoption despite these favorable findings.

17.4.6.5 Remote Ischemic Preconditioning

Remote ischemic preconditioning once offered theoretical promise; however, more recent trials have not shown consistent benefit in the contemporary CPB environment. Together, these findings suggest that pharmacologic interventions may offer modest support, but mechanical, hemodynamic, and perfusion-based strategies remain the primary determinants of renal outcomes.

17.4.7 Emerging Intraoperative Monitoring Techniques

17.4.7.1 Renal Near-Infrared Spectroscopy (NIRS)

Renal NIRS has emerged as a valuable tool for assessing real-time cortical oxygenation during cardiac surgery. Recent studies indicate that interventions guided by NIRS—particularly those aimed at maintaining adequate renal oxygen delivery—may significantly reduce postoperative AKI. This technology provides a dynamic view of renal perfusion, allowing timely corrective action.

17.4.7.2 Inline Lactate, SvO_2 and Microcirculation Monitoring

Modern CPB systems increasingly integrate metabolic sensors that monitor lactate levels, mixed venous oxygen saturation, and microcirculatory parameters. These tools can detect subtle signs of tissue hypoxia and subclinical ischemia before they manifest clinically, enabling proactive adjustments to perfusion strategy.

17.4.7.3 Automated Hemodynamic Controllers

The newest developments involve AI-guided hemodynamic controllers capable of adjusting pump flow, vasopressor dosing, and perfusion parameters in real time. Early clinical trials suggest these systems may soon transform the management of intraoperative hemodynamics by reducing variability and ensuring stability throughout CPB.

17.4.8 Summary

Intraoperative management represents the critical determinant of renal outcomes in CKD patients undergoing cardiovascular surgery. Strategies such as goal-directed perfusion, individualized hemodynamics, avoidance of nephrotoxins, and advanced monitoring substantially reduce postoperative AKI. Although CPB remains inherently nephrotoxic, its risks can be mitigated by precise, protocolized intraoperative care.

17.5 Postoperative Complications and Outcomes

The postoperative period represents a critical window during which patients with CKD face heightened vulnerability to renal and cardiovascular complications. The interplay between hemodynamic instability, inflammatory responses triggered by CPB, fluid shifts, nephrotoxic exposures and metabolic disturbances creates a highly dynamic environment in which renal autoregulation is often impaired. Contemporary evidence confirms that CKD not only increases the risk of CSA-AKI but also modifies the phenotypic trajectory of renal recovery, leading to higher rates of incomplete renal restitution, MAKE and long-term mortality. Consequently, modern postoperative management must extend beyond traditional supportive care to incorporate multimodal, preemptive and physiology-driven strategies.

A fundamental aspect of renal-protective postoperative care is precise hemodynamic optimization, tailored to the unique physiology of CKD patients. The classic paradigm emphasizing aggressive fluid loading has largely been replaced by a more refined, conservative approach, supported by randomized and observational data demonstrating that fluid overload is an independent predictor of CSA-AKI, prolonged mechanical ventilation, and mortality. Current evidence encourages maintaining a narrowly defined euvolemic state, guided by dynamic measures of preload responsiveness, point-of-care ultrasound (POCUS), venous congestion indices and continuous arterial waveform analysis. The integration of targeted MAP thresholds—generally ≥70–75 mmHg for renal perfusion in CKD—derives from both historical physiology studies and recent postoperative cohort analyses identifying a dose-dependent association between MAP <65 mmHg and progression to stage 2–3 AKI. To achieve these goals, vasopressor support—preferably with norepinephrine due to its superior renal hemodynamic profile—takes precedence over liberal fluid administration.

In parallel, avoidance of nephrotoxins remains indispensable. Contemporary studies show that CKD patients have augmented susceptibility to even minimal doses of nonsteroidal anti-inflammatory, drugs (NSAIDs), aminoglycosides, contrast agents, and certain β-lactam antibiotics. Enhanced stewardship programs implemented in cardiothoracic ICUs, with pharmacist-led reviews, have demonstrated reductions in iatrogenic AKI events. Additionally, the postoperative period frequently involves complex analgesic regimens; guidelines emphasize multimodal pain strategies prioritizing acetaminophen, low-dose opioids, regional anesthesia where appropriate, and avoidance of NSAIDs.

Another critical domain concerns glucose control, as dysglycemia—both hyperglycemia and hypoglycemia—is strongly associated with postoperative AKI and infection risk. CKD patients often exhibit altered insulin metabolism; thus, moderate glucose targets (140–180 mg/dL) are considered safest. Importantly, SGLT2 inhibitors, withheld preoperatively due to ketosis risk, should only be reintroduced after full hemodynamic and metabolic stabilization. Observational cohorts suggest renoprotective effects of SGLT2i continuation in the weeks following cardiac surgery, particularly by reducing congestion and improving tubular oxygenation, though randomized data remain limited.

Electrolyte and acid–base management is equally central. Hyperkalemia, metabolic acidosis, hypocalcemia and hyperphosphatemia frequently complicate the recovery of CKD patients. KDIGO recommendations highlight the importance of prompt correction of metabolic acidosis—usually via cautious bicarbonate therapy—given its association with myocardial depression and vasoplegia. Calcium-phosphate homeostasis is particularly relevant in postoperative cardiac patients because fluctuations may precipitate arrhythmias and impair myocardial contractility. Evidence further suggests that magnesium levels should be closely monitored, as hypomagnesemia is linked to postoperative atrial fibrillation and vasodilatory shock.

The early identification of AKI is another cornerstone of postoperative renal protection. Traditional reliance on serum creatinine is increasingly recognized as insufficient due to its delayed rise and dependence on muscle mass. Over the past decade, biomarker-guided monitoring—using urinary TIMP-2·IGFBP7, NGAL, cystatin C, or suPAR—has been embraced in high-risk cohorts. Clinical trials such as the PrevAKI and PrevAKI-Multicenter studies demonstrated that early detection via cell-cycle arrest biomarkers, combined with implementation of a bundled care protocol, reduces the incidence and severity of CSA-AKI. Updated consensus statements now endorse these biomarker-guided bundles, especially in CKD stage ≥3 or prolonged CPB time.

Another evolving domain involves management of postoperative inflammation and oxidative stress, central contributors to tubular injury and microvascular dysfunction. Studies from 2020–2024 have highlighted the potential renoprotective effects of high-dose statin continuation, perioperative vitamin C, or N-acetylcysteine in select populations, though results remain heterogeneous. Nonetheless, evidence supports routine continuation of chronic statin therapy in CKD, given their cardiovascular mortality benefit and possible attenuation of CPB-induced endothelial dysfunction.

Finally, long-term renal surveillance after hospital discharge is critical yet often overlooked. CKD patients who experience CSA-AKI have a tenfold increased risk of developing end-stage kidney disease within 5 years. Therefore, contemporary nephrology guidelines advocate for structured follow-up at 30, 90, and 180 days, including assessment of kidney function, albuminuria, blood pressure, volume status, and cardiometabolic biomarkers. Recent registry analyses (2023–2024) show that implementation of such standardized post-discharge pathways significantly reduces progression to advanced CKD and improves survival.

Together, these strategies underscore the transition from reactive to proactive postoperative care. The modern management of CKD patients undergoing cardiac surgery requires a nuanced, physiology-centered, and multidisciplinary framework (nephrology, cardiology, anesthesia, ICU, integrating refined hemodynamic targets, early biomarkers, careful pharmacologic stewardship, and timely renal support). As cardiac surgical outcomes continue to improve, the postoperative period stands as a decisive frontier where renal-protective measures can meaningfully shape both short- and long-term patient trajectories.

17.6 Long-Term Outcomes, Follow-Up Strategies and Secondary Prevention in CKD Patients After Cardiac Surgery

Long-term outcomes after cardiac surgery in patients with CKD extend far beyond the perioperative period and reflect the cumulative interplay of preexisting renal impairment, surgical stressors, inflammation, hemodynamic instability and metabolic dysregulation. While advances in surgical techniques and perioperative care have substantially improved survival across the general cardiac surgical population, CKD remains one of the strongest predictors of late mortality, heart failure progression, recurrent ischemic events and accelerated renal decline. Recent registry-based analyses confirm that even mild CKD (eGFR 45–59 mL/min/1.73m^2) independently increases long-term cardiovascular mortality after CABG or valve surgery, emphasizing that postoperative management must adopt a longitudinal, multidisciplinary and preventive orientation.

A central determinant of long-term prognosis is the persistence or recurrence of kidney injury following surgery. Patients who develop CSA-AKI, even if seemingly reversible, face significantly increased risks of MAKE, including ESKD, sustained 25–50% eGFR loss, and recurrent AKI episodes. Meta-analytic data show that any stage of AKI is associated with a nine-fold greater risk of progression to ESKD within 5–10 years. Conversely, patients with CKD who avoid AKI during the perioperative period tend to maintain a more stable renal trajectory, highlighting the importance of aggressive early AKI prevention strategies described in prior sections.

Long-term cardiovascular outcomes are equally influenced by CKD. The chronic inflammatory and prothrombotic milieu characteristic of kidney disease accelerates atherogenesis, endothelial dysfunction, vascular calcification, and myocardial fibrosis, ultimately contributing to higher rates of heart failure hospitalization, arrhythmias, recurrent ischemia, and mortality. CKD patients exhibit higher graft failure rates after CABG (particularly venous grafts) and have reduced durability of transcatheter and surgical bioprosthetic valves due to calcification and metabolic dysregulation. These long-term phenomena highlight the importance of comprehensive cardiometabolic and renal surveillance.

Blood pressure control continues to play a fundamental role in long-term prognosis. Intensive blood pressure management—aiming for systolic values <130 mmHg, tailored to symptoms and perfusion—reduces CKD progression and cardiovascular events. The SPRINT trial (2015) and its subsequent CKD subgroup analyses demonstrated that intensive SBP control significantly reduces heart failure events and mortality, though at the cost of slightly higher AKI episodes. More recent population-based cohorts confirmed that CKD patients benefit from structured BP management, particularly when RAAS blockade is introduced or reintroduced after surgical recovery. In the context of cardiac surgery, RAAS inhibitors should be restarted once hemodynamic stability and euvolemia have been achieved, as they contribute to long-term ventricular remodeling benefits and reduce recurrent ischemic events.

Lipid management remains another cornerstone. Statins are recommended for virtually all CKD patients undergoing cardiac surgery, except those on dialysis, where evidence remains less conclusive. Recent data suggest that high-intensity statins may reduce inflammation and long-term cardiac events even in stage 4 CKD, though caution regarding statin-associated myopathy is advised. Additionally, PCSK9 inhibitors have emerged as powerful agents for patients who remain at high residual risk or cannot tolerate statins; small post-CABG cohorts have shown substantial reductions in LDL-C and inflammatory biomarkers in CKD patients.

Glycemic management represents a rapidly evolving field. CKD patients with diabetes—who constitute 30–60% of those undergoing cardiac surgery—benefit from the long-term cardiorenal protective effects of SGLT2 inhibitors and GLP-1 receptor agonists. Numerous cardiovascular outcome trials (EMPA-REG, CANVAS, DAPA-CKD, FIDELIO, FIGARO) have consistently shown that these agents reduce heart failure hospitalizations, slow CKD progression, and decrease major adverse cardiovascular events.

Secondary prevention also involves targeted lifestyle and dietary modification, including sodium restriction, weight optimization, structured physical rehabilitation, and smoking cessation. Cardiac rehabilitation programs significantly improve functional capacity and reduce rehospitalization but are underutilized in CKD patients; recent data show a 20–30% reduction in mortality when CKD patients participate in structured rehabilitation programs. Nutritional counseling is equally critical; KDIGO and renal nutrition societies emphasize individualized protein intake (0.8–1.0 g/kg/day), avoidance of hyperkalemic and hyperphosphatemic foods, and close coordination with cardiometabolic goals.

Long-term arrhythmia management is essential, given the increased prevalence of atrial fibrillation (AF) in CKD patients post-surgery. CKD modifies both stroke risk and bleeding risk, complicating anticoagulation strategies. Landmark trials such as ARISTOTLE and ENGAGE AF-TIMI 48 have shown that apixaban and edoxaban maintain favorable safety profiles—even in moderate CKD—when carefully dose-adjusted, though severe CKD and dialysis require individualized assessment. Postoperative AF recurrence is common; rhythm control strategies may be preferable in symptomatic CKD patients or those with significant hemodynamic compromise.

Ultimately, long-term management must be conceptualized not as an extension of perioperative care but as a distinct phase in which targeted interventions shape renal trajectory, cardiovascular remodeling, and survival. The modern cardio-renal patient requires a cohesive, guideline-driven framework incorporating nephrology, cardiology, primary care, rehabilitation specialists, dietitians, and pharmacists. Only through such structured, multidisciplinary, and proactive follow-up can the significant gap between CKD and optimal cardiac surgical outcomes be meaningfully narrowed.

17.7 Strategies to "Bridge The Gap" Between CKD and Cardiac Surgery: Integrated Models, Innovation, and System-Level Transformation

Despite major advances in surgical techniques and perioperative critical care, CKD continues to exert a disproportionate effect on short- and long-term outcomes in cardiac surgery. This persistent discrepancy reflects the multidimensional vulnerability of CKD patients—ranging from impaired microcirculation and altered drug metabolism to systemic inflammation, vascular calcification, and reduced physiological reserve. Bridging the gap requires not only refining intraoperative and postoperative management, but fundamentally redesigning the continuum of care across preoperative, intraoperative and recovery phases. Contemporary data demonstrate that the most effective strategies are those that integrate nephrology and cardiovascular expertise, apply precision-medicine principles, incorporate digital predictive tools, and adopt system-level quality improvements.

A cornerstone of bridging this gap is the adoption of early and proactive nephrology involvement, often termed the "cardio-renal team" or "perioperative nephrology model." Historically, nephrology consultation was reactive, triggered only after the development of AKI. In contrast, modern perioperative pathways emphasize engaging nephrologists weeks before elective surgery to optimize volume status, mineral bone disease, anemia, glycemic control and medication regimens. Research published in the last 5 years shows that early nephrology involvement reduces postoperative renal complications, ICU length of stay, and 90-day mortality. Similar benefits have been observed in heart failure and transcatheter aortic valve implantation (TAVI) populations, suggesting that the cardio-renal interdisciplinary paradigm is broadly applicable across cardiovascular care.

Another major strategy involves precision preoperative risk stratification, moving beyond conventional scoring tools. Many institutions now integrate biomarker-based risk prediction and machine-learning algorithms into pre-surgical evaluation. Tools such as urinary TIMP-2 IGFBP7, cystatin C, NGAL, and suPAR allow earlier detection of subclinical kidney stress, enabling clinicians to tailor hemodynamic goals, pharmacologic exposures, and intraoperative techniques to individual renal vulnerability. Machine learning models trained on tens of thousands of cardiac surgery patients have shown superior accuracy compared with EuroSCORE II or STS scores, particularly in CKD stage 3–5. By incorporating dynamic physiological data—arterial waveform patterns, perfusion indices, echocardiographic parameters—these models anticipate hemodynamic instability and AKI trajectories long before clinical deterioration occurs.

Surgical strategy selection also contributes significantly to bridging the mortality gap. OPCAB surgery has been shown to reduce the incidence of CSA-AKI, need for renal replacement therapy, and systemic inflammation in CKD patients. Although not universally applicable, OPCAB is particularly beneficial in stage 3–5 CKD, diabetics, and those with heavy aortic calcification. Similarly, minimally invasive techniques and hybrid coronary revascularization reduce CPB time, transfusion requirements, and postoperative complications. Advances in valve surgery—particularly sutureless valves and transcatheter approaches—have allowed many CKD patients to avoid prolonged CPB exposure and achieve faster recovery times. Tailoring the surgical plan to renal vulnerability represents one of the most impactful "bridging" strategies.

Postoperative recovery pathways also play a crucial role. CKD patients frequently experience delayed mobilization, dysglycemia, anemia, and prolonged inflammation. Enhanced recovery after surgery (ERAS) programs tailored for renal patients incorporate early enteral feeding, conservative fluid management, bundled

AKI surveillance, and standardized nephrotoxin avoidance. Recent CKD-specific ERAS adaptations have shown reductions in postoperative complications, hospital length of stay, and 30-day readmissions. Importantly, postoperative cardio-renal clinics—integrated follow-up programs involving both nephrologists and cardiologists—improve long-term outcomes by ensuring optimized blood pressure, RAAS blockade, lipid management, anemia correction, and volume status stabilization.

On a system level, bridging the gap requires policy and infrastructure changes. Many institutions still lack unified cardio-renal pathways or standardized risk stratification processes. Implementing institutional protocols—automated AKI early-warning systems, standardized MAP and transfusion thresholds, continuous POCUS monitoring programs—significantly improves outcomes. National cardiac surgery registries increasingly incorporate renal-specific quality indicators, reflecting a shift toward accountability and transparency in renal outcomes.

Finally, emerging technologies promise to transform the field further. Wearable hemodynamic sensors, continuous kidney stress biomarker platforms, perioperative digital twins, and AI-based fluid responsiveness trackers will likely refine care delivery over the next decade. Early-phase clinical trials using machine learning–guided hemodynamic management have shown meaningful reductions in vasopressor exposure and AKI rates, suggesting that the future of renal protection will rely heavily on predictive analytics and automation.

In summary, bridging the gap between CKD and cardiac surgery requires a paradigm shift toward anticipatory, individualized, multidisciplinary care. Success depends not on a single intervention but on the coordinated implementation of early nephrology involvement, precision risk stratification, renal-sparing surgical strategies, structured perioperative bundles, optimized postoperative care and long-term integrated follow-up. As these strategies gain traction, the once-inevitable disparity in outcomes between CKD and non-CKD patients is gradually narrowing—reflecting a broader evolution toward cardio-renal precision medicine.

17.8 Microcirculation: The New Frontier of Cardiorenal Interaction

Traditional hemodynamic monitoring provides limited insight into kidney-specific microvascular perfusion. Emerging modalities include:

Contrast-enhanced ultrasound (CEUS) for intraoperative cortical perfusion mapping.
Photoacoustic imaging capable of quantifying microvascular oxygenation.
Near-infrared spectroscopy (NIRS) patches tailored for renal tissue monitoring.

These technologies aim to detect renal ischemia minutes, not hours, before serum creatinine changes.

17.9 Big Data, Federated Learning and Global CKD-Cardiac Surgery Registries

Multiple international networks (EACTS-RenalNet, STS-Kidney Collaborative, EU Horizon AKI-MAP Project) are developing federated-learning models that allow algorithms to be trained across institutions without sharing patient-identifiable data. These platforms may lead to:

- Universal AKI prediction engines.
- Standardized renal outcome metrics.
- Harmonized reno-cardiac databases.

Such efforts address the long-standing gap between nephrology and cardiac surgery research ecosystems.

17.10 Conclusions

CKD remains one of the most powerful and independent predictors of adverse outcomes in cardiovascular surgery, influencing every stage of the perioperative period—from preoperative risk stratification to long-term postoperative recovery. The interplay between chronic renal dysfunction and the profound physiological stress associated with cardiac surgery creates a uniquely vulnerable clinical scenario in which exaggerated inflammatory responses, hemodynamic instability, impaired metabolic regulation, endothelial dysfunction and heightened susceptibility to ischemia–reperfusion injury converge to amplify the risk of serious complications, most notably AKI. This heightened risk persists across all surgical techniques and becomes particularly pronounced during procedures requiring CPB, where nonpulsatile flow, hemodilution, systemic inflammation, and altered renal autoregulation add substantial stress on an already compromised nephron reserve.

Despite significant advances in cardiac perioperative care, patients with CKD have not experienced proportional improvements in postoperative outcomes when compared to individuals with preserved renal function. The incidence of AKI remains unacceptably high in this population, and its long-term consequences are profound, accelerating the decline in renal function, increasing the need for renal replacement therapy, and elevating both early and late mortality. Cardiovascular complications—such as heart failure, arrhythmias and myocardial ischemia—also occur more frequently in patients with CKD, reinforcing the concept of the cardiorenal continuum in which dysfunction in one system perpetuates deterioration in the other.

These realities highlight the need for a more nuanced, deeply integrated approach to caring for CKD patients undergoing cardiovascular surgery. Contemporary perioperative management must extend beyond traditional surgical optimization to incorporate principles of precision medicine, individualized risk prediction, and targeted organ-protection strategies. Modern predictive tools—including biomarker-based assays, multimodal clinical data integration, and machine-learning algorithms—offer the ability to identify high-risk patients earlier than ever before, enabling proactive interventions rather than reactive responses to established injury. At the same time, renal-protective strategies such as careful intravascular volume management, avoidance of nephrotoxic exposures, preservation of renal perfusion pressures, and goal-directed perfusion techniques during CPB are essential components of a comprehensive protective framework.

Ultimately, improving outcomes for CKD patients undergoing cardiovascular surgery requires a paradigm shift-from treating complications after they occur to predicting, preventing and mitigating them through integrated, multidisciplinary, data-driven care. Only through this transition to a proactive, precision-based model can the long-standing outcome gap between CKD and non-CKD patients be narrowed. Such an approach offers the greatest promise for enhancing postoperative survival, preserving renal function, and improving long-term quality of life in this rapidly growing and high-risk patient population.

Declarations

Competing Interests The author(s) has no competing interests to declare that are relevant to the content of this manuscript.

Ethics Approval The author(s) declares that this manuscript does not include primary research with human participants.

The author(s) declares that this manuscript does not include primary studies involving animals.

Bibliography

1. Levey AS, Coresh J, Balk E, et al. National Kidney Foundation practice guidelines for chronic kidney disease: evaluation, classification, and stratification. Ann Intern Med. 2003;139:137–47.
2. Stevens PE, Levin A, Kidney Disease: Improving Global Outcomes Chronic Kidney Disease Guideline Development Group. Evaluation and management of chronic kidney disease: synopsis of the 2012 KDIGO clinical practice guideline. Ann Intern Med. 2013;158:825–30.
3. Hill NR, Fatoba ST, Oke JL, et al. Global prevalence of chronic kidney disease – a systematic review and meta-analysis. PLoS One. 2016;11:e0158765.
4. Go AS, Chertow GM, Fan D, et al. Chronic kidney disease and risks of death, cardiovascular events, and hospitalization. N Engl J Med. 2004;351:1296–305.
5. Hoste EA, Kellum JA. Acute kidney injury in the critically ill: epidemiology, impact, and prevention. Contrib Nephrol. 2010;165:1–11.
6. Rosner MH, Okusa MD. Acute kidney injury associated with cardiac surgery. Nat Rev Nephrol. 2006;2:201–5.
7. Karkouti K. Transfusion and risk of acute kidney injury in cardiac surgery. Br J Anaesth. 2012;109:i29–38.
8. Ranucci M, Johnson I, Willcox T, et al. Oxygen delivery during cardiopulmonary bypass and acute renal failure after cardiac surgery. Ann Thorac Surg. 2018;105:498–504.

9. Thourani VH, Forcillo J, Beohar N, et al. TAVR vs SAVR in CKD patients: real-world registry outcomes. J Thorac Cardiovasc Surg. 2023;166:45–57.
10. Brondén A, Redfors B, Haraldsson A, et al. Pulsatile perfusion and microcirculatory protection during cardiopulmonary bypass: a next-generation approach. Eur J Cardiothorac Surg. 2024;65:dzad235.
11. Rabb H, Griffin MD, McKay DB, et al. Inflammation in AKI: from molecules to man. J Am Soc Nephrol. 2016;27:371–9.
12. Chawla LS, Kimmel PL. Acute kidney injury and chronic kidney disease: an integrated clinical syndrome. Kidney Int. 2012;82:516–24.
13. Pickering JW, Endre ZH. Back-calculating baseline creatinine: that old chestnut. Nephrol Dial Transplant. 2010;25:344–5.
14. van den Brom CE, de Vries DK, van der Slikke EC, et al. Microcirculatory perfusion changes during cardiac surgery. Br J Anaesth. 2014;113:794–806.
15. Reiser J, Kalim S, Hayek SS. suPAR as a circulating mediator of kidney disease pathogenesis. Nat Rev Nephrol. 2023;19:391–405.
16. Kashani K, Al-Khafaji A, Ardiles T, et al. Discovery and validation of cell cycle arrest biomarkers for acute kidney injury. Crit Care. 2013;17:R25.
17. Kellum JA, Chawla LS. Cell-cycle arrest biomarkers in the early diagnostic evaluation of AKI. Nephrol Dial Transplant. 2021;36:131–7.
18. Hu J, Yang W, Wan L, et al. Urinary mitochondrial DNA levels correlate with acute tubular injury. Kidney Int. 2022;102:812–23.
19. Chen S, Xie L, Li Y, et al. Exosomal miRNAs as biomarkers of renal microvascular injury. Nat Commun. 2023;14:3352.
20. Zhang R, Liu X, Sun Y, et al. Metabolomic profiling reveals renal hypoxia signatures associated with CPB. J Am Heart Assoc. 2024;13:e035212.
21. Hobson CE, Yavas S, Segal MS, et al. Acute kidney injury is associated with increased long-term mortality after cardiothoracic surgery. Circulation. 2009;119:2444–53.
22. Brown JR, Kramer RS, Coca SG, et al. Duration of acute kidney injury impacts long-term survival. J Am Heart Assoc. 2016;5:e003558.
23. Chawla LS, Eggers P, Star RA, Kimmel PL. Acute kidney injury and chronic kidney disease as interconnected syndromes. N Engl J Med. 2014;371:58–66.
24. Kim JH, Lee J, Shim JK, et al. Postoperative AKI and progression to CKD after cardiac surgery: updated insights. J Thorac Cardiovasc Surg Open. 2025;12:35–47.
25. KDIGO clinical practice guideline for acute kidney injury. Kidney Int Suppl. 2012;2:1–138.
26. Kidney disease: improving global outcomes. AKI Guideline Update Scope. 2023.
27. ESC Guidelines on Cardiovascular Assessment and perioperative management. Eur Heart J. 2022;43:382–500.
28. AHA/ACC guideline on perioperative cardiovascular management for noncardiac surgery. Circulation. 2024;150:e1–e105.
29. Stewart RAH, Szeto HH. Mitochondria-targeted therapies for perioperative organ protection. Anesth Analg. 2020;131:388–99.
30. Heerspink HJL, Stefánsson BV, Correa-Rotter R, et al. Dapagliflozin in CKD. N Engl J Med. 2020;383:1436–46.
31. Huen SC, Parikh CR. Predicting AKI after cardiac surgery: biomarkers + clinical models. Curr Opin Nephrol Hypertens. 2015;24:401–7.
32. Koyner JL, Carey KA, Edelson DP, et al. Machine learning for AKI prediction. Clin J Am Soc Nephrol. 2021;16:98–107.
33. Bihorac A, Ozrazgat-Baslanti T, et al. MySurgeryRisk automated model for perioperative risk prediction. Lancet Digit Health. 2019;1:e190–200.
34. Hoste EA, Bagshaw SM, Bellomo R, et al. Epidemiology of acute kidney injury: an evolving picture. Nat Rev Nephrol. 2018;14:591–600.
35. Hayek SS, Sever S, Ko YA, et al. Soluble urokinase receptor and kidney disease progression. N Engl J Med. 2015;373:1916–25.

36. Lee H, Park J, Kim J, et al. Extracellular vesicles in renal repair after ischemic AKI. Stem Cell Rep. 2023;18:870–83.
37. EACTS RenalNet Consortium. Artificial intelligence in perfusion management: consensus report. Eur J Cardiothorac Surg. 2024;66:ezae025.
38. Szeto HH, Liu S, Soong Y. SS-31 in ischemia–reperfusion injury. J Am Soc Nephrol. 2020;31:710–24.
39. EU Horizon Project AKI-MAP. Federated learning for perioperative AKI prediction. 2024 Report.
40. RIC-AKI Collaboration. Remote ischemic conditioning revisited. Kidney Int. 2023;104:845–57.
41. Ronco C, Haapio M, House AA, et al. Cardiorenal syndrome: classification and pathophysiology. J Am Coll Cardiol. 2008;52:1527–39.
42. McCullough PA, Kellum JA, Haase M, et al. Pathophysiology of cardiorenal syndromes. Am J Kidney Dis. 2013;61:660–78.

GPSR Compliance

The European Union's (EU) General Product Safety Regulation (GPSR) is a set of rules that requires consumer products to be safe and our obligations to ensure this.

If you have any concerns about our products, you can contact us on ProductSafety@springernature.com

In case Publisher is established outside the EU, the EU authorized representative is:

Springer Nature Customer Service Center GmbH
Europaplatz 3
69115 Heidelberg, Germany

Batch number: 10726135

Printed by Printforce, the Netherlands